Pancreatitis

TOPICS IN GASTROENTEROLOGY

Series Editor: **Howard M. Spiro, M.D.**
Yale University School of Medicine

PANCREATITIS
Peter A. Banks, M.D.

A Continuation Order Plan is available for this series. A continuation order will bring delivery of each new volume immediately upon publication. Volumes are billed only upon actual shipment. For further information please contact the publisher.

Pancreatitis

Peter A. Banks, M.D.

*Associate Professor of Medicine at Tufts University
School of Medicine; Chief of Gastroenterology at
St. Elizabeth's Hospital of Boston; Lecturer in
Medicine at Harvard Medical School; and Assistant
Physician at Beth Israel Hospital, Boston, Massachusetts.*

PLENUM MEDICAL BOOK COMPANY
New York and London

Library of Congress Cataloging in Publication Data

Banks, Peter A
  Pancreatitis.

  (Topics in gastroenterology)
  Bibliography: p.
  Includes index.
  1. Pancreatitis. I. Title. II. Series. [DNLM: 1. Pancreatitis. WI805 B218p]
RC858.P35B36   616.3'7   78-11341
ISBN-13: 978-1-4613-2909-1   e-ISBN-13: 978-1-4613-2907-7
DOI: 10.1007/ 978-1-4613-2907-7

© 1979 Plenum Publishing Corporation

Softcover reprint of the hardcover 1st edition 1979

227 West 17th Street, New York, N.Y. 10011

Plenum Medical Book Company is an imprint of Plenum Publishing Corporation

To my Father

DR. BENJAMIN M. BANKS

Clinician, Teacher, Humanitarian

Foreword

It is with much pleasure that I introduce this first volume in a series of *Topics in Gastroenterology* aimed at the intelligent clinician. Dr. Peter Banks is first and foremost a clinician and teacher and therefore an ideal lead-off author. His very helpful review of pancreatitis is based not only on a thorough assimilation of clinical and experimental evidence but also on his long clinical practice in university hospitals and in private practice. Dr. Banks understands what we clinicians need to know about the pathophysiology of this challenging disorder. I found much practical information in this volume to help me in thinking about my own patients, and I recommend it with enthusiasm.

Howard M. Spiro, M.D.

Preface

In the preparation of this book, I have made a special effort to provide detailed clinical information on the care of the patient with pancreatitis. The usefulness of newer diagnostic tests such as amylase/creatinine clearance ratio, ERCP, diagnostic ultrasound, and C-T scan has been carefully evaluated. Particular attention has been devoted to the management of the more difficult therapeutic problems such as severe protracted pancreatitis, pancreatitis of unknown etiology, pancreatic pseudocyst, and pancreatic insufficiency. Points of controversy regarding medical and surgical alternatives in the treatment of acute and chronic pancreatitis have been reviewed with specific recommendations for therapy. In all discussions, emphasis has been placed on basic physiological principles that govern treatment. A comprehensive and current bibliography accompanies each chapter.

Many clinicians and investigators have contributed to the field of pancreatitis. I would like to express my deep appreciation and gratitude to two physicians in particular who are well represented in the bibliography: Dr. Henry D. Janowitz, who stimulated my interest in the pancreas during my years of training with him, and Dr. Howard M. Spiro, the editor of this series, who read the manuscript with great care and offered many important and helpful suggestions. I would also like to thank my secretary, Miss Ann Marie O'Rourke, who typed the several revisions of the manuscript with patience and diligence. Finally, this book could not have been completed without the understanding and support of my wife and children.

Peter A. Banks, M.D.

Boston

Contents

CHRONIC PANCREATITIS

ACUTE PANCREATITIS

ACUTE PANCREATITIS

1

General Considerations

1.1 ANATOMY

Embryologically, the pancreas arises from a large dorsal endodermal bud and a smaller ventral endodermal bud. Following rotation of the ventral bud posteriorly and the duodenum to the right, the two buds then fuse. The ventral component contributes most of the head of the pancreas. The larger dorsal bud forms the remainder of the gland.

The fully developed pancreas contains endocrine components (islet cells) and exocrine components (acini and excretory ducts). It does not possess a distinct connective tissue capsule. Instead, it is covered by a relatively thin layer of loose connective tissue. A network of connective tissue extends from the surface into the parenchyma subdividing the gland into small lobules.

The total length of the pancreas varies between twelve and twenty centimeters, its weight is 60 to 120 gm, width 3 to 5 cm, and maximal thickness 2 to 3 cm. The head of the pancreas nestles within the concavity of the duodenum at the level of the second lumbar vertebra. The *uncinate process* projects from the lower portion of the head. The neck, body, and tail extend in an oblique fashion upward to the level of the twelfth thoracic vertebra. The tail of the pancreas lies just anterior to the superior pole of the left kidney and is in close proximity to the spleen. The pancreas lies posterior to the stomach separated by the lesser sac. The mesocolon of the transverse colon extends from the anterior inferior surface of the pancreas to the transverse colon. During acute pancreatitis, inflammatory exudate may extend to the transverse colon by this route, and the lesser omental sac may fill with fluid displacing the stomach anteriorly and the transverse colon in a caudal direction.

The pancreas lies directly anterior to the inferior vena cava and aorta near the midline. The splenic artery and vein lie immediately behind the neck and body of the pancreas in a horizontal position. The distal portion of the common bile duct usually passes through the substance of the head of the pancreas before entering the duodenum. During acute pancreatitis, thrombosis of the splenic vein may lead to varices of the lower esophagus and fundus of the stomach, and compression of the intrapancreatic portion of the common bile duct may cause jaundice.

The islets of Langerhans contain cell types that are capable of producing a variety of hormones, including glucagon by α cells, insulin by β cells, somatostatin by D cells, gastrin by non-α non-β cells, and possibly vasoactive intestinal polypeptide by non-α non-β cells. The secretion of glucagon and insulin has major physiologic significance. The physiologic role of somatostatin has not as yet been defined, and in health neither gastrin nor vasoactive intestinal polypeptide is secreted in quantity from islet cells. Hormone-secreting tumors have been documented from each of these cell types, including the well-known insulinoma and gastrinoma, the less common syndrome of pancreatic cholera (whether caused by vasoactive intestinal polypeptide,[1-3] or some other hormone[4]), the distinctly rare glucagonoma,[5,6] and now one report of a somatostatinoma.[7]

The exocrine portion of the pancreas is composed of small groups of acini separated into lobules by a connective tissue stroma. Each acinus drains into a small pancreatic duct. These small ducts form a network of larger ducts assuming a herring-bone pattern until eventually all pancreatic secretion drains into the major excretory ducts of Wirsung and Santorini. The acini are composed of tall columnar epithelium. The very small ductules that drain acini (called centroacinar cells) contain somewhat flattened epithelial cells. The cells of the ductal epithelium become progressively taller in the form of columnar cells as smaller ducts coalesce to become larger ducts. The main duct of Wirsung extends from the tail of the pancreas near its posterior surface to the duodenum at the ampulla of Vater. The accessory duct of Santorini springs from the main duct in the region of the neck of the pancreas and then courses independently in a more ventral direction before entering the duodenum approximately 2 cm above the main duct of Wirsung. There is considerable variation in the size, shape, and position of the pancreatic ducts. In one study, only 24% of patients had a functional accessory duct that drained into the minor papilla.[8] If the flow of pancreatic juice is obstructed in the main duct near the duodenum, the presence of a functioning accessory duct would permit the flow of pancreatic juice from the main duct into the accessory duct and from there into the duodenum.

In perhaps 60% to 70% of adults, the main pancreatic duct of Wirsung joins the common bile duct before emptying into the duodenum via the ampulla of Vater. This arrangement (called a "common channel") may be important in the development of pancreatitis associated with biliary tract disease. Among adults who do not have a common channel, the common bile duct and pancreatic duct enter the duodenum side by side via separate orifices.

1.2 PHYSIOLOGY

Pancreatic acini secrete enzymes which are important for the digestion of dietary carbohydrate, fat, and protein. Pancreatic ductules secrete a bicarbonate-rich fluid which carries the enzymes quickly into the duodenum. It is important that the milieu within ducts and within the duodenum remain alkaline because pancreatic enzymes are rendered inactive in the presence of acid (as are bile salts).

1.2.1 Stimulation of Pancreatic Secretion

Pancreatic secretion is stimulated by the vagus nerve and by a variety of hormones [gastrin from the antrum of the stomach and cholecystokinin-pancreozymin (CCK-PZ) and secretin from the small intestine]. Stimulation of the vagus nerve results in the secretion of pancreatic enzymes from acinar tissue but does not stimulate ductules to secrete bicarbonate. Gastrin has a moderately strong stimulatory effect on pancreatic enzyme secretion and a very weak stimulatory effect on pancreatic bicarbonate secretion. CCK-PZ is a very strong stimulant of pancreatic enzyme secretion and a weak stimulant of pancreatic bicarbonate secretion. Secretin plays essentially no role by itself in pancreatic enzyme secretion, but is a very strong stimulant of bicarbonate secretion from pancreatic ductules.

Interrelationships among these stimulants of pancreatic secretion and the mechanisms of pancreatic secretion are extremely complex and are the subject of several fine reviews.[9-18] The sight, smell, or chewing of food (the cephalic phase) probably stimulates the pancreas directly to secrete enzymes via vagal pathways, but the major influence of vagal stimulation on pancreatic secretion is by way of the stomach. Vagal impulses from the cephalic phase stimulate the release of gastrin from the antrum. Gastrin stimulates pancreatic enzyme secretion directly and also stimulates acid secretion from gastric parietal cells. When acid reaches the duodenum, it stimulates the release of secretin and to a much lesser extent CCK-PZ. Vagal impulses also stimulate parietal cells directly to secrete acid.

Once food reaches the stomach, the gastric phase of gastric and pancreatic secretion takes place. Distention of the fundus and antrum of the stomach stimulates the release of gastrin from the antrum and the secretion of acid from parietal cells. Vagal reflexes are thought to be responsible for these effects.[19,20] Gastrin is also released by products of protein digestion.[21] Parietal cells are stimulated directly to secrete acid by intraluminal calcium.[22]

The intestinal phase of pancreatic secretion is the most important. When the pH of the duodenum is reduced to 4.5 or lower, secretin is released.[23-25] A traditional view has been that acid is the sole stimulant of secretin release, but recent evidence suggests that certain fatty acids may also stimulate the release of secretin.[26,27] The threshold for release of secretin by acid is an important one to remember. In the treatment of acute pancreatitis, all efforts must be made to maintain an intraduodenal pH above 4.5 in order to avoid the stimulation of pancreatic secretion by secretin. Acid in the duodenum appears to be a weak stimulant of CCK-PZ release,[26,28] as well as a strong stimulant of secretin release. Only a few types of food in the duodenum cause CCK-PZ release. Neither carbohydrate[25,29] nor neutral fat[27] stimulates pancreatic secretion. Fatty acids are potent stimulants of CCK-PZ release. Fatty acids with carbon chains 16 and 18 carbons long (representative of dietary fat) are much more potent stimulants of CCK-PZ release than are fatty acids with chain lengths of only 8 or 10 carbons.[27,30] For this reason, medium chain triglyceride (MCT) oil (which contains 68% C-8, 24% C-10, and less than 5% longer than C-10) would stimulate less pancreatic enzyme secretion than dietary fat and could prove useful in the dietary treatment of chronic relapsing pancreatitis. Certain neutral amino acids (especially phenylalanine and tryptophan), a few oligopeptides, and some polypeptides stimulate CCK-PZ release.[31-33] Intraluminal calcium is a potent stimulant of CCK-PZ release.[34] It is possible, but as yet unproven, that the vagus in the duodenum contributes to pancreatic secretion by influencing the release of hormones or by stimulating the pancreas directly. Stimulants of CCK-PZ release are extremely potent in their action. Emulsified fatty acids and calcium release sufficient amounts of CCK-PZ from the duodenum to provide maximal enzyme secretion from the pancreas[34,35]; a mixture of select amino acids provides an intermediate enzyme response.[13,35]

It may be of some physiologic importance that secretin and CCK-PZ are each found in reasonably abundant quantities in both the duodenum and jejunum, and that bicarbonate and enzyme outputs are of equal magnitude when either segment is perfused with a proper stimulant.[36-39] The abundance of CCK-PZ in duodenum and in jejunum allows for digestion of food throughout the upper small intestine. It also allows for at least some pancreatic stimulation following the surgical creation of a gastroje-junostomy. Ordinarily, most gastric acid is completely neutralized in the first portion of the duodenum, and for this reason, the additional amounts of secretin in the distal duodenum and jejunum would presumably have limited importance except for the purpose of neutralization of acid following a gastrojejunostomy.

1.2.2 Response of the Pancreas to a Meal

The many ways in which pancreatic acinar tissue is stimulated to release its enzymes ensures proper digestion of food. Pancreatic enzyme secretion in response to a test meal is sustained at a maximal level as long as food continues to enter the duodenum.[13,40] In general, gastric emptying proceeds more slowly with solid meals that are high in calories than with liquid meals.[13,40] It is for this reason that solid meals tend to stimulate the release of pancreatic enzymes for longer periods of time than liquid meals. An important principle based on these observations is that the dietary treatment for resolving pancreatitis should include relatively small liquid meals with modest amounts of calories, principally carbohydrate with minimal amounts of fat and protein.

Whereas the presence of acid in the duodenum under experimental conditions clearly causes secretion of pancreatic bicarbonate by releasing intraduodenal secretin,[25] in at least one report intraduodenal pH remained above 4.5 and serum secretin levels did not increase above baseline values in response to a meal.[25] As a result of this and other similar reports, the question has been seriously raised as to whether secretin has an important physiologic role during the digestive process.[38] It is likely that small amounts of secretin are released during digestion as a result of some acid reaching the duodenum.[35,41,42] While this amount of secretin by itself would exert only a small influence on pancreatic bicarbonate secretion, there is now evidence that the physiologic action of secretin on pancreatic ductules is markedly augmented by the presence of CCK-PZ, and similarly the physiologic action of CCK-PZ on pancreatic acinar tissue is augmented by secretin.[43-45] As such, hormonal stimulation of ductules by secretin plus CCK-PZ results in a markedly enhanced secretion of fluid and bicarbonate that is far in excess of a simple additive effect. In similar fashion, hormonal stimulation of acinar tissue by CCK-PZ plus secretin results in a marked increase in enzyme output. It is therefore important during the dietary treatment of resolving pancreatitis to prevent stimulation of both secretin and CCK-PZ because each potentiates the major physiologic action of the other.

1.2.3 Composition of Pancreatic Juice

(a) *Electrolytes.* The concentrations of sodium and potassium in pancreatic juice are essentially equal to their concentrations in plasma and are independent of the rate of secretion. Bicarbonate concentration of pancreatic juice increases markedly in response to stimulation of pancreatic ductules by secretin. As bicarbonate concentration increases, chloride concentration is reduced in reciprocal fashion. There is essentially no ionized calcium in pancreatic juice. Calcium that is present in pancreatic juice is bound to pancreatic enzymes.

The flow of pancreatic juice is reduced by the intravenous administration of a variety of agents including acetazolamide (Diamox),[46] antidiuretic hormone (ADH),[47] anticholinergic agents,[48,49] glucagon,[50] and somatostatin.[51,52] Although it is certainly desirable to reduce the flow of pancreatic juice in the treatment of acute pancreatitis, there are no controlled studies which support the value of these agents.

(b) *Pancreatic Enzymes.* Proteolytic enzymes are secreted as proenzymes. The major proteolytic enzymes are trypsinogen, chymotrypsinogen, and elastase (which are called endopeptidases because they cleave peptide bonds of dietary protein that occupy internal positions), and procarboxypeptidase-A and procarboxypeptidase-B (which are called exopeptidases because they cleave the peptide bond of the end amino acid). At least one trypsin inhibitor is secreted in pancreatic juice to prevent the premature activation of trypsin within pancreatic ducts. When pancreatic proteolytic enzymes reach the duodenum, enterokinase activates trypsinogen to trypsin. Once this initial step takes place, there is a cascade of activation of the remaining proteolytic enzymes by activated trypsin. Activated trypsin also autocatalyzes trypsinogen to trypsin and thereby makes available an abundant supply of this enzyme to catalyze the other proteolytic enzymes.

The major lipolytic enzymes are lipase and phospholipase-A and -B. Lipase is secreted in active form but does not damage pancreatic acinar cells or ductules. Phospholipase-A and -B require activation by a small amount of trypsin. Lipase quickly cleaves two fatty acids from dietary triglyceride leaving a 2-monoglyceride. The cleavage of the third fatty acid proceeds somewhat more slowly.

Amylase is secreted in active form but is nontoxic to the pancreas. It hydrolyzes starch to maltose.

1.2.4 Cellular Processes in Pancreatic Secretion

The mechanism by which pancreatic ductules secrete bicarbonate remains unclear. Carbonic anhydrase is present in ductular epithelium and presumably plays a role.

The primary event in the action of CCK-PZ on acinar cells is the release of calcium from membrane-bound compartments.[53] Several interesting questions have been raised regarding cellular processes involved in the secretion of pancreatic enzymes. A traditional view has been that enzymes must be prepackaged as zymogens before extrusion. It now appears likely that pancreatic secretion of enzymes may occur in the absence of zymogen granules.[54,55] Another traditional view is that the secretion of pancreatic enzymes tends to be parallel (that is, the ratio of the various enzymes during secretion remains constant). While there is still some evidence for parallel secretion of digestive enzymes,[56] increasing evidence both in man,[57-59] and in the experimental animal,[60-62] suggests that secretion of pancreatic enzymes is nonparallel, and that in man, the composition of diet may strongly influence the composition of pancreatic enzymes that are secreted.[63]

There is ample evidence that fasting or hormonal deprivation causes atrophy of the pancreas,[64] and that gastrin in particular is a trophic hormone for the pancreas.[65,66] During total parenteral nutrition in the experimental animal, serum gastrin levels are reduced and pancreatic atrophy occurs unless infusions of exogenous pentagastrin are administered.[65]

REFERENCES

1. Said SI, Faloona GR: Elevated plasma and tissue levels of vasoactive intestinal polypeptide in the watery-diarrhea syndrome due to pancreatic, bronchogenic and other tumors. N Engl J Med 293:155–160, 1975.
2. Graham DY, Johnson CD, Bentlif PS, et al: Islet cell carcinoma, pancreatic cholera, and vasoactive intestinal polypeptide. Ann Intern Med 83:782–785, 1975.
3. Thomas ML, Lamb GHR, Barraclough MA: Angiographic demonstration of a pancreatic "vipoma" in the WDHA syndrome. Am J Roentgenol 127:1037–1039, 1976.
4. Kahn CR, Levy AG, Gardner JD, et al: Pancreatic cholera: Beneficial effects of treatment with streptozotocin. N Engl J Med 292:941–945, 1975.
5. McGavran MH, Unger RH, Recant L, et al: A glucagon-secreting alpha-cell carcinoma of the pancreas. N Engl J Med 274:1408–1413, 1966.
6. Yoshinaga T, Okuna G, Shinji Y, et al: Pancreatic A-cell tumor associated with severe diabetes mellitus. Diabetes 15:709–713, 1966.
7. Ganda OP, Weir GC, Soeldner JS, et al: "Somatostatinoma": A somatostatin-containing tumor of the endocrine pancreas. N Engl J Med 296:963–967, 1977.
8. Kreel L, Sandin B, Slavin G: Pancreatic morphology, a combined radiological and pathological study. Clin Radiol 24:154–161, 1973.
9. Scratcherd T, Case RM: The secretion of electrolytes by the pancreas. Am J Clin Nutr 26:326–339, 1973.
10. Beck IT: The role of pancreatic enzymes in digestion. Am J Clin Nutr 26:311–325, 1973.
11. Brooks FP: The neurohumoral control of pancreatic exocrine secretion. Am J Clin Nutr 26:291–310, 1973.

12. Rayford PL, Miller TA, Thompson JC: Secretin, cholecystokinin and newer gastroin-
    testinal hormones. *N Eng J Med* 294:1093–1100, 1976.
13. Di Magno EP, Go VLW: The clinical application of exocrine pancreatic function tests.
    Dis Mon September : 3–36, 1976.
14. Lenninger S: The autonomic innervation of the exocrine pancreas. *Med Clin North Am*
    58:1311–1318, 1974.
15. Scratcherd T: Pancreatic function tests: the physiological background. *Gut* 16:648–663,
    1975.
16. Harper AA: The control of pancreatic secretion. *Gut* 13:308–317, 1972.
17. Janowitz HD: Pancreatic secretion of fluid and electrolytes. Pages 925–931 in *Handbook
    of Physiology*. Section 6: Alimentary Canal. Volume 2, *Secretion*. Charles F. Code ed.
    American Physiologic Society, Washington, DC, 1967.
18. Singh M, Webster PD, III: Neurohormonal control of pancreatic secretion. *Gastroenter-
    ology* 74:294–309, 1978.
19. Richardson CT, Walsh JH, Hicks MI, et al: Studies on the mechanisms of food-stimu-
    lated gastric acid secretion in normal human subjects. *J. Clin Inves* 58:623–631, 1976.
20. Debas HT and Grossman MI: Chemicals bathing the oxyntic gland area stimulate acid
    secretion in dog. *Gastroenterology* 69:654–659, 1975.
21. Preshaw RM, Cooke AR, Grossman MI: Stimulation of pancreatic secretion by a hu-
    moral agent from the pyloric gland area of the stomach. *Gastroenterology* 49:617–622,
    1965.
22. Holtermuller KH, Goldsmith RS, Sizemore GW, et al: Dissociation of gastric acid and
    serum gastrin responses to intraluminal calcium in man: influence of calcitonin and
    parathyroid hormone. *Gastroenterology* 67:1101–1106, 1974.
23. Meyer JH, Way LW, Grossman MI: Pancreatic bicarbonate response to various acids in
    duodenum of the dog. *Am J Physiol* 219:964–970, 1970.
24. Meyer JH, Way LW, Grossman MI: Pancreatic response to acidification of various
    lengths of proximal intestine in the dog. *Am J Physiol* 219:971–977, 1970.
25. Rhodes RA, Tai H-H, Chey WY: Observations on plasma secretin levels by radioimmu-
    noassay in response to duodenal acidification and to a meat meal in humans. *Am J Dig
    Dis* 21:873–879, 1976.
26. Debas HT, Grossman MI: Pure cholecystokinin: pancreatic protein and bicarbonate
    response. *Digestion* 9:469–481, 1973.
27. Meyer JH and Jones RS: Canine pancreatic responses to intestinally perfused fat and
    products of fat digestion. *Am J Physiol* 226:1178–1187, 1974.
28. Barbezat GO, Grossman MI: Release of cholecystokinin by acid. *Proc Soc Exp Biol
    Med* 148:463–467, 1975.
29. Boden G, Essa N, Owen OE, et al: Effects of intraduodenal administration of HC1 and
    glucose on circulating immunoreactive secretin and insulin concentrations. *J Clin Invest*
    53:1185–1193, 1974.
30. Malagelada J–R, DiMagno EP, Summerskill WHJ, et al: Regulation of pancreatic and
    gallbladder functions by intraluminal fatty acids and bile acids in man. *J Clin Invest*
    58:493–499, 1976.
31. Meyer JH, Kelly GA, Spingola LJ, et al: Canine gut receptors mediating pancreatic
    responses to luminal L-amino acids. *Am J Physiol* 231:669–677, 1976.
32. Meyer JH, Kelly GA, Jones RS: Canine pancreatic response to intestinally perfused
    oligopeptides. *Am J Physiol* 231:678–681, 1976.
33. Meyer JH, Kelly GA: Canine pancreatic responses to intestinally perfused proteins and
    protein digests. *Am J Physiol* 231:682–691, 1976.
34. Holtermuller KH, Malagelada J-R, McCall JT, et al: Pancreatic, gallbladder, and gastric

responses to intraduodenal calcium perfusion in man. *Gastroenterology* 70:693–696, 1976.

35. Go VLM: Coordination of the digestive sequence. *Mayo Clin Proc* 48:613–616, 1973.
36. DiMagno EP, Go VLW, Summerskill WHJ: Intraluminal and postabsorptive effects of amino acids on pancreatic enzyme secretion. *J Lab Clin Med* 82:241–248, 1973.
37. Buffa R, Solcia E, Go VLW: Immunohistochemical identification of the cholecystokinin cell in the intestinal mucosa. *Gastroenterology* 70:528–532, 1976.
38. Wormsley KG: Is secretin secreted? *Gut* 14:743–751, 1973.
39. Wormsley KG: Response to duodenal acidification in man. *Scand J Gastroenterology* 5:353–360, 1970.
40. Brunner H, Northfield TC, Hofmann AF, et al: Gastric emptying and secretion of bile acids, cholesterol, and pancreatic enzymes during digestion. *Mayo Clin Proc* 49:851–860, 1974.
41. Wormsley KG: The pathophysiology of duodenal ulceration. *Gut* 15:59–81, 1974.
42. Llanos OL, Konturek SJ, Rayford PL, et al: Pancreatic bicarbonate, serum gastrin, and secretin responses to meals varying in pH. *Am J Physiol* 233:E41–E46, 1977.
43. Meyer JH, Spingola LJ, Grossman MI: Endogenous cholecystokinin potentiates exogenous secretin on pancreas of dog. *Am J Physiol* 221:742–747, 1971.
44. Grossman MI, Konturek SJ: Gastric acid does drive pancreatic bicarbonate secretion. *Scand J Gastroenterology* 9:299–302, 1974.
45. Meyer JH, Grossman MI: Comparison of D– and L-phenylalanine as pancreatic stimulants. *Am J Physiol* 222:1058–1063, 1972.
46. Banks PA and Sum PT: Mode of action of acetazolamide on pancreatic exocrine secretion. *Arch Surg* 102:505–508, 1971.
47. Banks PA, Rudick J, Dreiling DA, et al: Effect of antidiuretic hormone on pancreatic exocrine secretion. *Am J Physiol* 215:361–365, 1968.
48. Dreiling DA, Janowitz HD: Inhibitory effect of new anticholinergics on the basal and secretin-stimulated pancreatic secretion in patients with and without pancreatic disease. *Am J Dig Dis* 5:639–654, 1960.
49. Bock OAA, Bank, S, Marks IN, et al: Effect of propantheline bromide and pipenzolate bromide upon exocrine pancreatic secretion. *Gastroenterology* 55:199–203, 1968.
50. Dyck WP, Texter EC, Lasater JM, et al: Influence of glucagon on pancreatic exocrine secretion in man. *Gastroenterology* 58:532–539, 1970.
51. Hanssen LE, Hanssen KF, Myren J: Inhibition of secretin release and pancreatic bicarbonate secretion by somatostatin infusion in man. *Scand J Gastroenterol* 12:391–394, 1977.
52. Domschke S, Domschke W, Rosch W, et al: Inhibition by somatostatin of secretin-stimulated pancreatic secretion in man: a study with pure pancreatic juice. *Scand J Gastroenterol* 12:59–63, 1977.
53. Shelby HT, Gross LP, Lichty P, et al: Action of cholecystokinin and cholinergic agents on membrane-bound calcium in dispersed pancreatic acinar cells. *J Clin Invest* 58:1482–1493, 1976.
54. Rothman SS: Enzyme secretion in the absence of zymogen granules. *Am J Physiol* 228:1828–1834, 1975.
55. Rothman SS: Secretion of new digestive enzyme by pancreas with minimal transit time. *Am J Physiol* 230:1499–1503, 1976.
56. Steer ML, Glazer G: Parallel secretion of digestive enzymes by the in vitro rabbit pancreas. *Am J Physiol* 231:1860–1865, 1976.
57. Goldberg DM, Wormsley KG: The interrelationships of pancreatic enzymes in human duodenal aspirate. *Gut* 11:859–866, 1970.

58. Dagorn JC, Sahel J, Sarles H: Nonparallel secretion of enzymes in human duodenal juice and pure pancreatic juice collected by endoscopic retrograde catheterization of the papilla. *Gastroenterology* 73:42–45, 1977.

59. Robberecht P, Cremer M, Christophe J: Discharge of newly synthesized proteins in pure juice collected from the human pancreas. *Gastroenterology* 72:417–420, 1977.

60. Rothman SS, Isenman LD: Secretion of digestive enzyme derived from two parallel intracellular pools. *Am J Physiol* 226:1082–1087, 1974.

61. Rothman SS: Independent secretion of different digestive enzymes by the pancreas. *Am J Physiol* 231:1847–1851, 1976.

62. Rothman SS, Wells H: Enhancement of pancreatic enzyme synthesis by pancreozymin. *Am J Physiol* 213:215–218, 1967.

63. Tandon BN, Banks PA, George PK, et al: Recovery of exocrine pancreatic function in adult protein-calorie malnutrition. *Gastroenterology* 58:358–362, 1970.

64. Webster PD, III, Black O, Jr., Mainz DL, et al: Pancreatic acinar cell metabolism and function. *Gastroenterology* 73:1434–1449, 1977.

65. Johnson LR, Lichtenberger LM, Copeland EM, et al: Action of gastrin on gastrointestinal structure and function. *Gastroenterology* 68:1184–1192, 1975.

66. Johnson LR: The trophic action of gastrointestinal hormones. *Gastroenterology* 70:278–288, 1976.

Etiology of Acute Pancreatitis

2.1 BILIARY TRACT DISEASE

Biliary tract disease is associated with 30% to 75% of all cases of pancreatitis. Some patients with gallstones develop acute pancreatitis in association with symptoms of acute cholecystitis. Others develop pancreatitis in the context of gallstones within the common bile duct causing pain (biliary colic), sepsis, and jaundice. Still others develop acute pancreatitis without any symptoms suggestive of acute cholecystitis or active disease within the common bile duct. These various clinical presentations have at least two features in common: (1) all usually cause mild edematous pancreatitis which resolves completely, although in some instances an episode may progress into severe hemorrhagic pancreatitis associated with serious complications; and (2) once the biliary tract disease has been eliminated by surgery, the patient usually experiences no further episodes of acute pancreatitis.

The manner in which biliary tract disease predisposes to acute pancreatitis has intrigued physicians. There is experimental evidence that acute cholecystitis may cause acute pancreatitis by the transmission of toxic or infectious material via lymphatic communications between the biliary tract and the pancreas.[1] It is not clear whether this mechanism occurs in man.

Several reports have helped considerably in our understanding of why some patients with active disease within the common bile duct develop pancreatitis, whereas others do not.[2,3] In these reports, patients who were jaundiced and experienced coexisting pancreatitis invariably passed gallstones in their stool, whereas patients who were jaundiced but did not experience pancreatitis rarely passed gallstones. A logical formulation is that when gallstones migrate from the gallbladder into the common bile duct and from the common bile duct through the ampulla of

Vater into the gut lumen, they are apt to cause episodes of pancreatitis. This formulation is reinforced by the observation that exacerbations of pancreatitis were associated with the passage of additional gallstones in the stool.[2,3] Thus far, the stools of patients who develop pancreatitis in association with either asymptomatic cholelithiasis or acute cholecystitis have not been similarly examined. If the passage of gallstones represents a common link in pancreatitis associated with all forms of biliary tract disease, gallstones should be present in the stool in these clinical situations as well.

It is of interest to re-read Opie's communications in 1901. In his first article,[4] he noted at autopsy a stone in the distal common bile duct of a patient who died of severe pancreatitis associated with a pancreatic abscess. He reasoned that the stone had at one time produced temporary obstruction of the duct of Wirsung causing pancreatitis. In the context of the concept of migration of gallstones causing pancreatitis,[2,3] it is more likely that the gallstone that was responsible for the fatal pancreatitis had already been passed into the duodenum, and that stones retained within the common bile duct may precipitate additional episodes of pancreatitis.[2,3] In his second publication,[5] he reported a case of fatal hemorrhagic pancreatitis associated with a stone that was impacted in the ampulla of Vater. He reasoned that the impacted stone enabled bile to reflux from the common bile duct into the pancreatic duct causing pancreatitis. It is likely that the temporary impaction of a gallstone in the ampullary region causes regurgitation of bile into the pancreatic duct. A permanent impaction as demonstrated by Opie occurs very rarely.

There are several potential problems with the "reflux" theory, but there are also considerable data that support it. From an anatomic standpoint, regurgitation of bile into the pancreatic duct would depend on the presence of a common channel joining the distal common bile duct with the pancreatic duct, since if the pancreatic duct and the common bile duct enter the duodenum separately, the impaction of a gallstone in the ampullary region would not influence flow in the adjacent separate pancreatic duct. Proponents of the "common channel" theory have produced evidence that as many as 70% of people have a common channel (as did the patient reported by Opie) and would be at risk to the development of pancreatitis following the regurgitation of bile into the pancreatic duct.

Another troublesome point is that the musculature of the duodenum surrounding the sphincter of Oddi also surrounds the orifice of the pancreatic duct, and spasm of the sphincter of Oddi that might occur with an impacted stone could actually isolate the pancreatic duct from the common bile duct rather than favor regurgitation of bile into the pancreatic duct.[6] However, additional evidence suggests that the constricting mechanisms are complex and that obstruction of the distal common bile duct may occur without simultaneous constriction of the pancreatic duct.[7]

A third problem is that in only a very few cases (perhaps only 5%) of pancreatitis associated with biliary tract disease is a gallstone actually demonstrated to be impacted in the ampulla of Vater. Such an arrangement would probably cause reflux of bile at high pressure. For the vast majority of patients who do not have a stone impacted at the ampulla of Vater, reflux of bile would presumably take place at more physiologic pressures, and chemical alterations of bile would be required to produce pancreatitis. There is considerable evidence that in health bile refluxes from time to time from the common bile duct into the pancreatic duct, and that in the presence of biliary tract disease reflux of "toxic" bile at physiologic pressures could be the cause of acute pancreatitis.[8] For example, infected bile infused at low pressures into the pancreatic duct of the dog causes severe destructive changes in the epithelium of the pancreatic duct associated with severe parenchymal necrosis.[9] The presence of *Escherichia coli* may cause pancreatic damage by itself or may convert one or more components of bile into toxic ingredients that damage the pancreas.[8,9]

One might anticipate that if a gallstone were to lodge even temporarily in the ampullary region prior to migration into the small intestine and cause pancreatitis by promoting reflux of bile into the pancreatic duct, there would be abnormalities of liver function tests, such as elevation of serum alkaline phosphatase. The fact that liver function tests are frequently entirely normal in acute pancreatitis associated with acute cholecystitis and acute pancreatitis associated with asymptomatic cholelithiasis would appear to militate against the concept of transient impaction of a gallstone in the ampullary region. On the other hand, two recent experiments indicate that even complete biliary obstruction for up to 2 hr in the rat does not produce an elevation of serum alkaline phosphatase levels.[10,11] Accordingly, migration of a gallstone causing temporary impaction in the ampullary region remains a reasonable hypothesis to explain pancreatitis associated with biliary tract disease.

2.2 ALCOHOL

Alcohol in responsible for at least 30% of cases of pancreatitis in the United States, and in some series as many as 60% to 90% of cases.[12,13] The explanation that has usually been offered for these figures has focused on known physiologic effects of alcohol. Alcohol stimulates the secretion of at least some acid from the stomach. When acid at a pH of less than 4.5 comes in contact with duodenal mucosa, secretin is released causing a flow of pancreatic juice. Alcohol also increases sphincteric resistance at the choledochoduodenal junction (but apparently does not cause an actual inflammation of the ampulla of Vater or duodenum). Pancreatitis would presumably occur because of secretion associated with obstruction to flow.

There are major flaws in this line of reasoning. First, the amount of acid secreted in response to alcohol may be minimal. Second, the effect of alcohol on the flow of pancreatic secretion is variable. For example, in both man and the experimental animal, the administration of alcohol intravenously inhibits rather than stimulates pancreatic secretion.[14-16] Third, spasm of the sphincter of Oddi is not apt to produce significant obstruction of the pancreatic duct. Finally, if alcohol caused pancreatitis simply by producing both secretion and obstruction to flow, it should not be difficult to document pancreatitis among young people who consume excessive amounts of alcohol on an intermittent basis. Yet, when an attempt was made to document alcoholic pancreatitis among college students, no cases were found.[17]

In recent years, attention has focused on possible metabolic effects of alcohol on the pancreas.[8] Evidence has accumulated as a result of scientific efforts by Professor Henri Sarles that the earliest recognizable changes in the pancreas caused by alcohol are the precipitation of protein plugs within pancreatic ductules and subsequent obstruction of ducts by these precipitates.[14,18,19] These changes, which have been observed in both man and the experimental animal, occur at first in scattered fashion but then become more diffuse. The precipitation of protein plugs leads to additional morphologic changes including ductular dilatation, ductular proliferation, dilatation of acinar tissue, focal atrophy and erosion of ductal epithelium at points of contact with plugs, desquamation of epithelium resulting in intraluminal debris, and ductal sclerosis which may obliterate the lumen of the duct. Ducts may therefore be obstructed by protein plugs, desquamation of epithelium, debris, and sclerosis. In time, the protein plugs may calcify and form intraductal stones. The main pancreatic duct is at first normal but in time becomes involved with the same process.

Chemical analysis has revealed that the protein plugs are composed of pancreatic enzymic protein. A number of factors appear to be required for the secretion of pancreatic enzymes in concentrated fashion and their inspissation within small ductules. There is a dietary requirement for protein and lipid without which protein plugs do not form in the experimental animal despite copious alcoholic ingestion.[10,20] The need for a high-protein, high-lipid diet would presumably be to ensure adequate pancreatic enzyme secretion. A deficiency in enzyme secretion, as occurs for example in protein-calorie malnutrition,[21] would probably prevent this phenomenon. Hyperconcentration of enzymes, which may favor inspissation, has been related also to an apparent decrease in secretin release caused by the chronic use of alcohol.[22] Other factors that may be important in the inspissation of enzymic protein are an increase in mucopolysaccharide,[23] and premature activation of zymogens within ductules.[24]

Experimentally, protein plugs have been recovered from pancreatic juice in the dog after only 3 months of chronic alcohol ingestion.[22,25] In man, at least 5 to 10 years of heavy drinking are required before the first clinical episode of alcoholic pancreatitis.[17,26,27] During this interval, the deposition of protein plugs and associated histologic damage take place such that at the time of the first clinical episode, widespread histologic damage has already occurred.[17] The amount of alcohol that may be consumed on a regular basis during these many years is not clearly defined. Several recent articles place this amount in the vicinity of 150 to 180 gm/day.[20,28,29] The long interval of steady alcohol consumption that is required before the first clinical expression of the illness is underscored by the fact that most patients develop their first attack of alcoholic pancreatitis between the ages of 30 and 40.[1,27,30]

Other suggestions have been made to explain the relationship between alcohol ingestion and pancreatitis. One in particular relates the ingestion of alcohol to an enhanced reflux of duodenal contents through the ampulla of Vater into the pancreatic duct.[31] If duodenal reflux were an important feature of alcoholic pancreatitis in man, a single episode of alcohol ingestion could cause pancreatitis, but appears not to. Another suggestion is that alcohol might stimulate the secretion of secretin from the duodenum.[32] Additional studies have suggested that if alcohol does cause the release of secretin, it may do so via the release of gastric acid rather than as a direct effect.[33] In either case, this effect would not be sufficient to cause acute pancreatitis in the absence of ductal obstruction by protein plugs. Finally, it is possible that lipid abnormalities associated with the ingestion of alcohol cause pancreatitis. This relationship is discussed in the following section.

2.3 HYPERLIPIDEMIA

The association of pancreatitis with a disturbance of lipid metabolism has long been appreciated. Two forms have been recognized. In one, a disorder of lipid metabolism has been thought to occur on a familial basis and to persist indefinitely. In the other, the disorder has been considered to be a temporary sequel of an episode of pancreatitis that would disappear once there was clinical improvement.[34]

It is now becoming clear that disorders of lipid metabolism in pancreatitis cannot be defined this simply. It is true that there are patients with a familial disturbance of lipid metabolism who on rare occasions develop recurrent episodes of acute pancreatitis.[35] The types that have been identified are Types 1, 4, and 5 according to the Fredrickson classification. In Type 1, the excessive triglycerides are in the form of chylomicrons. Serum chylomicrons are normally increased after meals but should return to normal levels 12 to 14 hr after the last meal. The presence of excessive chylomicrons in serum imparts a diffuse cloudy appearance to the serum. If the serum is then refrigerated overnight, chylomicrons rise to the surface forming a creamy layer leaving a clear layer below. In Type 5, the chemical basis for the abnormality is an increased serum level of both chylomicrons and endogenous triglycerides. The endogenous triglycerides are transported in serum as very low density lipoproteins (VLDL). When the serum of a patient with Type 5 hypertriglyceridemia is refrigerated overnight, a creamy layer appears on top (caused by chylomicrons) and turbid serum appears below (caused by very low density lipoproteins). On very rare occasions, Type 4 hyperlipoproteinemia may cause acute pancreatitis. Type 4 has as its chemical basis an increased level of endogenous triglycerides.

Patients with a familial form of hyperlipidemia causing pancreatitis are frequently diagnosed in childhood or during early adult life. When one excludes for the moment these relatively few patients with easily diagnosed familial hyperlipidemia, there is left a considerable number of patients with pancreatitis whose lipid disorder became evident during an episode of pancreatitis and who were not initially thought to have a familial form of the disorder. One early speculation was that pancreatitis itself may cause a transient lipid disorder in man as well as in the rabbit.[36] The difficulty with this concept was the realization that the only patients with an associated lipid disorder were those with alcoholic pancreatitis.[12,37,38] Patients with pancreatitis associated with biliary tract disease, hyperparathyroidism, hereditary pancreatitis, and trauma did not develop a lipid disorder. A number of suggestions have been made to explain the development of hyperlipidemia in association with alcoholic pancreatitis.[37,39] Whatever the specific reason, a crucial observation was that serum triglyceride levels in most of these patients did not return completely to normal as had been expected during an asymptomatic interval.[12,37,38] The concept that has since evolved is that a lipid disorder associated with alcoholic pancreatitis is likely to have an underlying genetic mechanism such that even during an asymptomatic period the patient maintains a slightly to moderately elevated level of serum triglycerides. Moderate alcoholic ingestion may then cause a substantial increase in serum triglyceride levels in a fashion that does not occur unless there is a preexisting disorder of lipid metabolism.[40]

The vast majority of patients with alcoholic pancreatitis do not exhibit a disorder of lipid metabolism. Among those that are documented to have an elevated triglyceride level during an episode of alcoholic pancreatitis, it is likely that pancreatitis was caused by many years of alcohol abuse and the lipid abnormality is simply a marker of alcoholic ingestion. However, a very high triglyceride level induced by alcohol may contribute to pancreatic inflammation and may by itself induce acute pancreatitis.[12] The importance of this observation is that acute pancreatitis may occur on the basis of sporadic alcohol consumption if serum triglyceride levels become markedly elevated.

The incidence of lipid abnormalities in alcoholic pancreatitis is variable. In one report, the figure was 12%;[37] in another, 38%.[41] In another study, 22% of patients with acute pancreatitis (several of whom consumed at least some alcohol) were found to have an associated Type 5 hyperlipidemia.[42]

In addition to patients with well-recognized familial hyperlipidemia and patients in whom a genetic predisposition is uncovered by the use of alcohol, there is another group of patients who have been found to have a lipid abnormality associated with pancreatitis. These are patients utilizing estrogen therapy.[43,44,45] Most if not all of these patients have a persistent disorder of lipid metabolism following discontinuation of the medication with serum triglyceride levels remaining indefinitely in a slightly to moderately elevated range. The types of lipid disorder that have been documented have been Type 4,[43] and Type 5.[44,45] Estrogen therapy is capable of causing an increase in serum triglyceride level from moderate levels to an extremely elevated level in excess of 3000 mg/100 ml.[46] The mechanism appears to be an increase in hepatic biosynthesis of very low density lipoproteins.[47] The discovery that a Type 4 hyperlipidemia is capable of causing acute pancreatitis is thought to be related to the very high levels of triglyceride that can be induced by estrogens as compared to the lower levels of serum triglyceride among most patients with Type 4 disease.[43]

An interesting feature of pancreatitis associated with a disorder of lipid metabolism is the frequency with which serum amylase levels remain normal despite both clinical and at times surgical evidence of acute pancreatitis. Those features are described in detail in Chapter 6 (measurement of serum amylase).

The manner in which an elevated triglyceride level causes pancreatitis among patients with familial hyperlipidemia, among some patients with alcohol-induced hyperlipidemia, and among patients with estrogen-induced hyperlipidemia is unclear. Experimental evidence suggests that pancreatic lipase may convert triglycerides within the pancreas into toxic free fatty acids which then cause acute pancreatic inflammation.[48]

It is now known that hyperlipidemia may be responsible not only for acute pancreatitis but also the development of pancreatic insufficiency.[44,49-51] One patient has developed severe pancreatic exocrine insufficiency associated with familial Type 1 hyperlipoproteinemia in the absence of clinical pancreatitis.[51] Another, whose chronic pancreatitis was thought to be related to hyperlipidemia, required pancreatic surgery for relief of pain.[52]

2.4 HEREDITARY PANCREATITIS

There is documentation of at least 21 families and 106 family members with hereditary pancreatitis.[53] Thus far, all patients have been white with an equal number of males and females. The genetic pattern of this disorder appears to be transmitted as an autosomal dominant trait. Symptoms usually occur at an early age, occasionally in infancy and generally by ages 10–12. Most episodes of pancreatitis subside within a few days without major complications. Occasionally, an attack is quite severe and leads to a serious complication, such as a pseudocyst. In general, the prognosis is favorable despite recurrences of acute pancreatitis that occur at intervals of several months to several years.

The cause is unknown. At least half of the cases have been associated with large intraductal stones located within pancreatic ducts in the head of the pancreas and occasionally in the body and tail of the pancreas as well. At times there is advanced pancreatic fibrosis with relative sparing of islet cells. Despite the high incidence of intraductal calcification, steatorrhea and diabetes in association with hereditary pancreatitis are usually relatively mild. Pancreatic function studies have shown marked impairment of volume flow, and impairment of bicarbonate concentration and enzyme secretion.[53,54]

Approximately one-half of patients with hereditary pancreatitis have undergone surgery, but no specific anatomic variation has been found that explains this illness. Endoscopic retrograde pancreatography has failed to reveal an abnormality of pancreatic ducts that is specific for hereditary pancreatitis.[54] A reasonable view is that an undefined metabolic disturbance causes severe pancreatic damage in this illness. Two of the original cases described in 1952 were documented to have an associated aminoaciduria. Since that time, detailed studies on numerous patients have failed to confirm a specific defect in amino acid excretion in hereditary pancreatitis.

An increased incidence of pancreatic carcinoma has been reported among patients with hereditary pancreatitis. Two explanations have been offered. The first is that chronic pancreatitis in general may predispose to the development of pancreatic carcinoma. The second is that family members who do not have pancreatitis may be as susceptible to pancreatic carcinoma as patients with hereditary pancreatitis.[55] If this observation is correct, the development of pancreatic carcinoma in hereditary pancreatitis would indicate a familial predisposition not related specifically to the development of pancreatitis.

2.5 HYPERPARATHYROIDISM AND HYPERCALCEMIA

Approximately 7% to 19% of patients with hyperparathyroidism in the United States,[56,57] and 6.5% of such patients in Europe,[58] have been shown to develop acute pancreatitis. Patients with parathyroid adenoma, parathyroid carcinoma, and hyperplasia of the parathyroid gland are all susceptible to this complication.[56] The mechanisms that have been cited to explain the development of pancreatitis in hyperparathyroidism have included: obstruction of pancreatic ducts by stones, activation of trypsin by excess calcium within pancreatic secretion, and vasculitis within the pancreas.[8]

There are major problems with each of these proposed mechanisms. In regard to obstruction of pancreatic ducts by stones, it should be recalled that only 25% to 45% of patients with acute pancreatitis associated with hyperparathyroidism have demonstrable intraductal stones.[58] Therefore, the majority of patients clearly require an alternative explanation. Even among patients with intraductal stones, surgical correction of hyperparathyroidism usually prevents further episodes of acute pancreatitis.[56,57] The presence of intraductal stones does not appear to be critical for the initiation or perpetuation of pancreatitis associated with hyperparathyroidism.

Under certain conditions, the addition of calcium to human pancreatic juice may increase the conversion of trypsinogen to trypsin in an in vitro system.[59] Furthermore, an increased concentration of calcium in pancreatic juice has been associated with an increase in trypsin levels of pancreatic juice in the dog.[60] However, this association has not been demonstrated in man. The possibility that pancreatic juice calcium may be important in pancreatic disease will be discussed shortly.

Finally, there is one reported case of intravascular clotting associated with hyperparathyroidism and acute pancreatitis.[61] Since thrombi were found in the smaller vascular channels of both pancreas and kidney, these abnormalities may have been on the basis of disseminated intravascular coagulation secondary to pancreatitis rather than a specific effect of hyperparathyroidism or hypercalcemia on the pancreas.

It is tempting to speculate that parathormone itself rather than induced hypercalcemia causes pancreatitis. First, at least one patient has developed chronic pancreatitis with steatorrhea without symptoms of acute pancreatitis and without demonstrable intraductal stones.[62] Second, pancreatic inflammation has been produced in the experimental animal by inducing excess parathormone activity without the prior development of stones.[60] Third, almost all of the cases of pancreatitis in association with hypercalcemia have been on the basis of hyperparathyroidism. However, if parathormone is capable of causing acute pancreatitis, one might expect that chronic renal failure complicated by secondary hyperparathyroidism would also be associated with acute pancreatitis. One might also expect that the various tumors that secrete ectopic parathormone would cause acute pancreatitis. Thus far, neither of these associations has been noted.[63] One possible reason for this nonassociation is the fact that parathormone secreted by malignant tumors is immunologically distinct from parathormone secreted by parathyroid gland,[64] and may not damage the pancreas. Another possible explanation is that parathyroid excess in association with malignancy is usually of too short a duration to damage the pancreas.

Pancreatic exocrine function among patients with hyperparathyroidism has not been studied in detail. Thus far, among cases of hyperparathyroidism without evident pancreatitis, pancreatic function studies with the use of intravenous secretin have either been normal,[58,65,66] or have shown decreased enzyme output.[58,66] Among patients with acute or chronic pancreatitis associated with hyperparathyroidism, a reduction in bicarbonate concentration has been noted.[62,67–69] A decrease in volume response has also been noted.[68,69] Steatorrhea,[62,67] and diabetes[62] have also been reported.

Very few patients with hypercalcemia not associated with hyperparathyroidism develop pancreatitis. In most of the reports, there have been associated features that may have been responsible for the pancreatitis rather than the hypercalcemia. These features include severe seizure activity,[70] and use of Prednisone in a critically ill patient with multiple myeloma.[71] Other case reports are lacking in details.[72] Two recent reports of acute hypercalcemia induced by excessive intravenous calcium replacement are more convincing that induced hypercalcemia may cause acute pancreatitis.[73,74] In view of the large numbers of patients who have hypercalcemia associated with diseases other than hyperparathyroidism, it is interesting that the incidence of pancreatitis is extremely low if it occurs at all.

The way in which hypercalcemia may cause pancreatitis remains obscure. The obvious inference is that increased amounts of calcium gain access to pancreatic juice and either cause the development of intraductal stones, activate trypsin, or interfere with cellular processes in some unknown fashion. The secretion of calcium in pancreatic juice in health and disease is just beginning to be understood. Several points are of interest. Pancreatic juice calcium concentration cannot be increased simply by increasing serum calcium in acute experiments.[75,76] In response to intravenous cholecystokinin-pancreozymin (CCK-PZ) there is a marked increase in pancreatic juice calcium concentration and pancreatic juice enzyme concentration.[76-80] The calcium that appears in association with enzyme secretion is part of the amylase molecule. In response to intravenous secretin, intraductal calcium concentration falls to very low levels paralleling very low concentrations of pancreatic-juice enzymes.[77] In chronic pancreatitis, intravenous CCK-PZ may fail to cause an increased pancreatic enzyme concentration and an increased pancreatic-juice calcium concentration.[79,80] This response is not unexpected, since in chronic pancreatitis there is considerable acinar damage and decreased enzyme secretion. However, in chronic pancreatitis, varieties of abnormalities of pancreatic juice calcium have been noted, including an increased basal pancreatic juice calcium concentration.[65,80-82] In the absence of pancreatic enzymes, it is likely that an increased pancreatic juice calcium concentration in chronic pancreatitis signifies an entry of calcium from either interstitial sources or the serum. If this is ionized calcium, its presence may enhance the calcification of intraductal debris or protein plugs.

In summary, hypercalcemia does not readily lead to increased concentration of calcium in pancreatic juice. Chronic pancreatitis may be associated with increased calcium concentration in pancreatic juice. Once the pancreas is damaged, the usual mechanisms that prevent the entry of ionized serum calcium and possibly other constituents of serum may become impaired. Whether the increased pancreatic juice calcium in this state contributes to pancreatic disease is speculative. There are several varieties of pancreatic diseases including diabetes mellitus[82] and pancreatic carcinoma[83] that are associated with increased pancreatic juice calcium concentration without causing either pancreatitis or intraductal stones.

2.6 STRUCTURAL ABNORMALITIES

2.6.1 Common Bile Duct and Ampullary Region

Choledochal cysts invariably cause abdominal pain, frequently but not invariably are associated with an abdominal mass and jaundice,[84] and on rare occasion cause acute pancreatitis.[85]

The region of the distal common bile duct and ampulla may be obstructed by parasitic infestations[86] and by gallstones wedged in the ampullary region. There is one case of a pedunculated polyp of the ampulla of Vater that prolapsed into the main pancreatic duct causing pancreatitis.[87] There is increasing awareness of the association of recurrent acute pancreatitis with a condition termed stenosis of the sphincter of Oddi.[88-94] In some instances, symptoms have begun early in childhood suggestive of a congenital abnormality. In others, symptoms have begun in adult life. Most patients have experienced recurrent severe abdominal pain. The etiology of inflammatory changes of the sphincter of Oddi (including at times severe fibrosis) is not clear in all cases. Some patients undoubtedly have these changes as a complication of biliary tract disease probably as a result of passage of gallstones through the sphincter of Oddi into the duodenum.[2] Other patients with no disorder of gallbladder or common bile duct develop stenosis of the sphincter of Oddi for unknown reasons. The difficulties in diagnosis of this entity and the surgical correction will be described in detail in Chapter 8.

2.6.2 Duodenum

It would appear logical that the reflux of duodenal contents into the pancreatic ducts could be an important cause of pancreatitis.[95] A major attraction of this thesis is the fact that trypsin usually does not become activated until it reaches the duodenum, where enterokinase catalyzes this transformation. Once this takes place, activated trypsin then autocatalyzes additional amounts of trypsin from trypsinogen and also activates the remaining proteolytic enzymes from their inactive precursors.

There is considerable experimental evidence attesting to the fact that reflux of duodenal contents may be associated with severe pancreatitis.[8] For example, a severe form of pancreatitis can be induced experimentally following the formation of a closed duodenal loop and generation of high intraduodenal pressures. The variables that appear to be responsible for pancreatitis in this model include the presence of activated trypsin and bacteria, vascular ischemia, and the very high pressures at which duodenal fluid is regurgitated into the pancreatic duct via the ampulla of Vater. The importance of bacteria in this model is underscored by the fact that the incidence of hemorrhagic pancreatitis can be reduced if the bacterial flora within the closed duodenal loop are suppressed by antibiotics. However, even in germ-free dogs, hemorrhagic pancreatitis ensues as long as there is vascular compromise to the loop.

The relationship of duodenal reflux to the development of pancreatitis remains uncertain. For example, in the dog, when vascular compromise of a closed duodenal loop is prevented, pancreatitis can also be prevented. In addition, there is evidence that pressure relationships in the dog may favor the reflux of duodenal contents into the pancreatic ducts without apparent ill effect.[96] Furthermore, in man, following sphincteroplasty of both the ampulla of Vater and the duct of Wirsung, barium can be seen to reflux not only into the common bile duct but also into the pancreatic duct without ill effect. For these reasons, one would anticipate that structural abnormalities of the duodenum would rarely be associated with acute pancreatitis in man.

Acute and chronic pancreatitis have been reported in association with an annular pancreas.[8,97,98] The precise cause of the pancreatitis is not entirely clear. Since the pancreatic tissue usually encircles the duodenum proximal to the ampulla of Vater, there is no intraduodenal obstruction that might force duodenal contents into the pancreatic duct.[99] One suggestion that has been made is that the pancreatic duct within the encircling annular pancreas might become stretched or angulated in a way that would cause inflammation of at least this portion of the pancreas.

Several cases of large intraluminal duodenal diverticula have been reported in association with acute pancreatitis.[100,101] Some intraluminal diverticula appear to be large enough to cause significant duodenal obstruction in the vicinity of the ampulla of Vater. One might also suspect that there would be significant stasis of intraduodenal contents leading to bacterial overgrowth. Regurgitation of duodenal fluid containing bacteria might be injurious to the pancreas whereas regurgitation of relatively sterile contents (such as after a sphincteroplasty) might be harmless.

Duodenal diverticula in the vicinity of the ampulla of Vater have been noted with increasing frequency. In one report, the insertion of the common bile duct and pancreatic duct into a duodenal diverticulum was noted in 3% of patients.[102] Pancreatitis has been noted in association with this anatomic variation.[103]

Examples of significant duodenal obstruction that may be associated with acute pancreatitis include afferent loop obstruction, superior mesenteric artery obstruction of the duodenum, and carcinoma obstructing the duodenum.[104] It should be kept in mind that duodenal obstruction may cause an increase in serum amylase without pancreatitis if there is extra-vasation of amylase-rich duodenal fluid into the peritoneal cavity and resorption into the blood stream.

On occasion, a patient with regional enteritis involving the duodenum has developed pancreatitis.[105] The evidence for an association is convincing on the basis of characteristic clinical presentation and operative findings.[105] Reflux of barium from the duodenum to the pancreas and biliary ducts has been noted. The reflux could have been caused by a fistulous communication between the diseased duodenum and pancreatic duct or possibly by destruction of the sphincter of Oddi by the inflammation. If regurgitation of duodenal contents causes pancreatitis in this clinical entity, it is likely that duodenal juice is altered (such as by overgrowth with bacteria) to account for the development of pancreatitis since under other circumstances (such as following a sphincteroplasty), barium can be seen to reflux into the pancreatic duct without causing pancreatitis. Another mechanism of pancreatitis in regional enteritis of the duodenum and ileum would be the development of gallstones, a well-recognized complication of regional enteritis involving the terminal ileum.

2.6.3 Pancreatic Duct

Pancreatic ductal obstruction beyond the sphincter of Oddi is an unusual cause of acute pancreatitis in man. Obstruction of the main pancreatic duct causing acute pancreatitis has occurred in association with a variety of tumors, including ductal adenocarcinoma,[106,107] islet cell tumors,[107,108] and carcinoma metastatic to the pancreas.[109] Tumor-induced pancreatitis may lead to the development of pancreatic pseudocysts,[107,109] and amylase-rich ascitic fluid due to extravasation of pancreatic juice from a pseudocyst.[109]

A stricture of the orifice of the duct of Wirsung may cause severe recurrent pancreatitis and on rare occasion chronic calcific pancreatitis.[110]

The cause of acute pancreatitis in association with severe pancreatic ductal obstruction is perhaps best explained by rupture of pancreatic ductules and acini. This phenomenon has been documented in man[109] and in the experimental animal[111] in response to severe obstruction. Another mechanism documented in one patient with ductal obstruction caused by a carcinoma of the pancreas is premature intraductal activation of pancreatic zymogens.[112] Activated enzymes could be forced through disrupted ducts to cause severe inflammation of acinar and interstitial structures or might even sift through normal clefts located between acinar cells and thereby reach interstitial tissue if the obstruction is not severe enough to cause actual ductal disruption.[113]

There are probably many important variables in the effect of ductal obstruction on the pancreas. Acute obstruction in man in association with trauma to the pancreas may cause severe pancreatitis.[114] On the other hand, ligation of the pancreatic duct draining the residual tail of the pancreas following pancreaticoduodenectomy for carcinoma may result in no significant acute pancreatitis.[115] Furthermore, partial ductal obstruction such as by a solitary stone in the pancreatic duct near the head of the pancreas may not cause important symptomatology during life.[116]

On the basis of extensive experimentation involving ductal ligation, it is evident that ligation of the pancreatic duct followed by stimulation of pancreatic secretion may cause extensive edema of the pancreas,[117] at times relatively severe inflammation with fat necrosis,[118] but not hemorrhagic pancreatitis.[117,118] The variables that may convert pancreatic edema into pancreatic necrosis include ischemia,[119] variation of the completeness of ductal obstruction, and variation in intensity of pancreatic secretion.[120] Complete ligation of the pancreatic duct in the experimental animal results in prompt histologic changes within the first week including ductal and lymphatic distention, interstitial edema,[121] and destruction of acinar and ductal cells.[122] In the absence of ischemia, intense pancreatic stimulation, and possibly other variables, the long-term effects of complete pancreatic ductal ligation are atrophy of acinar tissue and fibrosis.[123] Although islet cells may appear normal,[123] there may be impairment of insulin secretion.[124]

2.7 IATROGENIC CAUSES

2.7.1 Medications

A variety of medications are generally listed as causes of acute pancreatitis. A basic difficulty is the uncertainty whether a medication or some other factor is responsible for the condition. For example, patients receiving various diuretic agents have been reported to develop pancreatitis, including Chlorothiazide,[125,126] Chlorthalidone,[127] and Frusemide (Lasix).[128] In each instance, there was a delay of several weeks to several months before the development of pancreatitis. Many of the patients were elderly with either severe congestive heart failure or severe hypertension. Hypovolemia induced by the diuretic rather than a toxic property of the diuretic itself may have led to severe hypotension and ischemia of the pancreas. It is also possible that the cause of the pancreatitis was totally unrelated to the use of the medication. In one case report, for example, there was a background of significant alcohol intake;[138] in another, patients were pregnant.[126] One recent report offers quite convincing evidence that Furosemide not only caused the initial pancreatitis but also a second episode which followed a second administration of the medication.[129]

Furosemide increases the volume and bicarbonate output of the pancreas in man in response to a steady-state infusion of secretin.[130] This augmentation of volume and bicarbonate would presumably occur under basal conditions as well, but this physiologic action of Furosemide is probably not the one that causes pancreatitis. Thiazides such as hydrochlorothiazide and chlorthalidone have the capacity for causing a necrotizing vasculitis in the skin,[131] and chlorothiazide has been shown to produce inflammatory changes in the pancreases of mice.[132] Whatever capacity thiazides have in damaging the pancreas, case reports of pancreatitis are few and far between.

Other medications reported to cause acute pancreatitis are glucocorticoid agents. Again, it is difficult to evaluate individual case reports that document pancreatitis in association with the use of steroid agents, since diseases under treatment are usually capable of producing vascular injury (such as lupus erythematosis and polyarteritis nodosa). Pancreatitis on the basis of glucocorticoid usage was reported among six children, one or two of whom did not appear to have any underlying illness that could conceivably have been responsible for pancreatitis.[133] Recently, adrenocorticotropic hormone has been found to inhibit pancreatic enzyme secretion in man without affecting volume and bicarbonate secretion.[134] In this report, pure pancreatic juice was collected by external transduodenal drainage of the main pancreatic duct. This physiologic effect does not help explain possible toxicity of steroid agents on the pancreas.

Several reports have incriminated Phenformin in the development of pancreatitis.[135-138] Severe lactic acidosis occurred in most of the cases,[138] and may represent a common link. Lactic acidosis of various causes may also cause an elevation in serum amylase without pancreatitis.[139] The source of the hyperamylasemia has not been determined. Procaine-induced lupus erythematosis was associated with acute pancreatitis in one report.[140] Several drugs have been reported to be responsible for a syndrome of necrotizing angiitis in the pancreas and in other organs as well.[188]

The use of L-asparaginase has been associated with acute pancreatitis in two patients with leukemia.[141,142]

Salicylazosulfapyridine (Azulfidine) has caused pancreatitis and has also caused recurrences following rechallenge.[143] The use of azathioprine (Imuran) has been associated with acute pancreatitis in several instances.[144-146] Rechallenge with this medication caused a second episode of pancreatitis in all three reports. This would suggest that azathioprine causes at least some cases of acute pancreatitis following renal transplantation.

2.7.2 Endoscopic Retrograde Cholangiopancreatography

The insertion of an endoscope into esophagus, stomach, and duodenum is at times associated with an elevation of serum amylase concentration without evidence of pancreatitis. Since an elevation in serum amylase concentration may also occur when the insertion is limited to the esophagus and stomach, the likelihood is that there is release of amylase from salivary glands during the procedure and not amylase from the pancreas. Elevation of serum amylase during an endoscopic procedure is documented in as many as 25% to 50% of patients undergoing cannulation of the main pancreatic duct as part of an endoscopic retrograde cholangiopancreatography (ERCP).[147,148] In almost all instances, the elevation of serum amylase is not associated with clinical symptomatology and does not represent an episode of acute pancreatitis. The increase in serum amylase is probably caused by reflux of residual intraductal amylase into the interstitium of the pancreas and then into the systemic circulation. An alternative explanation would be release of amylase from salivary glands during the procedure.

On rare occasions the introduction of contrast material into the pancreas is associated not only with an increase in serum amylase but also with clinical manifestations of acute pancreatitis. The incidence of this complication is 1% to 3.5%.[148–152] The patients who appear to be most susceptible are those who have had a previous episode of pancreatitis,[149] those who have disease of the pancreas,[151] and those who are endoscoped by relatively inexperienced endoscopists.[149] The various factors that are associated with ERCP-induced acute pancreatitis include the speed and pressure of injection of contrast material, the volume injected, the number of injections into the pancreatic duct, and underlying pathology of pancreatic ducts.[152] The use of large volumes and excessive pressure tend to overdistend the pancreatic ducts and cause acinar opacification. Evidence is accumulating that postinjection pancreatitis occurs almost exclusively among patients with acinar opacification.[152] The incidence of postinjection pancreatitis can be reduced considerably by using small amounts of contrast material at physiologic pressures and utilizing careful fluoroscopic monitoring of the effects of injection. In one study with manometric control of injection pressure, the frequency of acinar filling was reduced to 2.4%, and there was no clinical evidence of acute pancreatitis.[153]

Thus far, there have been no fatalities from acute pancreatitis caused by ERCP, but five fatalities have occurred because filling of a pancreatic pseudocyst caused sepsis and pancreatic necrosis.[152,154] If a pseudocyst has been documented by diagnostic ultrasound, ERCP should be carried out only if absolutely necessary and only with extreme caution. However, it is reassuring to note that in almost all instances that a pseudocyst has been documented by ERCP, there have been no complications.[152]

Another serious complication of ERCP is trauma to the head of the pancreas during attempted injection of contrast material into the ampulla of Vater. In two patients, a localized mass lesion was produced that was suggestive of carcinoma at the time of surgery.[155] Submucosal injection into the wall of the duodenum during efforts to visualize the pancreatic ducts has on one occasion caused extravasation of dye into venous pathways that opacified the portal vein.[156] Even contrast material successfully injected into the pancreatic duct may gain almost instantaneous access to the systemic circulation with visualization of kidneys, ureter, and bladder.[152,157,158] The incidence of this occurrence has been reported at between 5%[158] and 35%.[152] Almost all patients with urographic visualization have also shown evidence of acinar opacification. The importance of urographic visualization is twofold. First, it may be taken as evidence for injection at excessive pressures or utilization of excessive volumes of contrast material. Second, since contrast material may gain access to the circulation, screening of the patient for possible allergy to the contrast material should be done prior to the performance of ERCP.

The past few years have witnessed attempts to manipulate the ampulla of Vater in patients with biliary tract calculi and sludge. These attempts have included endoscopic retrograde flush of the biliary tree, endoscopic dilatation of the ampulla of Vater, extraction of common duct stones with a balloon or basket inserted through the instrument, and endoscopic electrosurgical sphincterotomy.[159-161] In one series, electrosurgical papillotomy was attempted among 22 patients with no complications.[159] In another, there were three episodes of pancreatitis with 1 fatality among 265 patients[160]; in a third, there were 9 instances of nonfatal pancreatitis among 267 patients.[161] Assignment of the proper role of this therapeutic approach awaits further experience.

2.7.3 Postoperative Pancreatitis

Pancreatitis can be a serious and even lethal complication of surgery. In two published series, mortality as a result of postoperative pancreatitis was 24%[162] and 42%.[163] The vast majority of cases involved operations in the vicinity of the pancreas. The mechanisms that have been proposed to explain postoperative pancreatitis include direct trauma to the pancreas, interference with blood supply of the pancreas, and possibly a decrease in trypsin inhibitor level in pancreatic juice.[162] If the pancreas itself must be incised as part of an operative approach, the possibility of pancreatitis would presumably be enhanced because of direct injury.[84] Choledochal injury at the time of surgery may also lead to postoperative pancreatic complications including fistula between common bile duct and pancreas and pancreatic pseudocyst.[164]

The majority of cases of postoperative pancreatitis occur after surgery involving the stomach and biliary tract. The incidence following gastrectomy has been estimated at 0.8%[162] and after biliary tract surgery from 0.2%[162] to 4%.[163] There are several features which may increase the likelihood of pancreatitis following biliary tract surgery. These include common bile duct exploration,[163] and use of large dilators passed through the sphincter of Oddi as well as the use of a long-arm T tube.[162] Pancreatitis following surgery on the biliary tract occurs much more frequently among patients who have had clinical evidence of pancreatitis preoperatively (21%) as compared to those who did not (2%).[163] Operative cholangiography appears not to increase the risk of postoperative pancreatitis.[162,163]

From a clinical standpoint, it may be difficult to recognize the development of pancreatitis following abdominal surgery. Manifestations of pancreatitis including nausea and vomiting, abdominal pain, and abdominal tenderness may either be masked by the use of narcotic agents or misinterpreted as routine postoperative pain. An elevation of serum amylase in the postoperative period would appear to be a reasonable way to diagnose pancreatitis, but is not. In one recent study, the incidence of postoperative elevation of serum amylase was 10% of all patients, only half of whom underwent abdominal operations. None of the patients exhibited clinical evidence of pancreatitis.[165] In some instances, the elevation of serum amylase was caused by salivary isoamylase. A possible mechanism for release of salivary amylase is passage of an endotracheal tube. Among patients whose elevations were predominantly pancreatic and therefore suggestive of pancreatitis, there may indeed have been subclinical pancreatitis. Another explanation would be that the use of a narcotic agent caused spasm of the sphincter of Oddi and regurgitation of pancreatic amylase into the interstitium of the pancreas and then into the general circulation. This is probably the mechanism of the elevated serum amylase levels following ERCP and following the morphine-prostigmine test.

An elevation in serum amylase in the postoperative period should alert the clinician to the possibility of postoperative pancreatitis. The use of the amylase–creatinine clearance ratio and serum isoamylases in making the distinction between pancreatitis and spurious elevation of serum amylase will be described in Chapter 6.

2.7.4 Renal Transplantation

The incidence of pancreatitis following renal transplantation is 2% to 7%.[166-171] The mortality figures vary from 20% in one small series[166] to figures between 50% and 70%.[167,169,170] There is no particular type of renal disease that predisposes to posttransplantation pancreatitis. In some instances, pancreatitis occurs within a few days of a transplantation suggesting a form of postoperative pancreatitis. In most instances, however, pancreatitis occurs several months following surgery, at times 4 to 5 years following surgery. In one series, the average interval between transplantation and the development of pancreatitis was 216 days.[167]

Various factors may contribute to pancreatitis following transplantation. These include the use of medications such as azathioprine, adrenocorticosteroid agents, and L-asparaginase.[166] Various infectious agents have also been suggested. Cytomegalovirus has been noted within pancreatic tissue.[169,172] Other proposed mechanisms include postoperative hyperparathyroidism[169] and vasculitis.[169,172]

It is often quite difficult to establish a diagnosis of posttransplantation pancreatitis. Symptoms of abdominal discomfort including nausea and vomiting occur quite frequently among patients with uremia and do not necessarily indicate the development of pancreatitis. Serum amylase may be somewhat elevated on the basis of uremia alone. When serum amylase is elevated in excess of twice normal, pancreatitis should be suspected.[167]

Pathologically, posttransplantation pancreatitis may be associated with marked destruction of the pancreas including severe vasculitis,[172] hemorrhagic pancreatitis,[166] and pancreatic abscess and pseudocyst.[173]

2.8 PANCREATIC TRAUMA

2.8.1 Penetrating Injuries

The incidence of pancreatic injury during penetrating injuries to the abdomen has been estimated at 3%.[174] Adjacent viscera are almost always injured as well, particularly liver, stomach, colon, kidney, and duodenum. Surgical treatment of penetrating injury to the pancreas places emphasis on hemostasis, debridement of necrotic material, adequate drainage, and control of pancreatic secretion if there is ductal laceration. Methods of control of pancreatic secretion are included in the discussion of blunt trauma.

2.8.2 Blunt Trauma

The incidence of injury to the pancreas during blunt trauma to the abdomen has been estimated at 1% to 3%.[174] The vast majority of cases are caused by compression of the pancreas against the spine. The types of injury to the pancreas that may occur under these circumstances include contusion, laceration, subcapsular hematoma, complete transection of the pancreas, transection of the pancreatic duct, and combined injury to duodenum and head of the pancreas.[175] The types of blunt trauma that cause pancreatic injury include automobile accidents (either steering wheel injury or pedestrian injury),[176] handle bar injuries among children, physical assaults associated with blows to the abdomen, football injuries, and serious falls. At least one patient developed traumatic pancreatitis following an automobile accident in which the left lower thorax was struck causing a sheering force transmitted from the thorax.[177] It might be anticipated that vigorous external cardiac massage might also transmit a sheering force to the abdomen and be responsible for an occasional case of pancreatitis.

From a clinical standpoint, it may be extremely difficult to recognize injury to the pancreas following blunt trauma to the abdomen. Signs and symptoms suggestive of pancreatic injury are usually present, including abdominal pain and mild tenderness,[175] but these features might as easily indicate injury to other intraabdominal structures. The distinction of pancreatic trauma from important trauma to surrounding structures may be made if free air is discovered under the diaphragm on an upright abdominal x-ray (indicating a perforation) or if gastrograffin swallow reveals the presence of severe duodenal injury.[175]

A great deal of attention has focused on the possibility that measurement of serum amylase may be of diagnostic help. Unfortunately, in the context of blunt trauma to the abdomen, elevation of serum amylase appears to be entirely nonspecific.[176,178] Serum amylase may be elevated when no abdominal injury can be determined; it may be elevated on the basis of injury to an intraabdominal structure other than the pancreas (such as duodenum); and in only an occasional patient is an elevation of serum amylase indicative of pancreatic injury.

In the majority of patients with pancreatic injury caused by blunt abdominal trauma, there is significant intraabdominal injury to other organs as well (particularly the spleen, liver, and stomach).[174,179] Full inspection of intraabdominal organs is mandatory when surgery is performed, and the surgical approach is in many ways similar to the approach to penetrating abdominal trauma. Hemostasis must be secured. Necrotic tissue must be carefully debrided, pancreatic secretion controlled, and appropriate drainage undertaken.[175] Mortality from injury of the head of the pancreas is substantially greater than injury to body and tail because of the coexistence of significant duodenal damage. If there is substantial damage to the head of the pancreas and duodenum, a pancreaticoduodenectomy is required, but this operation should be reserved for the rare situation in which there is considerable devitalization of tissue. In general, a conservative approach is favored consistent with the above goals.

When the main pancreatic duct is severed either by blunt or penetrating trauma, pancreatic secretion must be controlled. The usual method is resection of body and tail of the pancreas distal to the transsection. On occasion, a Roux-en-Y drainage of the distal pancreatic duct is performed if resection of the distal pancreas is felt to be technically too difficult.[114] Resection is probably preferable especially since metabolic complications (steatorrhea and diabetes) generally do not occur if the portion of the pancreas that is resected lies to the left of the superior mesenteric vessels.[177] In general, mortality and morbidity are increased with increasing delay of surgery.[175] Mortality also tends to be high in patients subjected to pancreaticoduodenectomy.[180]

Mortality in penetrating injury to the pancreas varies between 14% and 25%.[174,178,179,181] In blunt trauma, the mortality has been reported as low as 0[178] to 10%.[174]

When pancreatic trauma is strongly suspected, a laparotomy is essential. If the indication for surgery is not clear but lingering abdominal symptoms suggest the possibility of pancreatic ductal injury, ERCP may define the presence of ductal stricture or a pseudocyst.[114]

2.9 VASCULAR DISEASES

2.9.1 Thrombi and Emboli

Since the collateral circulation of the pancreas is extensive, vascular disease would not be likely to cause pancreatitis unless the vascular insult is overwhelming or there is already severe compromise of the circulation (such as severe arteriosclerosis). Within the scope of these possibilities, a number of cases of pancreatitis secondary to vascular disease have been recorded.

Pancreatic necrosis may occur on the basis of embolization of blood clots in the heart to the pancreatic circulation.[86,182] Another form of embolization to the circulation of the pancreas associated with pancreatitis is atheromatous embolization.[183-185] In this condition, cholesterol plaques dislodged from the aorta embolize to the kidney (causing malignant hypertension), to peripheral arterioles (causing the purple-toe syndrome), and to the pancreas (causing acute pancreatitis). In one series of patients, the organ distribution of atheromatous embolization was kidney in 62% and pancreas in 52%.[183] The suggestion has been made that the use of anticoagulation may in some way facilitate the dislodging of cholesterol emboli.[184] Aortography may also facilitate the development of atheromatous embolization.[185] Cholesterol embolization should be suspected in an older patient with extensive arteriosclerotic disease of the aorta if abdominal pain occurs in association with evidence of peripheral arterial insufficiency and hypertension.

Platelet thrombi may develop in pancreatic vessels in systemic lupus erythematosis[186] and in thrombotic thrombocytopenic purpura.[187] Acute pancreatitis has occurred in both situations.

2.9.2 Vasculitis

Diffuse vascular injury to the pancreas may cause pancreatitis. The types of vascular injury are: necrotizing angiitis caused by drugs,[188] malignant hypertension,[182] and periarteritis nodosa.[86,182,186,189]

2.9.3 Severe Hypotension

Evidence is accumulating that severe hypotension especially in an older age group may be responsible for a form of ischemic pancreatitis. In one series of patients who died following cardiac surgery, the incidence of unsuspected pancreatitis at autopsy was 16%.[190] In another autopsy series, several patients were discovered to have unsuspected pancreatitis following a major cerebral vascular accident complicated by severe hypotension.[191] In a third report, several patients who had undergone prolonged cardiopulmonary bypass were found at autopsy to have developed pancreatitis presumably on the basis of a vascular complication.[192]

2.9.4 Miscellaneous

There are several reports suggesting that celiac artery compression may on rare occasion be associated with acute pancreatitis.[193,194] An ischemic cause would be unlikely in view of the collateral circulation.

A vascular etiology of pancreatitis should be strongly considered in an elderly patient with unexplained pancreatitis. Some of the cases of pancreatitis in association with diuretic therapy in older patients may have a vascular etiology (such as dehydration and hypovolemia).

2.10 INFECTIOUS AGENTS AND TOXINS

Acute pancreatitis may complicate viral hepatitis.[195-199] Most patients experienced no symptoms suggestive of acute pancreatitis, but were found to have evidence of pancreatitis after they died of fulminant hepatic failure. While it is possible that the virus itself caused coexisting pancreatitis, there may have been other causes of pancreatitis (including hypotension, bleeding disorders, uremia, massive doses of steroids, and seizure activity). In at least two instances, there is convincing evidence that the pancreatitis was caused by the virus. In one, the ascitic fluid contained considerable quantities of amylase;[196] in the other, there was convincing radiologic evidence of acute pancreatitis associated with viral hepatitis.[199]

Other viruses that cause acute pancreatitis include mumps,[200,201] Coxsackie virus,[202-204] echovirus,[203] and infectious mononucleosis.[205] Cytomegalovirus has been found in pancreatic acinar cells, but it is not known whether it causes acute pancreatitis.[206] The suggestion has been made that mycoplasma pneumonia infections may cause pancreatitis,[207] but additional studies have failed to reveal antibody rises among patients with acute pancreatitis.[208,209]

Clinorchis sinensis may be responsible for acute pancreatitis. Histologic changes among patients infected with this parasite include the presence of flukes crowding pancreatic ducts causing ductal dilatation, squamous metaplasia of pancreatic ducts, and periductal fibrosis.[210] A more recent communication documenting the association of *Clinorchis sinensis* with pancreatitis is marred somewhat by the heavy alcohol consumption of the patient.[211] Other parasitic infestations that may cause pancreatitis by obstruction of the sphincter of Oddi include ascaris and hydatid cysts.[86] In endemic areas, *Schistosoma mansoni* may produce a calcified granulomatous pancreatitis.

The capacity of toxins to produce acute pancreatitis is poorly understood. In Trinidad, the most frequent cause of pancreatitis is the sting of a scorpion.[212] Detailed clinical observations of patients stung by scorpions indicate that there may be severe damage to a variety of organs including the stomach, brain, kidney, liver, heart, and pancreas.[213] The sting may be lethal in younger age groups. Pancreatitis has been verified following the sting of a scorpion both at surgery and at autopsy in numerous individuals. There were several instances of pancreatic pseudocyst.[213] An interesting clinical feature of the disease among many patients has been excessive salivation.[212,213] It is quite likely that at least some of the cases of presumed pancreatitis, especially those without abdominal pain, develop elevation of serum amylase levels on the basis of salivary gland dysfunction.

2.11 OTHER CAUSES

2.11.1 Congenital Abnormalities

Congenital abnormalities of the sphincter of Oddi causing pancreatitis have been enumerated in previous sections. An additional anatomic variation is the occurrence of pancreatitis in an accessory pancreatic lobe containing an aberrant pancreatic duct that communicated with a gastric duplication.[214] Pancreatitis has been noted in the condition termed pancreas divisum, in which the two pancreatic ductal systems are completely separate and correspond to the original ventral and dorsal component.[215] Either the duct of Wirsung or the duct of Santorini may be the focus of pancreatitis.

2.11.2 Pancreatitis in Childhood

An episode of acute pancreatitis in childhood may occur on the basis of an infectious agent such as mumps,[216] or on the basis of abdominal trauma.[216] A frequent form of trauma is a handle bar injury from a bicycle. A child may experience intermittent abdominal discomfort for several weeks and even months before the correct diagnosis is made. On rare occasions, a child presents with an abdominal mass indicating the presence of a pancreatic pseudocyst, and it is only after detailed questioning that a prior episode of trauma can be recalled.

Recurrent episodes of acute pancreatitis are uncommon in the pediatric population. The differential diagnosis includes hereditary pancreatitis, hereditary hyperparathyroidism, hyperlipoproteinemia, ascariasis, and rarely cystic fibrosis.[217] On rare occasions, a pediatric patient develops severe chronic relapsing pancreatitis with evidence of fibrosis[218] and calcification[219] of uncertain etiology. Anatomic variations and abnormalities involving the sphincter of Oddi and the orifice of the duct of Wirsung may also cause recurrent pancreatitis in childhood.[110,216,218,220]

There is at least one case of intrapancreatic duodenal duplication causing recurrent pancreatitis in a child.[221] On rare occasion in a child or teenager, cholelithiasis is the etiologic factor for acute pancreatitis or acute recurrent pancreatitis.

2.11.3 Pancreatitis in Association with Pregnancy

More than 100 cases of pancreatitis have been reported in association with pregnancy.[222] Most of the episodes occur during the third trimester or in the postpartum period. A medical approach is generally favored unless a severe complication necessitates emergency surgery. The seriousness of pancreatitis during pregnancy is underscored by a fetal and maternal mortality of 20% each.[222]

The most frequent etiology is coexisting biliary tract disease. At times, the etiology is obscure. Increases in enzyme secretion during pregnancy have been documented in the dog,[223] but the significance of this change is unclear.

2.11.4 Miscellaneous

Relapsing acute pancreatitis has been documented in association with acute intermittent porphyria.[224] Acute and chronic pancreatitis has been associated with sclerosing cholangitis and sicca complex in a brother and sister.[225] Numerous examples of pancreatitis have been reported in association with accidental hypothermia[226–228]; severe hypotension may have contributed to the pancreatitis.

Finally, acute pancreatitis has been reported following a prolonged fast and subsequent dietary gluttony in an 18-year-old boy.[229] The initial speculation was that pancreatic secretions became inspissated within the ductal system during the fast and caused a functional obstruction to the brisk flow of pancreatic juice in response to food. Additional follow-up on this patient during the past 20 years has revealed that an anatomic abnormality present in the sphincter of Oddi was responsible for this initial episode of pancreatitis, and additional ones as well, until sphincteroplasty was performed.

REFERENCES

1. Weiner S, Gramatica L, Voegle LD, et al: Role of the lymphatic system in the pathogenesis of inflammatory disease in the biliary tract and pancreas. *Am J Surg* 119:55–61, 1970.

2. Acosta JM, Ledesma CL: Gallstone migration as a cause of acute pancreatitis. *New Engl J Med* 290:484–487, 1974.
3. Acosta JM, Rossi R, Ledesma CL: The usefulness of stool screening for diagnosing cholelithiasis in acute pancreatitis. *Am J Dig Dis* 22:168–172, 1977.
4. Opie EL: The relation of cholelithiasis to disease of the pancreas and to fat necrosis. *Am J Med Sci* 121:27–43, 1901.
5. Opie EL: The etiology of acute hemorrhagic pancreatitis. *Johns Hopkins Hosp Bul* 121:182–188, 1901.
6. Caroli J, Porcher P, Pequignot G, et al: Contribution of cineradiography to study of the function of the human biliary tract. *Am J Dig Dis* 5:677–696, 1960.
7. Jones SA, Steedman RA, Keller TB, et al: Transduodenal sphincteroplasty (not sphincterotomy) for biliary and pancreatic disease. *Am J Surg* 118:292–306, 1969.
8. Banks PA: Acute pancreatitis. *Gastroenterology* 61:382–397, 1971.
9. Konok GP Thompson AG: Pancreatic ductal mucosa as a protective barrier in the pathogenesis of pancreatitis. *Am J Surg* 117:18–23, 1969.
10. Corlette MB Mendes-Monteiro AC, Bismuth H, et al: Transient bile duct obstruction. *Arch Surg* 111:1017–1020, 1976.
11. Kaplan MM, Righetti A: Induction of rat liver alkaline phosphatase: the mechanism of the serum elevation in bile duct obstruction. *J Clin Invest* 49:508–516, 1970.
12. Cameron JL, Zuidema GD, Margolis S: A pathogenesis for alcoholic pancreatitis. *Surgery* 77:754–763, 1975.
13. Albo R, Silen W, Goldman L: A critical clinical analysis of acute pancreatitis. *Arch Surg* 86:1032–1038, 1963.
14. Sarles H: Chronic calcifying pancreatitis—chronic alcoholic pancreatitis. *Gastroenterology* 66:604–616, 1974.
15. Bayer M, Rudick J, Lieber CS, et al: Inhibitory effect of ethanol on canine exocrine pancreatic secretion. *Gastroenterology* 63:619–626, 1972.
16. Marin GA, Ward NL, Fischer R: Effects of ethanol on pancreatic and biliary secretions in humans. *Am J Dig Dis* 18:825–833, 1973.
17. Strum WB, Spiro HM: Chronic pancreatitis. *Ann Intern Med* 74:264–277, 1971.
18. Nakamura K, Sarles H, Payan H: Three-dimensional reconstruction of the pancreatic ducts in chronic pancreatitis. *Gastroenterology* 62:942–949, 1972.
19. Sarles H, Tiscornia O: Ethanol and chronic calcifying pancreatitis. *Med Clin North Am* 58:1333–1346, 1974.
20. Sarles H: An international survey on nutrition and pancreatitis. *Digestion* 9:389–403, 1973.
21. Tandon BN, Banks PA, George PK, et al: Recovery of exocrine pancreatic function in adult protein-calorie malnutrition. *Gastroenterology* 58:358–362, 1970.
22. Tiscornia OM, Singer M, de Olivera JPM, et al: Exocrine pancreas response to a test meal in the dog. *Am J Dig Dis* 22:769–774, 1977.
23. Wakabayashi A, Takeda Y: The behavior of mucopolysaccharide in the pancreatic juice in chronic pancreatitis. *Am J Dig Dis* 21:607–612, 1976.
24. Allan J, White TT: An alternate mechanism for the formation of protein plugs in chronic calcifying pancreatitis. *Digestion* 11:428–431, 1974.
25. Sarles H, Tiscornia O, Palasciano G, et al: Effects of chronic intragastric ethanol administration on canine exocrine pancreatic secretion. *Scand J Gastroenterol* 8:85–96, 1973.
26. Owens JL Jr, Howard JM: Pancreatic calcification: a late sequal in the natural history of chronic alcoholism and alcoholic pancreatitis. *Ann Surg* 147:326–338, 1958.
27. Marks IN, Bank S, Louw JH, et al: The clinical varieties of alcoholic pancreatitis in the south western Cape. *S Afr Med J* 39:1093–1095, 1965.

28. Bordalo O, Batista A, Noronha M, et al: Effects of ethanol on liver morphology and pancreatic function in chronic alcoholism. *M Sinai J Med* 41:722–731, 1974.
29. Sarles H: Alcoholism in pancreatitis. *Scand J Gastroenterol* 6:193–198, 1971.
30. Paloyan D, Simonowitz D: Diagnostic considerations in acute alcoholic and gallstone pancreatitis. *Am J Surg* 132:329–331, 1976.
31. Rosato EF, Butler CJ, Grossman R, et al: Effect of alcohol on duodenal-pancreatic reflux. *Am J Surg* 125:228–230, 1973.
32. Straus E, Urbach H-J, Yalow RS: Alcohol-stimulated secretion of immunoreactive secretin. *N Engl J Med* 293:1031–1032, 1975.
33. Llanos OL, Swierczek JS, Teichmann RK, et al: Effect of alcohol on the release of secretin and pancreatic secretion. *Surgery* 81:661–667, 1977.
34. Banks PA, Janowitz HD: Some metabolic aspects of exocrine pancreatic disease. *Gastroenterology* 56:601–627, 1969.
35. Fredrickson DS, Levy RI, Lees RS: Fat transport in lipoproteins—an integrated approach to mechanisms and disorders. *N Engl J Med* 276:34–44, 1967.
36. Kessler JI, Finkel M, Ho P-P, et al: Lipoprotein lipase inhibition in rabbits with experimental pancreatitis. *Proc Soc Exp Biol Med* 110:24–26, 1962.
37. Greenberger NJ, Hatch FT, Drummey GD, et al: Pancreatitis and hyperlipemia: a study of serum lipid alterations in 25 patients with acute pancreatitis. *Medicine* 45:161–174, 1966.
38. Cameron JL, Capuzzi DM, Zuidema Gd, et al: Acute pancreatitis with hyperlipemia. *Am J Med* 56:482–487, 1974.
39. Chait A, Mancini M, February A, et al: Clinical and metabolic study of alcoholic hyperlipidaemia. *Lancet* 2:62–64, 1972.
40. Ginsberg H, Olefsky J, Farquhar JW, et al: Moderate ethanol ingestion and plasma triglyceride levels. *Ann Intern Med* 80:143–149, 1974.
41. Cameron JL, Capuzzi DM, Zuidema GD, et al: Acute pancreatitis with hyperlipemia: the incidence of lipid abnormalities in acute pancreatitis. *Ann Surg* 177:483–489, 1973.
42. Farmer RG, Winkelman EI, Brown HB, et al: Hyperlipoproteinemia and pancreatitis. *Am J Med* 54:161–165, 1973.
43. Davidoff F, Tishler S, Rosoff C: Marked hyperlipidemia and pancreatitis associated with oral contraceptive use. *N Engl J Med* 289:552–555, 1973.
44. Bank S, Marks IN: Hyperlipaemic pancreatitis and the pill. *Postgrad Med J* 46:576–578, 1970.
45. Glueck CJ, Scheel D, Fishback J, et al: Estrogen-induced pancreatitis in patients with previously covert familial Type V hyperlipoproteinemia. *Metabolism* 21:657–666, 1972.
46. Molitch ME, Oill P, Odell WD: Massive hyperlipemia during estrogen therapy. *JAMA* 227:522–525, 1974.
47. Chan L, Jackson RL, O'Malley BW, et al: Synthesis of very low density lipoproteins in the cockerel. *J Clin Invest* 58:368–379, 1976.
48. Cameron JL: Lipid abnormalities and acute pancreatitis. *Hosp Pract* 12:95–101, 1977.
49. Salen S, Kessler JI, Janowitz HD: The development of pancreatic secretory insufficiency in a patient with recurrent pancreatitis and Type V hyperlipoproteinemia. *M Sinai J Med NY* 37:103–107, 1970.
50. Herfort K, Sobra J, Fric P, et al: Familial hyperlipoproteinemia and exocrine pancreas. *Scand J Gastroenterol* 6:139–143, 1971.
51. Krauss RM, Levy AG: Subclinical chronic pancreatitis in Type I hyperlipoproteinemia. *Am J Med* 62:144–149, 1977.
52. Silen W, Baldwin J, Goldman L: Treatment of chronic pancreatitis by longitudinal pancreaticojejunostomy. *Am J Surg* 106:243–258, 1963.

53. Kattwinkel J, Lapey A, di Sant 'Agnese PA, Edwards WA, et al: Hereditary pancreatitis: three new kindreds and a critical review of the literature. *Pediatrics* 51:55–69, 1973.

54. Perrault J, Gross JB, King JE: Endoscopic retrograde cholangiopancreatography in familial pancreatitis. *Gastroenterology* 71:138–144, 1976.

55. Case Records of the Massachusetts General Hospital. *N Engl J Med* 286:1353–1359, 1972.

56. Mixter CG, Keynes WM, Cope O: Further experience with pancreatitis as a diagnostic clue to hyperparathyroidism. *N Engl J Med* 266:265–272, 1962.

57. Ludwig GD, Chaykin LB: Pancreatitis associated with primary hyperparathyroidism. *Med Clin North Am* 50:1403–1418, 1966.

58. Schmidt H, Creutzfeldt W: Calciphylactic pancreatitis and pancreatitis in hyperparathyroidism. *Clin Orthop Relat Res* 69:135–145, 1970.

59. Haverback BJ, Dyce B, Bundy H, et al: Trypsin, trypsinogen and trypsin inhibitor in human pancreatic juice. *Am J Med* 29:424–433, 1960.

60. Kelley TR: Relationship of hyperparathyroidism to pancreatitis. *Arch Surg* 97:267–274, 1968.

61. Baer L, Neu HC: Intravascular clotting and acute pancreatitis in primary hyperparathyroidism. *Ann Intern Med* 64:1062–1065, 1966.

62. Warshaw AL, Heizer WD, Laster L: Pancreatic insufficiency as the presenting feature of hyperparathyroidism. *Ann Intern Med* 68:161–167, 1968.

63. Omenn GS, Roth SI, Baker WH: Hyperparathyroidism associated with malignant tumors of nonparathyroid origin. *Cancer* 24:1004–1012, 1969.

64. Reiss E: Hyperparathyroidism. *Adv Intern Med* 19:287–301, 1974.

65. Hansky J: Calcium content of duodenal juice. *Am J Dig Dis* 12:725–733, 1967.

66. Goebell H, Horn HD, Bode C, et al: Primarer hyperparathyreoidismus und exokrine Pankreasfunktion. *Klin Wochenschr* 48:810–819, 1970.

67. Kurlander DJ, Raskin HF, and Kirsner JB: Coexistence of pancreatitis and hyperparathyroidism. *Ann Intern Med* 58:1013–1016, 1963.

68. Dreiling DA, Mazure PA, Cohen N, et al: Newer horizons in the etiology of pancreatitis: metabolic and endocrinologic factors. *Am J Dig Dis* 7:112–126, 1962.

69. Mixter G, Hinton JW, Pfeffer RB: Pancreatitis in association with hyperparathyroidism. *NYJ Med* 58:3470–3474, 1958.

70. Leeson PM, Fourman P: Acute pancreatitis from vitamin-D poisoning in a patient with parathyroid deficiency. *Lancet* 1:1185–1186, 1966.

71. Meltzer LE, Palmon, FP, Paik YK, et al: Acute pancreatitis secondary to hypercalcemia of multiple myeloma. *Ann Intern Med* 57:1108–1012, 1962.

72. Aldis AS: Clinical experiences of the lesser known manifestations of hyperparathyroidism. *Proc R Soc Med* 54:489–492, 1961.

73. Manson RR: Acute pancreatitis secondary to iatrogenic hypercalcemia. *Arch Surg* 108:213–215, 1974.

74. Hochgelerent EL, David DS; Acute pancreatitis secondary to calcium infusion in a dialysis patient. *Arch Surg* 108:218–219, 1974.

75. McPherson RC, Pace WG: Calcium excretion by the pancreas in hypercalcemia. *Surg Forum* 12:372–373, 1961.

76. Zimmerman MJ, Moore EW, Dreiling DA, et al: Pancreatic juice ionized and total calcium in dogs in response to secretin, pancreozymin, and calcium infusions. *J Clin Invest* 50:103a, 1971.

77. Zimmerman MJ, Dreiling DA, Rosenberg IR, et al: Secretion of calcium by the canine pancreas. *Gastroenterology* 52:865–870, 1967.

78. Goebell H, Steffen C Bode C: Stimulatory effect of pancreozymin-cholecystokinin on calcium secretion in pancreatic juice of dogs. *Gut* 13:477–482, 1972.

79. Goebell H, Baltzer G, Schlott KA, et al: Parallel secretion of calcium and enzymes by the human pancreas. *Digestion* 8:336–346, 1973.
80. Goebell H, Bode C, Horn HD: Einflub von Secretin und Pankreozymin auf die Calciumsekretion im menschlichen Duodenalsaft bei normaler und gestorter Pankreasfunktion. *Klin Wochenschr* 48:1330–1339, 1970.
81. Nimmo J, Finlayson NDC, Smith AF, et al: The production of calcium and magnesium during pancreatic function tests in health and disease. *Gut* 11:163–166, 1970.
82. Gullo L, Sarles H, De Barros, Motto C, et al: Pancreatic secretion of calcium in healthy subjects and various diseases of the pancreas. *Rendic Gastroenterol* 6:35–44, 1974.
83. Warwick RRG, Tothill P, Percy-Robb IW, et al: The calcium concentration in pancreatic secretion in chronic pancreatitis and carcinoma of the pancreas. *Scand J Gastroenterol* 8:301–305, 1973.
84. Thomas CG, Zawacki JK, Ona FV, et al: Intrapancreatic choledochal cyst. *Gastroenterology* 71:1071–1074, 1976.
85. Cuschieri A and Davies RS: Acute pancreatitis complicating a choledochal cyst. *Br Med J* 3:698, 1969.
86. Pellegrini CA, Paloyan D, Acosta JM, et al: Acute pancreatitis of rare causation. *Surg Gynecol Obstet* 144:899–902, 1977.
87. Ohmori K, Kinoshita H, Shiraha Y, et al: Pancreatic duct obstruction by a benign polypoid adenoma of the ampulla of Vater. *Am J Surg* 132:662–663, 1976.
88. Nardi GL, Acosta JM: Papillitis as a cause of pancreatitis and abdominal pain. *Ann Surg* 164:611–621, 1966.
89. Nardi GL: Remediable chronic pancreatitis. *Surg Clin North Am* 54:613–620, 1974.
90. Nardi GL: Papillitis and stenosis of the sphincter of Oddi. *Surg Clin North Am* 53: 1149–1160, 1973.
91. Cattell RB, Colcock BP, Pollack JL: Stenosis of the sphincter of Oddi. *N Engl J Med* 256:429–435, 1957.
92. Jones SA, Smith LL, Gregory G: Sphincteroplasty for recurrent pancreatitis. *Ann Surg* 147:180–190, 1958.
93. White TT: Indications for sphincteroplasty as opposed to choledochoduodenostomy. *Am J Surg* 126:165–170, 1973.
94. Delmont J, ed: The Sphincter of Oddi. Third Gastroenterological Symposium, S. Karger, Basel, 1977.
95. McCutcheon AD: A fresh approach to the pathogenesis of pancreatitis. *Gut* 9:296–310, 1968.
96. Owyang C, Dozois RR, DiMagno EP, et al: Relationships between fasting and postprandial pancreaticoduodenal pressures, pancreatic secretion, and duodenal volume flow in the dog. *Gastroenterology* 73:1046–1049, 1977.
97. Lloyd-Jones W, Mountain JC, Warren KW: Annular pancreas in the adult. *Ann Surg* 176:163–170, 1972.
98. Dodd GD, Nafis WA: Annular pancreas in the adult. *Am J Roentgenol* 75:333–342, 1956.
99. Alexander HC: Annular pancreas in the adult. *Am J Surg* 119:702–704, 1970.
100. Lawson TL: Intraluminal duodenal diverticulum. *Am J Dig Dis* 19:673–677, 1974.
101. Nosher JL, Seaman WB: Association of intraluminal duodenal diverticulum with acute pancreatitis. *Radiology* 115:21–22, 1975.
102. Nelson JA, Burhenne HJ: Anomalous biliary and pancreatic duct insertion into duodenal diverticula. *Radiology* 120:49–52, 1976.
103. Willox GL, Costopoulos LB: Entry of common bile and pancreatic ducts into a duodenal diverticulum. *Arch Surg* 98:447–450, 1969.

104. Dreiling DA, Kirschner PA, Nemser H: Chronic duodenal obstruction: a Mechano-vascular etiology of pancreatitis. *Am J Dig Dis* 5:991–1005, 1960.
105. Legge DA, Hoffman HN II, Carlson HC: Pancreatitis as a complication of regional enteritis of the duodenum. *Gastroenterology* 61:834–837, 1971.
106. Gambill EE: Pancreatitis associated with pancreatic carcinoma: a study of 26 cases. *Mayo Clin Proc* 46:174–177, 1971.
107. Waes LV, Maele VV, Demeulenaere L, et al: Carcinoma of the pancreas presenting as relapsing pancreatitis. *Am J Gastroenterology* 68:88–90, 1977.
108. Gambill EE: Pancreatic and ampullary carcinoma: diagnosis and prognosis in relationship to symptoms, physical findings, and elapse of time as observed in 255 patients. *South Med J* 63:1119–1122, 1970.
109. Niccolini DG, Graham JH, Banks PA: Tumor-induced acute pancreatitis. *Gastroenterology* 71:142–145, 1976.
110 White TT, Kavlie H: Congenital obstruction of the pancreatic duct at the duodenum. *Ann Surg* 178:194–196, 1973.
111. Herriott BA, Palmer AA: Rupture of small ducts and acini in the pancreas of the rat and guinea pig following major duct obstruction. *Aust J Exp Biol Med Sci* 44:143–156, 1966.
112. Allen BJ, Tournut R, White TT: Intraductal activation of pancreatic zymogens behind a carcinoma of the pancreas. *Gastroenterology* 65:412–418, 1973.
113. Anderson MC, Schiller WR: Microcirculatory dynamics in the normal and inflamed pancreas. *Am J Surg* 115:118–127, 1968.
114. Gougeon FW, Legros G, Archambault A, et al: Pancreatic trauma: a new diagnostic approach. *Am J Surg* 132:400–402, 1976.
115. Goldsmith HS, Ghosh BC, Huvos AG: Ligation versus implantation of the pancreatic duct after pancreaticoduodenectomy. *Surg Gynecol Obstet* 132:87–92, 1971.
116. Stobbe KC, ReMine WH, Baggenstoss AH: Pancreatic lithiasis. *Surg Gynecol Obstet* 131:1090–1099, 1970.
117. Popper HL, Necheles H: Edema of the pancreas. *Surg Gynecol Obstet* 74:123–124, 1942.
118. Lium R, Maddock S: Etiology of acute pancreatitis. *Surgery* 24:593–604, 1948.
119. Popper H, Necheles H, Russell KC: Transition of pancreatic edema into pancreatic necrosis. *Surg Gynecol Obstet* 87:79–82, 1948.
120. Hermann RE, Davis JH: The role of incomplete pancreatic duct obstruction in the etiology of pancreatitis. *Surgery* 48:318–329, 1960.
121. Hiatt N, Warner NE: Serum amylase and changes in pancreatic function and structure after ligation of pancreatic ducts. *Am Surg* 35:30–35, 1969.
122. Churg A, Richter WR: Early changes in the exocrine pancreas of the dog and rat after ligation of the pancreatic duct. *Am J Pathol* 63:521–534, 1971.
123. Little JM, Laurer C, Hogg J: Pancreatic duct obstruction with acrylate glue: a new method for producing pancreatic exocrine atrophy. *Am J Dig Dis* 81:243–249, 1977.
124. Ambromovage AM, Pairent FW, Howard JM: Pancreatic exocrine insufficiency: the effects of long-term pancreatic duct ligation on serum insulin levels and glucose metabolism in the dog. *Ann Surg* 177:338–343, 1973.
125. Johnston DH, Cornish AL: Acute pancreatitis in patients receiving chlorothiazide. *JAMA* 170:2054–2056, 1959.
126. Minkowitz S, Soloway HB, Hall JE, et al: Fatal hemorrhagic pancreatitis following chlorothiazide administration in pregnancy. *Obstet Gynecol* 24:337–342, 1964.
127. Jones MF, Caldwell JR: Acute hemorrhagic pancreatitis associated with administration of chlorthalidone. *N Engl J Med* 267:1029–1031, 1962.

128. Wilson AE, Mehra SK, Gomersall CR, et al: Acute pancreatitis associated with frusemide therapy. *Lancet* 1:105, 1967.
129. Call T, Malarkey WB, Thomas FB: Acute pancreatitis secondary to furosemide with associated hyperlipidemia. *Am J Dig Dis* 22:835–838, 1977.
130. Thomas FB, Sinar D, Caldwell JH, et al: Stimulation of pancreatic secretion of water and electrolytes by furosemide. *Gastroenterology* 73:221–225, 1977.
131. Bjornberg A, Gisslen H: Thiazides; a cause of necrotising vasculitis? *Lancet* 2:982–983, 1965.
132. Cornish AL, McClellan JT, Johnston DH: Effects of chlorothiazide on the pancreas. *N Engl J Med* 265:673–675, 1961.
133. Riemenschneider TA, Wilson JF, Vernier RL: Glucocorticoid-induced pancreatitis in children. *Pediatrics* 41:428–437, 1968.
134. Gullo L, Costa PL, Fontana G, et al: Effect of adrenocorticotropic hormone on pure exocrine pancreatic secretion in man. *Gastroenterology* 73:762–764, 1977.
135. Wilde H: Pancreatitis and phenformin. *Ann Intern Med* 77:324, 1972.
136. Levitan AA: Phenformin and pancreatitis. *Ann Intern Med* 78:306–307, 1973.
137. Graeber GM, Marmor BM, Hendel RC, et al: Pancreatitis and severe metabolic abnormalities due to phenformin therapy. *Arch Surg* 111:1014–1016, 1976.
138. Chase HS Jr. Mogan GR: Phenformin-associated pancreatitis. *Ann Intern Med* 87:314–315, 1977.
139. Conlay LA, Loewenstein JE: Phenformin and hyperamylasemia in lactic acidosis. *Ann Intern Med* 87:312–313, 1977.
140. Falko JM, Thomas FB: Acute pancreatitis due to procainamide-induced lupus erythematosus. *Ann Intern Med* 83:832–833, 1975.
141. Greipp PR, Brown JA, Grolnick HR: Defibrination in acute pancreatitis. *Ann Intern Med.* 76: 73–76, 1972.
142. Shaw MT, Barnes CC, Madden FJF, et al: L-Asparaginase and pancreatitis. *Lancet* 2:721, 1970.
143. Block MB, Genant HK, Kirsner JB: Pancreatitis as an adverse reaction to salicylazosulfapyridine. *N Engl J Med* 282:380–382, 1970.
144. Nogueira JR, Freedman MA: Acute pancreatitis as a complication of imuran therapy in regional enteritis. *Gastroenterology* 62:1040–1041, 1972.
145. Kawanishi H, Rudolph E, Bull FE: Azathioprine-induced acute pancreatitis. *N Engl J Med* 289:357, 1973.
146. Paloyan D, Levin B, Simonowitz D: Azathioprine-associated acute pancreatitis. *Am J Dig Dis* 22:839–840, 1977.
147. Cotton PB, Blumgart LH, Davies GT, et al: Cannulation of papilla of vater via fiberduodenoscope. *Lancet* 1:53–58, 1972.
148. Katon RM, Lee TG, Parent JA, et al: Endoscopic retrograde cholangiopancreatography (ERCP). *Am J Dig Dis* 19:295–306, 1974.
149. Nebel OT, Silvis SE, Rogers G, et al: Complications associated with endoscopic retrograde cholangiopancreatography. *Gastrointest Endosc* 22:34–36, 1975.
150. Zimmon DS: A diagnostic procedure of choice—endoscopic retrograde cholangiopancreatography (ERCP). *Cur Con Gastro* 1:3–8, 1976.
151. Zimmons DS, Falkenstein DB, Riccobono C, et al: Complications of endoscopic retrograde cholangiopancreatography. *Gastroenterology* 69:303–309, 1975.
152. Bilbao K, Dotter CT, Lee TT, et al: Complications of endoscopic retrograde cholangiopancreatography. *Gastroenterology* 70:314–320, 1976.
153. Kasugai T, Kuno N, Kizu M: Manometric endoscopic retrograde pancreatocholangiography. *Am J Dig Dis* 19:485–502, 1974.

154. Ammann RW, Deyhle P Butikofer E: Fatal necrotizing pancreatitis after peroral cholangiopancreatography. *Gastroenterology* 64:320–323, 1973.

155. Bloom GP, Fromm D, Rosenberg S, et al: Attempted retrograde cannulation of the ampulla: a probably cause of mass in the pancreas. *Ann Surg* 183:107–108, 1976.

156. Blackstone MO, Mizuno H: Reactive duodenal changes in chronic pancreatitis simulating the contiguous spread of pancreatic carcinoma. *Am J Dig Dis* 22:658–661, 1977.

157. Kaufman B, Gambescia R, Maldonado A, et al: Systemic absorption of contrast agent during endoscopic retrograde cholangiopancreatography. *Gastroent End* 22:175–176, 1976.

158 Sahel J and Sarles H: Endoscopic pancreatography and urograms. *Gastroenterology* 71:1109, 1976.

159. Zimmon DS, Falkenstein DB, Kessler RE: Management of biliary calculi by retrograde endoscopic instrumentation (lithocenosis). *Gastrointest End* 23:82–86, 1976.

160. Safrany L: Duodenoscopic sphincterotomy and gallstone removal. *Gastroenterology* 72:338–343, 1977.

161. Koch H, Rosch W, Schaffner O, et al: Endoscopic papillotomy. *Gastroenterology* 73:1393–1396, 1977.

162. White TT, Morgan A Hopton D: Postoperative pancreatitis. *Am J Surg* 120:132–137, 1970.

163. Bardenheier JA III, Kaminski DL, Willman VL: Pancreatitis after biliary tract surgery. *Am J Surg* 116:773–776, 1968.

164. Herrington JL Jr, Vasudeo P: Iatrogenic choledochal stricture with choledochopancreatic fistula and pseudocyst. *Arch Surg* 112:213–216, 1977.

165. Morrissey R, Berk JE, Fridhandler L, et al: The nature and significance of hyperamylasemia following operation. *Ann Surg* 180:67–71, 1974.

166. Corrodi P, Knoblauch M, Binswanger U, et al: Pancreatitis after renal transplantation. *Gut* 16:285–289, 1975.

167. Fernandez JA, Rosenberg JC: Post-transplantation pancreatitis. *Surg Gynecol Obstet* 143:795–798, 1976.

168. Woods JE, Anderson CF, Frohnert PP, et al: Pancreatitis in renal allografted patients. *Mayo Clin Proc* 47:193–195, 1972.

169. Johnson WC, Nabseth DC: Pancreatitis in renal transplantation. *Ann Surg* 171:309–314, 1970.

170. Penn I, Durst AL, Machado M, et al: Acute pancreatitis and hyperamylasemia in renal homograft recipients. *Arch Sug* 105:167–172, 1972.

171. Robinson DO, Alp MH, Grant AK, et al: Pancreatitis and renal disease. *Scand J Gastroenterol* 12:17–20, 1977.

172. Tilney NL, Collins JJ, Wilson RE: Hemorrhagic pancreatitis *N Engl J Med* 274:1051–1957, 1966.

173. Renning JA, Warden GD, Stevens LE, et al: Pancreatitis after renal transplantation. *Am J Surg* 123:293–296, 1972.

174. Thompson RJ Jr, Hinshaw DB: Pancreatic trauma. *Ann Surg* 163:153–160, 1966.

175. Lucas CE: Diagnosis and treatment of pancreatic and duodenal injury. *Surg Clin North Am* 57:49–65, 1977.

176. Olsen WR: The serum amylase in blunt abdominal trauma. *J Trauma* 13:200–204, 1973.

177. Richter RM, Burrows L, Dreiling DA: Isolated transection of the pancreas caused by blunt thoracic trauma. *J M Sinai Hosp NY* 32:660–662, 1965.

178. Barnett WO, Hardy JD, Yelverton RL: Pancreatic trauma. *Ann Surg* 163:892–901, 1966.

179. Stone HH, Stowers KB, Shippey SH: Injuries to the pancreas. *Arch Surg* 85:525–530, 1962.

180. Balasegaram M: Surgical management of pancreatic trauma. *Am J Surg* 131:536–540, 1976.

181. Nance FC, DeLoach DH: Pancreaticoduodenectomy following abdominal trauma. *J. Trauma* 11:577–585, 1971.

182. McKay JW, Baggenstoss AH, Wollaeger EF: Infarcts of the pancreas. *Gastroenterology* 35:256–264, 1958.

183. Probstein JG, Joshi RA, Blumenthal HT: Atheromatous embolization. *Arch Surg* 75:566–572, 1957.

184. Moldveen-Geronimus M, Merriam JC Jr: Cholesterol embolization. *Circulation* 35: 946–953, 1967.

185. Aach R, Kissane J: Chronic relapsing pancreatitis with cardiac and renal disease. *Am J Med* 53:335–342, 1972.

186. Pollak VE, Grove WJ, Kark RM, et al: Systemic lupus erythematosus simulating acute surgical condition of the abdomen. *N Engl J Med* 259:258–266, 1958.

187. Olsen H: Thrombotic thrombocytopenic purpura as a cause of pancreatitis. *Am J Dig Dis* 18:238–246, 1973.

188. Citron BP, Halpern M, McCarron M, et al: Necrotizing angiitis associated with drug abuse. *N Engl J Med* 283:1003–1011, 1970.

189. O'Neill PB: Gastrointestinal abnormalities in the collagen diseases. *Am J Dig Dis* 6:1069–1083, 1961.

190. Feiner H: Pancreatitis after cardiac surgery. *Am J Surg* 131:684–688, 1976.

191. Moberg, Svenhamn K, Wagermark J: Acute "idiopathic" pancreatitis. *Acta. Chir. Scand.* 134:369–372, 1968.

192. Panebicanco AC, Scott SM, Dart CH, et al: Acute pancreatitis following extracorporeal circulation. *Ann Thoracic Surg* 9:562–568, 1970.

193. Cleator IGM, Macpherson, AIS, Fraser GM: Coeliac artery compression. *J.R. Coll Surg Edinburgh* 16:96–99, 1971.

194. Watson WC and Sadikali F: Celiac axis compression. *Ann Intern Med* 86:278–284, 1977.

195. Geokas MC, Olsen H, Swanson V, et al: The association of viral hepatitis and acute pancreatitis. *Calif Med* 117:1–7, 1972.

196. Wands JR, Salyer DC, Boitnott JK, et al: Fulminant hepatitis complicated by pancreatitis. *Johns Hopkins Med J* 133:156–160, 1973.

197. Ham JM, Fitzpatrick P: Acute pancreatitis in patients with acute hepatic failure. *Am J Dig Dis* 18:1079–1083, 1973.

198. Lepore MJ, Stutman LJ, Bonanno CA, et al: Plasmapheresis with plasma exchange in hepatic coma. *Arch Intern Med* 129:900–907, 1972.

199. Achord JL: Acute pancreatitis with infectious hepatitis. *JAMA* 205:129–132, 1968.

200. O'Brien PK, Smith DS, Galpin OP: Acute pancreatitis and haemolytic anaemia associated with mumps-virus infection. *Br Med J* 2:1529, 1965.

201. Feldstein JD, Johnson FR, Kallick CA, et al: Acute hemorrhagic pancreatitis and pseudocyst due to mumps. *Ann Surg* 180:85–88, 1974.

202. Ursing B: Acute pancreatitis in coxsackie B infection. *Br Med J* 3:524–525, 1973.

203. Arnesio B, Eden T, Ihse I, et al: Enterovirus infection in acute pancreatitis. *Scan J Gastroenterol* 11:645–650, 1976.

204. Imrie CW, Ferguson JC, Sommerville RG: Coxsackie and mumpsvirus infection in a prospective study of acute pancreatitis. *Gut* 18:53–56, 1977.

205. Wislocki LC: Acute pancreatitis in infectious mononucleosis. *N Engl J Med* 275:322–323, 1966.
206. Case Records of the Massachusetts General Hospital. *N Engl J Med* 288:785–787, 1973.
207. Mardh PA, Ursing B: The occurrence of acute pancreatitis in mycoplasma pneumonia infection. *Scand J Infect Dis* 6:167–171, 1974.
208. Leinikki P, Pantzar P, Tykka H: Antibody response in patients with acute pancreatitis to mycoplasma pneumoniae. *Scand J Gastroenteral* 8:631–635, 1973.
209. Capner P, Lendrum R, Jeffries DJ, et al: Viral antibody studies in pancreatic disease. *Gut* 16:866–870, 1975.
210. McFadzean AJS, Yeung RTT: Acute pancreatitis due to Clonorchis sinensis. *Trans R Soc Trop Med Hyg* 60:466–470, 1966.
211. Shugar RA, Ryan JJ: *Clonorchis sinensis* and pancreatitis. *Am J Gastroenterol* 64:400–403, 1975.
212. Bartholomew C: Acute scorpion pancreatitis in Trinidad. *Br Med J* 1:666–668, 1970.
213. Waterman JA: Some notes on scorpion poisoning in Trinidad. *Trans R Soc Trop Med Hyg* 31:607–624, 1938.
214. Traverso LW, Damus PS and Longmire WP: Pancreatitis of unusual origin. *Surg Gynecol Obstet* 141:383–386, 1975.
215. Rosch W, Koch H, Schaffner O, et al: The clinical significance of the pancreas divisum. *Gastro Endos* 22:206–207, 1976.
216. Hendren WH, Greep JM, Patton AS: Pancreatitis in childhood. *Arch Dis Childhood* 40:132–145, 1965.
217. Shwachman H, Lebenthal E, Khaw K-T: Recurrent acute pancreatitis in patients with cystic fibrosis with normal pancreatic enzymes. *Pediatrics* 55:86–95, 1975.
218. Williams TE Jr, Sherman NJ, Clatworthy HW Jr: Chronic fibrosing pancreatitis in childhood. *Pediatrics* 40:1019–1023, 1967.
219. Dean RH, Scott HW Jr, Law DH IV: Chronic relapsing pancreatitis in childhood. *Ann Surg* 173:443–449, 1971.
220. Plechas NP: Chronic recurrent pancreatitis in childhood. *Arch Surg* 81:883–886, 1960.
221. Williams WH, Hendren WH: Intrapancreatic duodenal duplication causing pancreatitis in a child. *Surgery* 69:708–715, 1971.
222. Montgomery WH, Miller FC: Pancreatitis and pregnancy. *Obstet Gynecol* 35:658–663, 1970.
223. Rosenberg V, Rudick J, Robbiou M, et al: Pancreatic exocrine secretion during and after pregnancy. *Ann Surg* 181:47–50, 1975.
224. Kobza K, Gyr K, Neuhaus K, et al: Acute intermittent porphyria with relapsing acute pancreatitis and unconjugated hyperbilirubinemia without overt hemolysis. *Gastroenterology* 71:494–496, 1976.
225. Waldram R, Kopelman H, Tsantoulas D, et al: Chronic pancreatitis, sclerosing cholangitis, and sicca complex in two siblings. *Lancet* 1:550–552, 1975.
226. Maclean D, Murison J, Griffiths PD: Acute pancreatitis and diabetic detoacidosis in accidental hypothermia and hypothermic myxoedema. *Br Med J* 4:757–761, 1973.
227. Murphy E, Faul PJ: Accidental hypothermia in the elderly. *J Ir Med. Assoc* 53:4–8, 1963.
228. Duguid H, Simpson RG, Stowers JM: Accidental hypothermia. *Lancet* 2:1213–1221, 1961.
229. McDermott WV Jr, Bartlett MK, Culver PJ: Acute pancreatitis after prolonged fast and subsequent surfeit. *New Engl J Med* 254:379–380, 1956.

Pathophysiology of Acute Pancreatitis

Acute pancreatitis is caused by enzymatic autodigestion of the pancreas. Numerous experiments have been carried out in an effort to learn which enzymes are responsible. A favorite experimental design has been to reflux various enzymes into the pancreatic duct of experimental animals. Reflux of most materials at high pressure causes pancreatic injury. When reflux is achieved at more physiologic pressures, almost all the pancreatic enzymes except for amylase and carboxypeptidases are capable of causing pancreatic inflammation.[1] It is doubtful that these experiments conducted in animals bear a reasonable resemblance to acute pancreatitis in man.

Trypsin has traditionally been considered to be the most important enzyme in the pathophysiology of acute pancreatitis. Trypsin causes pancreatic edema when refluxed into the pancreatic duct of an animal, and causes a severe necrotizing pancreatitis if it is preincubated with blood.[2] However, the spectrum of pathologic changes caused experimentally by trypsin does not resemble human pancreatitis in that trypsin causes liquefaction necrosis with an abundant leukocyte infiltration whereas pancreatitis in man is characterized by coagulation necrosis associated at first with only a moderate leukocyte infiltration.[3,4] The concept that has evolved is that trypsin usually does not cause severe tissue destruction by itself but activates at least two other enzymes which are responsible for pancreatitis. Trypsin activates phospholipase-A and -B, which in turn convert lecithin of biliary secretion into lysolecithin. Lysolecithin destroys phospholipid layers of membranes and cells creating a picture of coagulation necrosis that is characteristic of acute pancreatitis in man.[3,4] Trypsin also activates elastase from its inactive proenzyme. Elastase causes severe vascular injury and may be the enzyme responsible for severe hemorrhage in pancreatitis.[5]

Since there are trypsin inhibitors within the pancreas and within pancreatic juice (as well as in plasma) and since trypsin itself is not activated until it comes into contact with enterokinase within the duodenum, consideration has been given to the concept that reflux of duodenal contents into the pancreatic duct is essential for the development of pancreatitis.[6] More recently, several studies have shown that pancreatic enzymes may be activated without exposure to the duodenum. For example, active chymotrypsin has been recovered from the pancreatic duct of a patient with an obstructing carcinoma of the pancreas[7,8]; pancreatic juice of patients with acute pancreatitis has been documented to contain active trypsin, chymotrypsin, and elastase.[9] The role of activated enzymes in causing pancreatic inflammation has finally been substantiated with the demonstration of active trypsin, chymotrypsin, and elastase within pancreatic exudate during experimental pancreatitis,[10] the recovery of elastase within ascitic fluid and plasma during experimental pancreatitis,[11] and the recovery of active trypsin, chymotrypsin, and elastase within the pancreas during experimental pancreatitis.[12] In summary, evidence is accumulating that trypsin is capable of being activated under certain circumstances without prior entry into the duodenum; that the activation of phospholipase-A and elastase by trypsin is capable of causing the full spectrum of pancreatic edema, pancreatic necrosis, and pancreatic hemorrhage; and finally, that these active enzymes are present in pancreatic tissue and pancreatic exudate.

The role of kallikrein and other vasoactive materials in pancreatitis has received close study. Data have accumulated suggesting that the activation of kallikrein by trypsin may cause hypotension, increased vascular permeability, and pain.[13] At least one vasoactive substance with a capacity for increasing capillary permeability has been recovered from pancreatic exudation in experimental pancreatitis.[14] Prostaglandin-like activity has been demonstrated in pancreatic venous blood and peritoneal exudation during experimental pancreatitis.[15] There may be a wide variety of vasoactive substances that increase vascular permeability within the pancreas, intensify pancreatic edema, and contribute to systemic hypotension.

During acute pancreatitis, the inflammatory process damages pancreatic ducts, acinar tissue, and interstitial tissue. An important consideration is the pathway by which activated pancreatic enzymes within pancreatic ducts gain access to interstitial tissue and its rich vascular network. A basic assumption is that active enzymes are present at some point in time within pancreatic ducts either by reflux from the duodenum or by spontaneous activation within the ducts; another possibility is that premature activation of enzymes takes place within acinar cells resulting in severe destruction of the tissue from within. Evidence has accumulated that even in the absence of ductal disruption, fluid within the pancreatic duct may gain access to pancreatic interstitial tissue by sifting through physiologic spaces located between acinar cells.[16,17]

During experimental pancreatitis, pancreatic interstitial tissue becomes quite edematous. Lymphatics that communicate with this tissue at first show an increased rate of lymph flow. As lymphatics become congested with red blood cells and tissue debris, flow decreases sharply, and tissue debris accumulates in capillaries and is carried via local pancreatic venous channels into the portal circulation. If lymphatic and venous pathways become severely congested, there may be marked intensification of interstitial edema.[16] Pancreatic arterioles may become markedly constricted thereby reducing blood flow within areas of maximal inflammation.[18] Reduction of circulation in areas of inflammation reduces levels of tissue proteinase inhibitors,[19] and also reduces the influx of proteinase inhibitors from the circulation. Impairment in circulation and actual vascular disruption have also been noted to involve ductal blood vessels.[20] Impairment of the microcirculation of the inflamed pancreas may be one of the critical factors that determines the severity of pancreatitis.[16,18,19]

The pathophysiology of pancreatitis in man probably involves one or more of the mechanisms outlined above. Some cases result from the reflux of either duodenal or biliary fluid into the pancreatic duct. In this situation, pancreatic tissue may be damaged directly as by bacteria, pancreatic enzymes may be activated by unknown mechanisms, or the reflux of duodenal fluid may already contain activated trypsin. Other cases are caused by obstruction of pancreatic ducts, either the main pancreatic duct in the case of a carcinoma or smaller ductules in alcoholic pancreatitis. Under these conditions, there may be premature activation of pancreatic enzymes. Still other cases result from direct damage to acinar tissue or possibly activation of enzymes, including pancreatitis caused by alcohol, drugs, fatty acids, infectious agents, and parathormone.

REFERENCES

1. Banks PA: Acute pancreatitis. *Gastroenterology* 61:382–397, 1971.
2. Anderson MC: Necrotizing properties of human blood following incubation with autologous pancreatic secretions. *J Surg Res* 5:239–244, 1965.
3. Creutzfelt W, Schmidt H: Aetiology and pathogenesis of pancreatitis. *Scand J Gastroenterol* 5 (sup 6):47–62, 1970.
4. Editorial: Mechanism of pancreatic autodigestion. *N Engl J Med* 283:487–488 1970.

5. Geokas MC, Rinderknecht K, Swanson V, et al: Pancreatic elastase and hemorrhagic pancreatitis. *Lab Invest* 19:235–239, 1969.
6. McCutcheon AD: A fresh approach to the pathogenesis of pancreatitis. *Gut* 9:296–310, 1968.
7. Allan BJ, Tournut R, White TT: Intraductal activation of pancreatic zymogens behind a carcinoma of the pancreas. *Gastroenterology* 65:412–418, 1973.
8. White TT, Allan BJ: Intrapancreatic activation of proteases in the etiology of pancreatitis and cancer of the pancreas. *Med Clin N Am* 58:1305–1310, 1974.
9. Geokas MC, Rinderknecht H: Free proteolytic enzymes in pancreatic juice of patients with acute pancreatitis. *Am J Dig Dis* 19:591–598, 1974.
10. Ohlsson K and Eddeland A: Release of proteolytic enzymes in bile-induced pancreatitis in dogs. *Gastroenterology* 69:668–675, 1975.
11. Kasahara K, Carballo Jr, Takada Y, et al: Elastase levels during bile-induced pancreatitis in dogs determined by radioimmunoassay. *Surg Gynecol Obstet* 141:347–351, 1975.
12. Rao KN, Tuma J, Lombardi B: Acute hemorrhagic pancreatic necrosis in mice. *Gastroenterology* 70:720–726, 1976.
13. Ofstad E: Formation and destruction of plasma kinins during experimental acute hemorrhagic pancreatitis in dogs. *Scand J Gastroenterol* 5 (sup 5):1–44, 1970.
14. Takada Y, Appert HE, Howard JM: Vascular permeability induced by pancreatic exudate formed during acute pancreatitis. *Surg Gynecol Obstet* 143:779–783, 1976.
15. Glazer G, Bennett A: Prostaglandin release in canine acute hemorrhagic pancreatitis. *Gut* 17:22–26, 1976.
16. Anderson MC, Schiller WR: Microcirculatory dynamics in the normal and inflamed pancreas. *Am J Surg* 115:118–127, 1968.
17. Pirola RC, Davis AE: Effect of pressure on the integrity of the duct-acinar system of the pancreas. *Gut* 11:69–73, 1970.
18. Papp M, Ungvari G, Nemeth PE, et al: The effect of bileinduced pancreatitis on intrapancreatic vascular pattern in dogs. *Scand J Gastroenterol* 4:681–689, 1969.
19. Herva P: Experimental biliary pancreatitis in dogs. *Scand J Gastroenterol* 5 (sup 8):1–63, 1970.
20. Schiller WR, Anderson MC: Microcirculation of the normal and inflamed canine pancreas. *Ann Surg* 181:466–470, 1975.

Pathology of Acute Pancreatitis

4.1 EDEMATOUS PANCREATITIS

The mildest form of acute pancreatitis is characterized by interstitial edema associated with a mild inflammatory exudate composed of either polymorphonuclear leukocytes or lymphocytes. Acinar tissue and ductular structures remain intact. There may be slight interstitial fibrosis. Occasionally there is a slight degree of fat necrosis. It is possible for this type of inflammatory process to recur on several occasions and resolve each time without residual histologic abnormality. This sequence is termed "relapsing acute pancreatitis" and is typical of the majority of instances of pancreatitis associated with biliary tract disease.

4.2 HEMORRHAGIC PANCREATITIS

A number of destructive forces are responsible for hemorrhagic pancreatitis.[1] First, there is destruction of pancreatic parenchyma in the form of coagulation necrosis (Figure 1). Inflammatory cells tend to confine themselves at first to the margins of necrotic areas. Once activated by trypsin, phospholipase-A constitutes a potent enzyme in this process. A second destructive force is necrosis of blood vessels. Pancreatic elastase is thought to be responsible for disruption and destruction of blood vessels. If destruction of blood vessels is particularly severe, extensive zones of pancreatic hemorrhage occur. A third destructive force is necrosis of fat by lipolytic enzymes. Fat cells are converted to necrotic areas surrounded by a rim of white blood cells (Figure 2). Fat necrosis takes

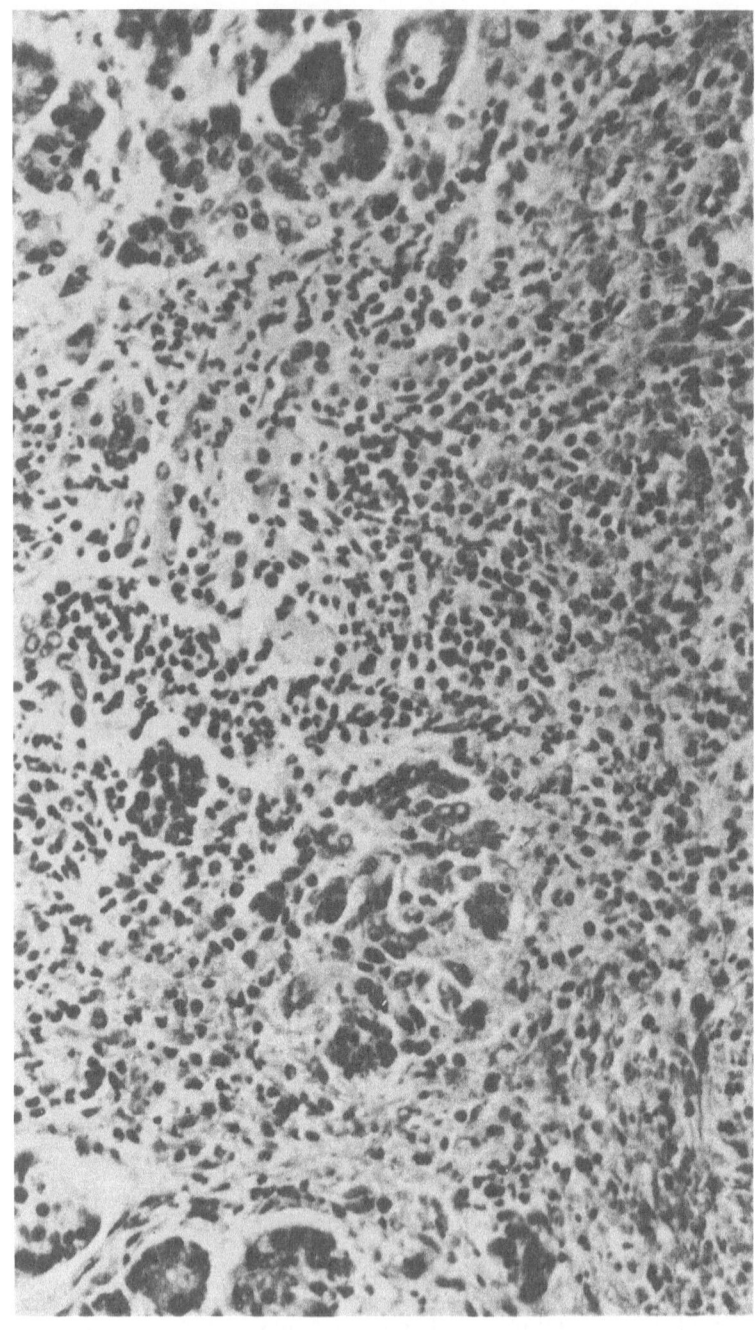

FIGURE 1 Histology of Acute Pancreatitis. A large coagulum contains remnants of viable acinar tissue, necrotic debris, and scattered polymorphonuclear leukocytes and round cells. Infiltration with leukocytes tends to be sparse at the onset of acute pancreatitis but more plentiful during a later phase.

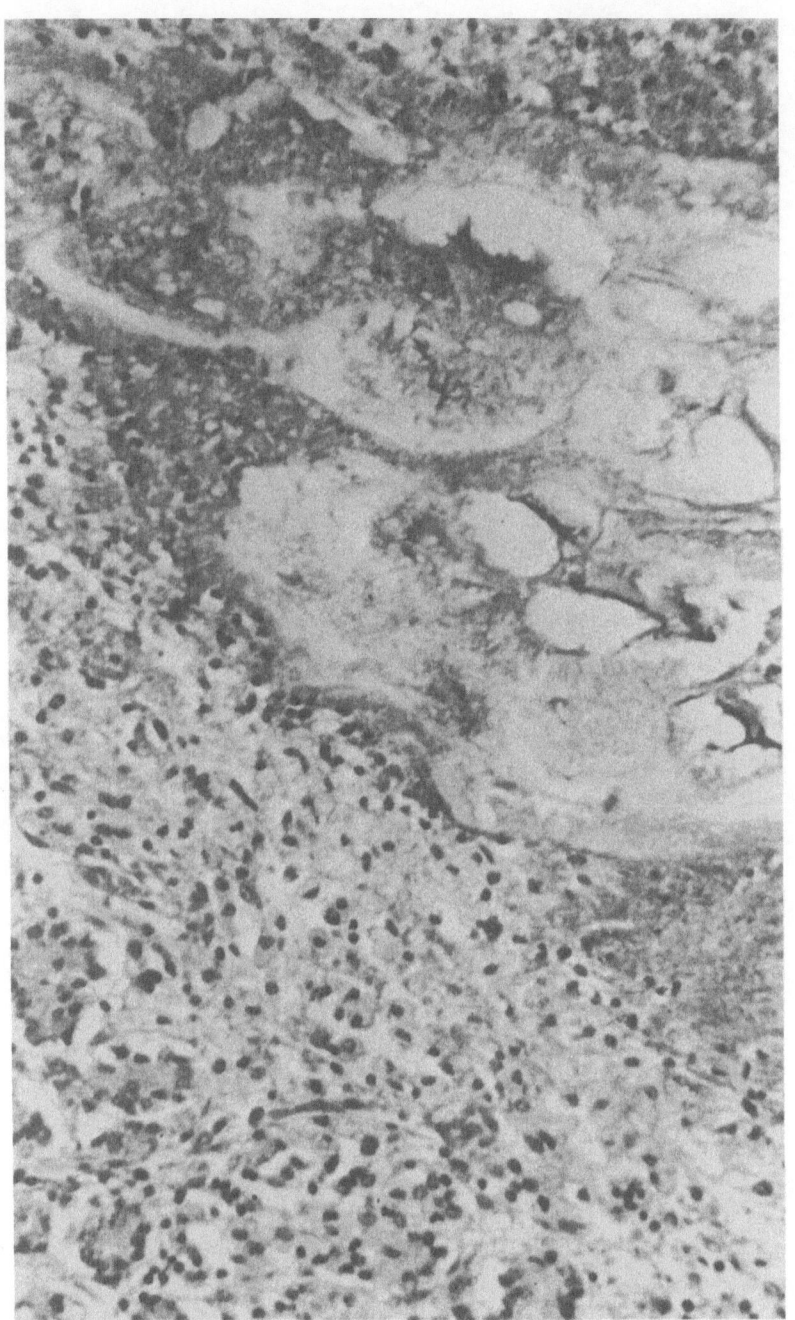

FIGURE 2 *Fat Necrosis in Acute Pancreatitis.* A large amorphous zone of fat necrosis is visible on the right. Inflammatory cells rim this zone but do not enter in quantity. Residual acinar tissue is visible at the upper left.

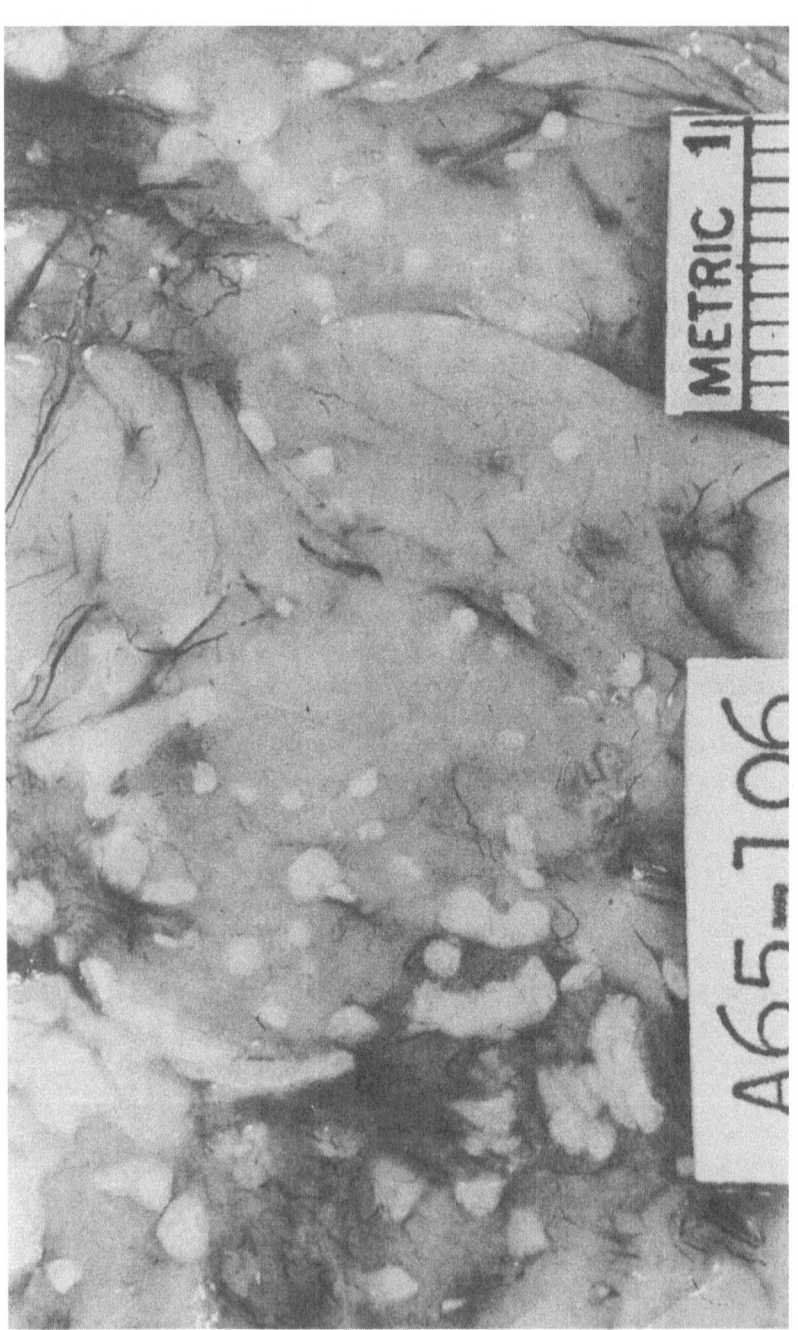

FIGURE 3 Fat Necrosis in Omentum in Acute Pancreatitis. Scattered whitish plaques are visible on omental tissue. Smaller plaques at the center coalesce into larger accumulations on both sides. The linear dark streaks are congested omental blood vessels.

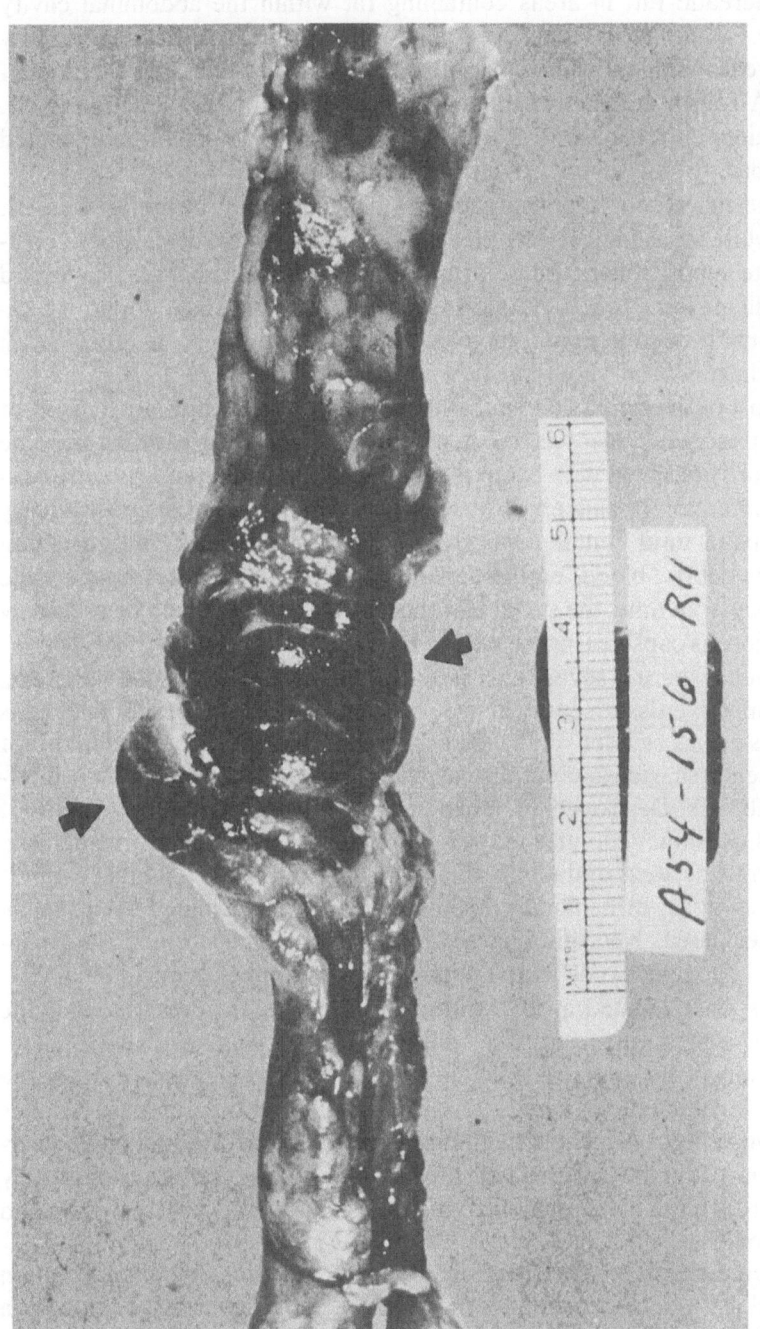

FIGURE 4 Pancreatic Pseudocyst. Gross specimen of pancreas at autopsy showing two discrete hemorrhagic pseudocysts in the center (arrows). The remainder of the pancreas shows evidence of acute and chronic inflammation with zones of hemorrhage (dark areas) interspersed with zones of necrosis (pale areas). (Courtesy of Dr. D. Antonioli.)

place in particular within the connective tissue septae of the pancreas, in peripancreatic fat, in areas containing fat within the abdominal cavity (Figure 3), and at times elsewhere as well. Free fatty acids liberated by lipase react with calcium to form calcium soaps within area of fat necrosis. A fourth destructive influence is the inflammatory reaction itself. The white cell response is in general less intense that might be expected on the basis of the severity of enzymatic destruction.

The macroscopic appearance of the gland may be quite mottled. Gray-white areas indicate the presence of parenchymal destruction; chalky-white deposits mark areas of fat necrosis; red areas that are friable and soft indicate zones of destruction associated with bleeding. Areas of relatively mild edema may merge with zones of frank necrosis with hemorrhage.

Most of the serious complications of acute pancreatitis are a result of severe pancreatic necrosis and hemorrhage. Necrotic areas may become secondarily infected with bacteria and develop into a relentless retroperitoneal infection (a pancreatic abscess). An area of necrosis may liquefy and expand until contained by surrounding structures. This coagulum contains debris, blood, and pancreatic juice and is termed a pancreatic pseudocyst. In time, the surface of this structure may develop a relatively tough fibrous capsule (Figure 4).

Even if there is severe necrosis and hemorrhage within the pancreas, the connective tissue septae may be reasonably well preserved. Islet cells at times are as severely damaged as are exocrine cells. The resolution of acute hemorrhagic pancreatitis may be associated with considerable interstitial fibrosis. Destroyed ductal and acinar cells are replaced by zones of fibrosis. Residual ductules may show evidence of squamous metaplasia. There may be areas of ductular dilatation and foci of ductular narrowing.

The impact of hemorrhagic pancreatitis is not confined to the retroperitoneal area. Necrotic pancreatic debris, enzymes, blood, and pancreatic juice may exude from the pancreas creating a chemical inflammatory response located at first within the lesser sac and the base of the transverse mesocolon but then spilling into the peritoneal cavity. Globules of oil appear in peritoneal fluid (chicken broth fluid) as a result of the action of pancreatic enzymes. Dissection of blood through tissue planes may cause areas of visible hemorrhage in the costovertebral angle (Turner's sign) or in the periumbilical area (Cullen's sign). Peritoneal fluid may pass through the diaphragm via lymphatics causing a pleural effusion and pneumonitis.

Hemorrhagic pancreatitis occurs only occasionally in association with biliary tract disease. It is more likely to occur in association with alcohol. With each succeeding bout of alcoholic pancreatitis, the likelihood of hemorrhagic pancreatitis becomes less as the pancreas becomes depleted of enzymes.

REFERENCE

1. Robbins SL: *Pathologic Basis of Disease.* Philadelphia, WB Saunders Co, 1974.

5

Clinical Manifestations of Acute Pancreatitis

There are no specific clinical features that readily distinguish pancreatitis from a variety of other illnesses. Abdominal pain occurs in almost all cases of acute pancreatitis. It may reach full intensity in a matter of minutes or more gradually over several hours. Pain is usually localized in the epigastrium. It is occasionally more intense to the left or right of the epigastrium, or diffuse in the upper abdomen. If pancreatic exudation spreads diffusely throughout the peritoneal cavity, abdominal discomfort may become generalized. On rare occasions, abdominal pain is restricted exclusively to the lower abdomen such that a diagnosis of acute pancreatitis is not even considered. Pain in the lower abdomen would presumably be caused by extension of pancreatic exudation through the mesentery of the small intestine to the region of the ileum and cecum.

The pain of pancreatitis is usually steady, boring, and penetrating. In approximately half the cases, it radiates straight through to the back. This type of radiation may occur whether pain develops quickly or gradually. It may be relieved somewhat by flexing the spine, by sitting forward with knees flexed against the chest, by squatting and clasping the knees to the chest, or by lying on one side with knees flexed. One characteristic feature of pain associated with acute pancreatitis is that it usually lasts for many hours and even several days rather than only a few minutes or a few hours.[1]

Most patients experience nausea and vomiting. The vomiting may be very severe and protracted ending in dry heaves. Vomiting of bilious material has been considered to be unusual in acute pancreatitis but may occur.[2,3] The relationship of abdominal pain to nausea and vomiting is variable. In some series of patients abdominal pain preceded nausea and vomiting[1]; in other series, abdominal pain occurred after the onset of nausea and vomiting.[4]

It might be anticipated that symptoms of acute pancreatitis would occur shortly after the ingestion of a meal or alcohol. For example, in pancreatitis associated with biliary tract disease, hormonal stimulation of gallbladder contraction by food might cause the migration of gallstones into the common bile duct and into the duodenum causing symptoms of pancreatitis shortly thereafter. In reality, it is difficult to establish such a time relationship, and in one series no time relationship could be identified.[3] Also, in alcoholic pancreatitis, hormonal stimulation of pancreatic secretion by either food or drink might be expected to cause prompt symptoms especially if there are multiple areas of ductular obstruction by protein plugs. At times, abdominal pain occurs promptly after a meal; at other times, symptoms of alcoholic pancreatitis may occur long after a meal or consumption of alcohol. In two large series of patients, the episode of alcoholic pancreatitis occurred on the afternoon after alcoholic overindulgence the previous evening.[1,5]

In very mild edematous pancreatitis, the patient is usually only moderately ill, and symptoms are suggestive of indigestion or "gastritis." The fact that a routinely drawn serum amylase is elevated may come as a surprise. Abdominal tenderness is usually confined to the epigastrium and is not severe. There may be no guarding whatsoever.

In severe edematous pancreatitis and in hemorrhagic pancreatitis, the patient often appears acutely and seriously ill. He may move restlessly in bed in an effort to relieve pain or may lie quietly if movement intensifies abdominal discomfort. The patient is not apt to be completely motionless as in the case of a perforated peptic ulcer. Temperature is usually between 99° and 102°. Pulse rate is usually greater than 100 beats/min. Respiratory rate may be increased. Hypertension may occur during the acute phase of the illness.[6] With clinical improvement, blood pressure returns to normal levels. If there is severe hypovolemia, the patient may be hypotensive.

The extremities may be cold and clammy. Scleral icterus may be present. Examination of the chest reveals limited diaphragmatic excursion if there is splinting of the diaphragm as a result of abdominal pain. Dullness to percussion and decreased breath sounds at either base may indicate the presence of a pleural effusion. The abdomen may be distended. Peristalsis is usually diminished and may be completely absent. An epigastric mass is occasionally palpated representing either a large pancreatic phlegmon or a pancreatic pseudocyst. Even when there is considerable muscular guarding in the upper abdomen, the lower abdomen generally remains soft and relatively nontender. Diffuse peritoneal irritation sometimes results in generalized abdominal signs and symptoms. Occasionally it leads to the development of a classic boardlike abdomen which is virtually indistinguishable on physical examination from a perforation such as a duodenal ulcer. In hemorrhagic pancreatitis, a bluish discoloration may be visible in the flanks (Turner's sign) or in the region of the umbilicus (Cullen's sign). The discoloration may represent dissection of blood to these areas, but at times occurs for unknown reasons even in the absence of intraperitoneal bleeding. It is important to note that these signs occur in other intraabdominal conditions as well, some associated with bleeding and others not, and are therefore not specific for acute pancreatitis.[7]

The presence of additional physical findings may be helpful in supporting a diagnosis of pancreatitis. Alcoholic pancreatitis would be suspected if the liver is enlarged and if there are stigmata of chronic liver disease such as thickening of palmar sheaths and spider angiomata. Pancreatitis secondary to acute cholecystitis would be suspected if there is severe abdominal tenderness and guarding in the upper right quadrant of the abdomen. Pancreatitis caused by hyperlipemia would be suggested by the presence of eruptive xanthoma of the skin and lipemic retinalis.[8-10] Parotid swelling would suggest pancreatitis associated with mumps. The presence of an infiltration on the lateral margins of the cornea (band keratopathy) would suggest pancreatitis in association with hypercalcemia.

On rare occasions, acute pancreatitis occurs without abdominal pain.[11-13] Under these circumstances, there is usually severe pancreatic necrosis and hemorrhage associated with shock and coma. Because of the absence of abdominal pain and significant abdominal tenderness, an accurate diagnosis may not be possible prior to autopsy.

Alcoholic pancreatitis is more common among males than females. The first clinical episode usually takes place prior to the age of 40.[1,4] Pancreatitis associated with biliary tract disease is more common among females and usually occurs in a slightly older age group.[4] Alcoholic pancreatitis is more likely to be associated with severe necrosis and hemorrhage than pancreatitis caused by biliary tract disease. Hemorrhagic pancreatitis is more likely to take place during an early episode of alcoholic pancreatitis than in a later episode.[2,14] From a clinical standpoint, the distinction between edematous and hemorrhagic pancreatitis may not be obvious early in the illness. The patient with edematous pancreatitis may also appear severely ill because of the intensity of the pain and the severe hypotension caused by pancreatic exudation.

REFERENCES

1. Marks IN, Bank S, Louw JH, et al: The clinical varieties of alcoholic pancreatitis in the South Western Cape. *S Afr Med J* 39:1093–1095, 1965.
2. Albo R, Silen W and Goldman L: A critical clinical analysis of acute pancreatitis. *Arch Surg* 86:174–180, 1963.
3. Pollock AV: Acute pancreatitis. *Br Med J* 1:6–14, 1959.
4. Olsen H: Pancreatitis. *Am J Dig Dis* 19:1077–1090, 1974.
5. Geokas MC, Van Lancker JL, Kadell BM, et al: Acute pancreatitis. *Ann Intern Med* 76:105–117, 1972.
6. Sankaran S, Lucas CE, Walt AJ: Transient hypertension with acute pancreatitis. *Surg Gynecol Obstet* 138:235–238, 1974.
7. Evans DM: Cullen's sign in perforated duodenal ulcer. *Br Med J* 1:154, 1971.
8. Bank S, Marks IN: Hyperlipeamic pancreatitis and the pill. *Postgrad Med J* 46:576–588, 1960.
9. Glueck CJ, Scheel D, Fishback J, et al: Estrogen-induced pancreatitis in patients with previously covert familial Type-5 hyperlipoproteinemia. *Metab Clin Exp* 21:657–666, 1972.
10. Molitch ME, Oill P, Odell WD: Massive hyperlipemia during estrogen therapy. *JAMA* 227:522–525, 1974.
11. Toffler AH, Spiro HM: Shock or coma as the predominant manifestation of painless acute pancreatitis. *Ann Intern Med* 57:655–659, 1962.
12. Dooner HP, Aliaga C: Painless acute necrotic pancreatitis. *Arch Intern Med* 116:828–831, 1965.
13. Read G, Braganza JM, Howat HT: Pancreatitis—a retrospective study. *Gut* 17:945–952, 1976.
14. Jordan GL, Spjut HJ: Hemorrhagic pancreatitis. *Arch Surg* 104:489–493, 1972.

6

Diagnosis of Acute Pancreatitis

6.1 AMYLASE

6.1.1 Metabolism of Amylase

Alpha amylase is an enzyme that splits the α-1, 4-glycosidic bonds of starch. Its optimal pH is 6.9. Its molecular weight is approximately 50,000. Chloride is required for optimal enzyme activity. Calcium is an integral part of the enzyme.

Careful analysis of human tissue homogenates reveals that a variety of tissues contain amylase activity, including the pancreas, salivary glands, fallopian tubes, ovary, lung, prostate, and possibly liver.[1,2] The isoenzymes of amylase from these tissues can be identified by using sophisticated techniques such as electrophoretic separation gels, chromatographic separation techniques, and isoelectric focusing. Amylase originating from the pancreas is designated as p-amylase; amylase originating from salivary glands is designated as s-amylase. There are several p-amylases from the pancreas and several s-amylases from salivary glands. The pancreas also produces a very small amount of s-type isoamylase.[3] Salivary glands produce exclusively s-isoamylase. Amylase activity in lung homogenates is s-isoamylase; that of female organs is both s-isoamylase and p-isoamylase.[1]

In health, at least one-half,[1] and probably more than one-half,[2,4-6] of total serum amylase is s-amylase; one-half or less than one-half is p-amylase. The only two organs that contribute to serum amylase in health are the salivary glands and the pancreas.[1]

The kidney normally removes 24% of serum amylase,[7] and the fact that most removal is by other means explains why serum amylase either remains normal or is only slightly elevated in renal insufficiency. An important measurement involving serum amylase is its clearance from the serum. Whereas the clearance of serum creatinine is in excess of 100 cc/min, the clearance of amylase is approximately 2 to 3 cc/min.[8-12] This is the reason that the ratio of amylase clearance to creatinine clearance is normally of the order of 3% (approximately $3/100 \times 100$).

6.1.2 Laboratory Measurement of Amylase

There are several methods of measuring amylase in biologic fluids. Saccharogenic methods measure the production of reducing sugars. In the iodometric technique (for example, the Caraway procedure), starches are hydrolyzed by amylase into colorless starch fragments. Iodine is then added. If residual unhydrolyzed starch is present, a colored starch-iodide complex is formed and can be measured. The decrease in absorbance is proportional to the amylase activity. When all the starch has been hydrolyzed, no further colored starch–iodide complexes are formed.

In the chromogenic method (an example of which is the Phadebas technique, Pharmacia, Piscataway, New Jersey), a dye is linked to an insoluble starch. As the starch is hydrolyzed by amylase, colored soluble starch fragments are formed and can be measured. The increase in absorbance is proportional to amylase activity.[13,14] Iodometric and chromogenic techniques both underestimate the quantity of amylase in urine.[14]

6.1.3 Causes of Increased Serum Amylase

(a) Pancreatic Diseases. In acute pancreatitis, serum amylase is usually but not invariably elevated.[12,15-17] An increase in serum amylase could result from either disruption of acinar tissue leading to pancreatic exudation into retroperitoneal and peritoneal spaces or obstruction to flow within pancreatic ducts leading to extravasation of amylase into lymphatic and venous pathways from the pancreas. In severe hemorrhagic pancreatitis, the serum amylase may be only minimally elevated or not elevated at all. Serum amylase remains normal during an exacerbation of chronic pancreatitis if acinar tissue had already been substantially destroyed.

Complications of acute pancreatitis are frequently but not always associated with an elevation of serum amylase. These complications include pancreatic pseudocyst, pancreatic ascites, and pancreatic abscess.

Occasionally, a pancreatic carcinoma is associated with an elevation of serum amylase. This may be due to obstruction to the flow of pancreatic juice leading to extravasation of fluid from pancreatic ductules into lymphatic and venous pathways and then into the systemic circulation. On rare occasions, an increase in serum amylase occurs either because the tumor secretes amylase or causes pancreatitis.

(b) Nonpancreatic Diseases with Surgicial Implications

Biliary Tract Disease. Biliary tract disease may cause an increase in serum amylase in the absence of pancreatitis. The mechanism appears to be transient obstruction to the flow of bile at the ampulla of Vater and subsequent regurgitation of pancreatic amylase via pancreatic ducts into venous and lymphatic pathways of the pancreas and then into the systemic circulation. This view is reinforced by the discovery that the additional amylase in circulation is p-isoamylase.[4] A normal amylase-creatinine clearance ratio would further support the belief that the increase in serum amylase is not associated with pancreatitis.[18]

Other Serious Intraabdominal Diseases. There are several serious intraabdominal conditions that may be associated with an elevation in serum amylase. The basis of an increase in serum amylase is leakage of intraluminal contents containing amylase through an ischemic, necrotic, or perforated hollow viscus with reabsorption of amylase from the peritoneal cavity into the systemic circulation.[13,19,20] These disorders include esophageal perforation, penetrating or perforated gastric or duodenal ulcer, acute cholecystitis, acute intestinal obstruction, obstruction of an afferent loop, intestinal ischemia or infarction, and peritonitis. Gynecological conditions associated with an elevation of serum amylase include ruptured ectopic pregnancy[13] and salpingitis.[21] Dissecting aortic aneurysm has also been reported to cause an elevation of serum amylase, but the mechanism is not clear.[13]

The importance of noting these conditions is that most if not all are associated with abdominal pain, most require surgical attention (frequently on an emergency basis), and many of them may be confused clinically with acute pancreatitis.

(c) Miscellaneous Conditions Associated with Elevated Serum Amylase

Diseases of the Salivary Glands. Diseases ot the salivary glands, including mumps, inflammation, and calculi obstructing salivary ducts, are associated with elevations of serum amylase.

Liver Disease. A number of patients have been documented with increased serum amylase levels in association with either alcoholic or nonalcoholic liver disease. The stages of liver disease have included acute, chronic active, and chronic (cirrhosis).[21-23] In two reports, the elevation of serum amylase was due exclusively to an increase in s-isoamylase, and there was clinical evidence of salivary gland dysfunction.[22,23] In the third report,[21] it was thought that the elevation of serum amylase was due either to an isoamylase that originated in the liver or alteration of normal serum amylase by liver disease. It is therefore important to keep in mind that an elevation of serum amylase in the context of liver disease (particularly alcoholic liver disease) need not mean coexisting pancreatitis.

Tumors. Various tumors have been identified which elaborate amylase and cause an elevation of serum amylase. These include papillary cystadenocarcinomas of the ovary, and carcinoma of lung, colon, and pancreas.[23-25]The isoamylase elaborated by tumors of lung and ovary have all been s-isoamylase[23-25]; colonic tumors have been either p-isoamylase or s-isoamylase[25]; pancreatic tumors were p-isoamylase in two cases and s-isoamylase in one.[25] The fact that a small amount of s-isoamylase is normally present in pancreatic tissue would presumably explain the presence of s-isoamylase in one carcinoma of the pancreas.[3]

Macroamylasemia. Occasionally, amylase with normal activity is complexed either with globulin (either IgA or IgG) or some other substance,[26] forming a macromolecular complex with a molecular weight of from 160,000 to in excess of 2,000,000. This molecule is too large to be filtered by the glomeruli, and, hence, levels of serum amylase are higher than normal and levels of urinary amylase are frequently lower than normal. The amylase that is bound is both s-isoamylase and p-isoamylase. The amylase that appears in urine is normal and represents the renal excretion of the unbound fraction of serum amylase.[27] Most people with macroamylasemia are healthy.[28,29] One patient has been described with acute intermittent porphyria[30]; another with intestinal malabsorption.[27] Macroamylasemia usually persists indefinitely but in one patient was transient.[30] Most cases of macroamylasemia that have been observed have been associated with elevations of serum amylase,[27,29-31] but it is now known that individuals with normal serum amylase may also have macroamylasemia.[28]

The diagnosis of macroamylasemia is suggested by a persistingly elevated serum amylase in the absence of signs or symptoms of pancreatitis. The diagnosis is further supported by a normal or low urinary clearance of amylase (in the presence of normal renal function). Interestingly and appropriately, when one patient with macroamylasemia developed acute pancreatitis, the clearance of amylase increased, and the amylase-creatinine clearance ratio was diagnostic for acute pancreatitis.[31]

Renal Insufficiency. The normal clearance of serum amylase is on the order of 2–3 ml/min.[8-12] In renal insufficiency, the clearance of amylase is reduced as creatinine clearance decreases.[8-11] Serum amylase may be slightly elevated in renal insufficiency but usually not more than twice normal.[8-11,32] There is no consistent relationship between elevations of

BUN and increases in serum amylase.[8] An important conclusion is that a serum amylase more than twice normal in a context of uremia should alert the clinician to search for a cause other than renal insufficiency.

Miscellaneous. There are various other disorders which on rare occasions may be associated with hyperamylasemia.[13]

Diabetic ketoacidosis is occasionally associated with an increase in serum amylase. The usual clinical assumption has been that the increased serum amylase reflects acute pancreatitis without pain, and that the diabetic ketoacidosis is a metabolic consequence of severe pancreatitis. It has recently been reported that increase in serum amylase in diabetic ketoacidosis was invariably s-isoamylase, indicating that its source was an organ other than the pancreas and that there was no underlying pancreatitis.[33]

An increase in serum amylase in the postoperative period may signify either postoperative pancreatitis or an increase in s-isoamylase possibly as a result of irritation of salivary glands during endotracheal intubation.

An increased serum amylase has been recorded following the use of high-dose intravenous steroids[34] and following the use of intravenous secretin as part of a clinical trial.[35] Serum amylase may be increased in prostatic diseases.[36]

Patients who undergo successful endoscopic retrograde cannulation of the pancreatic duct may have an increase in serum amylase without demonstrable pancreatitis. The isoamylase that increases is usually pancreatic.[37] It is presumed that p-isoamylase is refluxed via pancreatic ducts into the interstitium of the pancreas and then into the systemic circulation. Serum amylase may also be increased with the use of narcotics such as morphine for pain and following the provocative morphine-prostigmine test.[38] The mechanism may be the same.

6.1.4 Causes of Persistently Elevated Serum Amylase

Acute pancreatitis may persist for an extended period of time and may be associated with a prolonged elevation of serum amylase. Complications of pancreatitis (including pseudocyst, ascites, and abscess) and carcinoma of the pancreas may be associated with a persistingly elevated serum amylase.

The varieties of nonpancreatic diseases with surgical implications would not be expected to cause sustained elevations of serum amylase. Salivary gland tumors, inflammations, or calculi may all be associated with prolonged serum amylase elevations. The same would be true of certain tumors, renal insufficiency, and macroamylasemia.

6.1.5 Usefulness of the Amylase–Creatinine Clearance Ratio

(a) *Basic Considerations.* Measurement of serum amylase is useful but not specific for acute pancreatitis. A further disadvantage of serum amylase is that it may be elevated only transiently in acute pancreatitis. It has been found that after acute pancreatitis, urinary amylase tends to remain elevated after serum amylase returns to normal.[11,39] It was further shown that the usefulness of measuring urinary amylase and amylase clearance could be enhanced by measuring creatinine clearance simultaneously and expressing the result as a ratio (the amylase-creatinine clearance ratio). An important reason for including creatinine clearance in the equation is that in the presence of renal insufficiency the clearance of amylase decreases as the creatinine clearance decreases. For example, a normal amylase clearance of 3 cc/min should increase to at least 6 cc/min during acute pancreatitis; however, if there is coexisting renal insufficiency, the figure might be reduced to 3 cc/min (a "normal" level). Simultaneous measurement of creatinine clearance resolves this problem. For example, if the normal amylase clearance is 3 cc/min and if the normal creatinine clearance is of the order of 100 cc/min, the normal ratio of amylase clearance to creatinine clearance is 3%. If acute pancreatitis is associated with renal insufficiency, the creatinine clearance may be reduced from 100 to 50 cc/min. If the amylase clearance is thereby reduced from 6 to 3 cc/min, the ratio remains 6% (3/50 × 100), which is diagnostic of acute pancreatitis.

At first, it seemed reasonable to obtain timed outputs of urine in order to perform the clearance measurements (samples after 2, 12, or 24 hr). A much easier way to obtain the necessary data is to collect a specimen of serum and urine simultaneously and to measure amylase and creatinine concentration in serum and in urine. Volume and time are canceled by this instantaneous clearance. The amylase-creatinine clearance ratio would then be formulated on the basis of the following equation:

$$\frac{UA/SA}{UC/SC} \times 100 = \frac{UA \times SC}{UC \times SA} \times 100$$

where UA is urinary amylase, SA is serum amylase, UC is urinary creatinine, and SC is serum creatinine.

There is general agreement that the amylase–creatinine clearance ratio is normally 1–4%.[4,9–11,40–42] The technique utilized to measure amylase greatly determines whether the ratio is closer to 1% or 4%.[14] Suffice it to say that an amylase–creatinine clearance ratio of greater than

6% is diagnostic of acute pancreatitis by all currently available techniques.

The initial explanation for the increase of amylase–creatinine clearance ratio in acute pancreatitis was the fact that pancreatic amylase is cleared 80% faster than salivary amylase,[43] and that in acute pancreatitis most of the amylase in serum and urine originates from the pancreas.[5,40] It appears that this is not the full explanation since in acute pancreatitis the clearance of total amylase may be far in excess of the normal clearance of p-isoamylase. It has been found that in acute pancreatitis the clearances of both p-isoamylase and s-isoamylase are far in excess of normal, and both then contribute to the increase in amylase clearance in acute pancreatitis. The explanation is as follows. In health, serum amylase is first filtered by glomeruli and then reabsorbed by a tubular mechanism.[4,40,44] In acute pancreatitis, this tubular reabsorptive mechanism is inhibited thereby permitting excretion of increased amounts of both p-isoamylase and s-isoamylase.[40] Since most of the amylase in serum in acute pancreatitis is p-isoamylase, the total clearance approximates the enhanced clearance of p-isoamylase (which as stated is far in excess of the normal clearance of p-isoamylase).

(b) Diagnostic Specificity in Association with an Elevated Serum Amylase. In acute pancreatitis, serum amylase is usually increased, and the amylase–creatinine clearance ratio should also be increased because of inhibition of renal tubular reabsorption of amylase. In disease that may masquerade as acute pancreatitis, serum amylase may also be elevated, but the amylase–creatinine clearance ratio should remain normal because there is no renal tubular defect. If an amylase–creatinine clearance ratio is "normal" and fails to confirm an obvious diagnosis of acute pancreatitis, there are several possible explanations. The first is that the patient does not have acute pancreatitis. The second is that the test may have been done incorrectly. For example, if samples of blood and urine are not obtained at the same time, a valid clearance is not obtained, and the results should be discarded. Third, the "normal" ratio may in fact be accurate and supportive of a diagnosis of acute pancreatitis in accordance with the following explanation. Originally, the normal amylase–creatinine clearance ratio was reported to be approximately 3%; a value of 6% or higher was considered to be diagnostic for acute pancreatitis. It is now known that the technique for measuring amylase may greatly influence the amylase–creatinine clearance ratio both in health and in acute pancreatitis.[14] For example, when a saccharogenic technique is utilized, "normal" amylase–creatinine clearance ratio is approximately 2%, and a ratio of 6% or higher is diagnostic for acute pancreatitis. However, when the Phadebas chromogenic method is utilized, the "normal" value is approximately 1%, and a ratio of 3% or higher is diagnostic of acute pancreatitis. Similarly, when the iodometric technique of Caraway is used, "normal" ratio is approximately 1.5% and increases to 5% or higher in acute pancreatitis.[14] It is clear that the clinician must know which assay technique is utilized since a ratio of 3% may be diagnostic of acute pancreatitis with one technique but normal with another. A ratio of 6% or higher is diagnostic of acute pancreatitis with all techniques.

It is not known whether the amylase–creatinine clearance ratio is consistently elevated in the important complications of acute pancreatitis that are often associated with an increased serum amylase, including pancreatic ascites, pancreatis abscess, and pancreatic pseudocyst. If acute inflammation of the pancreas subsides but a pseudocyst persists, serum amylase may remain elevated, yet the amylase–creatinine clearance ratio may be normal. The probable explanation for the normal ratio is that the renal tubular defect responsible for an increased ratio disappears with resolution of acute inflammation. In carcinoma of the pancreas, the amylase–creatinine clearance ratio has been found to be normal.[41]

Among the variety of abdominal conditions that masquerade as acute pancreatitis and cause an elevated serum amylase, there have been numerous observations that the amylase–creatinine clearance ratio remains normal and thus distinguishes these illnesses from pancreatitis.[4,18,45,46] Thus far, among the miscellaneous nonpancreatic diseases associated with an increase in serum amylase, including salivary gland disease and macroamylasemia, the amylase–creatinine clearance ratio is either normal or appropriately low.[11,21,22,27,31,47] In one patient with an increased serum amylase owing to a carcinoma of the lung, the clearance of amylase was normal.[24] Published reports of amylase–creatinine clearance ratios in uremia have been variable. In two reports, the ratio increased in severe uremia[10,32]; in one, the ratio was unaffected by moderate or severe renal disease.[9] The influence of renal insufficiency on amylase–creatinine clearance ratio may be quite complex whether the serum amylase is elevated or not.[48]

(c) *Diagnostic Specificity of Amylase–Creatinine Clearance Ratio in Association with a Normal Serum Amylase.* In resolving acute pancreatitis, the amylase–creatinine clearance ratio may remain elevated for several days after serum amylase returns to normal.[11] In acute pancreatitis associated with hyperlipemia, amylase–creatinine clearance ratio may be diagnostic of acute pancreatitis even if serum amylase is normal[49]; a circulating inhibitor of serum amylase may be responsible for the normal serum amylase.[50]

Aside from these two clinical situations in which an increased amylase–creatinine clearance ratio is supportive of pancreatitis at a time that the serum amylase is normal, there are, unfortunately, several situations in which the ratio may be increased in the absence of discernible pancreatitis. First, an increased ratio has been reported in association with a normal serum amylase following common bile duct exploration.[51] It is possible that these patients indeed had subclinical pancreatitis without an elevation in serum amylase or that there was transient impairment of reabsorption of amylase by the kidney owing to factors other than acute pancreatitis. Second, patients with extensive burns and diabetic ketoacidosis have been reported with an elevated ratio associated with a normal serum amylase.[52] Again, transient renal impairment of amylase reabsorption may possibly be responsible for this effect.

Another possible explanation for an increased ratio in diabetic ketoacidosis is the fact that a high serum concentration of acetoacetate may falsely elevate the measurement of serum creatinine.[53] Since serum creatinine is in the numerator of the standard equation, a false elevation of serum creatinine would increase the ratio. Third, in uremia, an increased ratio may occur on the basis of tubular dysfunction among patients with normal serum amylase concentration as well as among those with an increased serum amylase. Unpublished data from our laboratory indicate that even mild impairment of renal function (not enough to increase the serum amylase) may cause an increased amylase–creatinine clearance ratio.[54]

In summary, there are several situations in which an elevated amylase–creatinine clearance ratio is not indicative of acute pancreatitis. For this reason, the measurement of the amylase–creatinine clearance ratio may have very limited usefulness if the serum amylase is normal (except in the situation of hyperlipemia associated with pancreatitis).

6.1.6 Usefulness of Isoamylase Determination

Diagnostic usefulness of isoamylases is limited by the fact that this measurement is not readily available. Acute pancreatitis would be characterized by a marked predominance of p-isoamylase in both serum and urine.[2,4–6,21,23,55,57] Other disorders involving the pancreas would presumably also have a predominance of p-isoamylase in serum (such as pancreatic pseudocyst), but have not been studied.

A predominance of p-isoamylase in serum has been demonstrated after retrograde cannulation of pancreatic duct,[37] and in association with biliary tract calculi in the absence of discernible pancreatitis.[4] In these two situations, pancreatic amylase may gain access to the circulation by refluxing into the pancreatic duct and then into the venous and lymphatic pathways draining the pancreas. Disorders of the salivary glands are associated with an increased s-isoamylase in serum[2,6,47]; tumors show an increase of either salivary or pancreatic isoamylase depending on which amylase is secreted by the tumor; and macroamylasemia shows a predominance of either salivary or pancreatic isoamylase.[58] In one report, isoamylase determination was normal in uremia.[10] Observations from our laboratory suggest that pancreatic isoamylase (which usually is less than 50% of total serum amylase) is increased in mild uremia.[54]

The major use of serum isoamylase determination would be to confirm that an elevation of serum amylase originates from the pancreas. Aside from a rare tumor that elaborates p-isoamylase, and aside from the uremic state which may be associated with an excess of p-isoamylase, a marked excess of p-isoamylase in serum indicates a disease of the pancreas. The choices would be pancreatitis, a complication of pancreatitis, pancreatic carcinoma, reflux of pancreatic juice secondary to retrograde cannulation, or reflux of pancreatic juice associated with biliary tract calculi.

Determination of isoamylases may also be worthwhile if the serum amylase is normal. For example, in chronic pancreatitis, total serum amylase may be normal but p-isoamylase lower than normal which would be indicative of severe acinar injury.[6,56,59,60] Furthermore, if the serum amylase is normal but the amylase–creatinine clearance ratio is increased, determination of serum isoamylase may reveal a pattern that is inconsistent with acute pancreatitis (such as a predominance of salivary isoamylase in diabetic ketoacidosis).[33]

6.1.7 Diagnostic Usefulness of Amylase Measurements in Other Fluids

(a) Pleural and Pericardial Fluid. Acute pancreatitis may be associated with a pleural effusion. The amylase content of the effusion is usually higher than the serum amylase and at times strikingly so. Amylase reaches pleural fluid both by lymphatic pathways and by extravasation through the diaphragm. Serum amylase is usually but not invariably increased when pleural fluid amylase is increased.[61]

An increase of amylase in pleural fluid is not diagnostic of pancreatitis or a complication of pancreatitis. Varieties of primary and metastatic tumors have been associated with an increase in pleural fluid amylase.[13,61] Rupture of the esophagus may increase both serum and pleural fluid amylase.[19,61] The isoamylase that has been recovered from pleural fluid has been s-isoamylase.[13,19] On rare occasions, pneumonia may cause an increase of pleural fluid amylase.[13,61]

Amylase has been recovered from pericardial fluid in a patient with acute pancreatitis.[62]

(b) Peritoneal Fluid. Ascites caused by acute pancreatitis is accompanied by a high amylase content. Serum amylase is usually but not invariably elevated. The syndrome of chronic pancreatic ascites also produces a high amylase content even if serum amylase is normal. The differential diagnosis of an elevated amylase content of ascites includes pancreatitis, chronic pancreatic ascites in association with a leaking pseudocyst or pancreatic ductal rupture, pancreatic carcinoma, intraabdominal malignancy that secretes amylase (such as ovarian tumor), and a perforation of a hollow viscus (such as a perforated duodenal ulcer).

6.1.8 Serum Amylase in Acute Pancreatitis

Serum amylase is frequently but not invariably elevated during the course of acute pancreatitis.[12,15,16] It may be increased within hours of the onset of symptoms and almost always within the first 24 hr. It usually returns to normal by the third to sixth day of illness.[39,63,64] Serum amylase levels do not correlate with the severity of pancreatitis.[63,65] For example, mild edematous pancreatitis may cause extremely high levels of serum amylase in excess of 1,000 units/ml. On the other hand, severe hemorrhagic pancreatitis may be associated with minimal or no elevation of serum amylase. Serum amylase levels do not correlate well with specific etiologies of pancreatitis. Markedly increased levels may occur in edematous pancreatitis of any etiology; slight increases of amylase elevation may reflect either severe overwhelming pancreatitis or extremely mild edematous pancreatitis of any etiology.

Serum amylase levels are not helpful in distinguishing pancreatitis from diseases that masquerade as pancreatitis. A surgical condition such as a perforated duodenal ulcer may be associated with a slight or substantial increase of serum amylase.

In summary, an increase of serum amylase supports but does not confirm a clinical impression of pancreatitis. Determination of amylase–creatinine clearance ratio and serum isoamylases at times provides additional valuable information.

6.2 LIPASE

Serum lipase should be measured more frequently. Older methodologies that required at least 24 hr of incubation have been replaced by newer more rapid techniques.[15,66] Traditional thinking has been that, in pancreatitis, increases of serum lipase occur later than increases in amylase but are then sustained for longer periods of time. This thinking may be in error. Increases of serum lipase tend to parallel those of serum amylase;

indeed, a rise in serum lipase occurs as frequently and perhaps more frequently than increases in serum amylase during acute pancreatitis.[12,15,16,18,20,66] In some instances, serum lipase is increased before amylase,[15,20] and abnormal levels persist for a longer interval than amylase.[16,20]

In pancreatitis associated with hyperlipidemia, serum lipase, as well as serum amylase, was found to be normal in at least one study.[67] It is not as yet known whether serum lipase invariably remains normal under these circumstances. Serum lipase may be increased among a variety of intraabdominal conditions that masquerade as acute pancreatitis, including common bile duct stones,[18,20] acute cholecystitis,[20] intestinal infarction and perforation,[20] and severe peptic ulcer disease.[20,45]

Serum lipase remains normal in a variety of disorders associated with an increase of serum amylase, including disorders of salivary glands, tumors that secrete amylase (such as carcinoma of the lung),[24] and macroamylasemia. Serum lipase levels in uremia have not been scrutinized.

Lipase has been recovered in peritoneal fluid in pancreatitis.[68,69] Since measurement of ascitic fluid amylase yields very valuable information, it is doubtful that measurement of ascitic fluid lipase would add additional important information unless the ascites were caused by an intraabdominal malignancy that secreted amylase. Under this circumstance, ascitic fluid amylase would be elevated but lipase would not.

In summary, in acute pancreatitis, serum lipase and amylase are usually elevated, the amylase–creatinine clearance ratio is increased, and isoamylase determination reveals a predominance of p-isoamylase. In nonpancreatic diseases with surgical implications, serum lipase and amylase may be elevated, the amylase–creatinine clearance ratio is normal, and ordinarily there is not a predominance of p-isoamylase unless there is regurgitation of pancreatic juice in biliary tract disease. Among miscellaneous conditions associated with elevated serum amylase, serum lipase remains normal in most, amylase–creatinine clearance ratio remains normal in all, and serum isoamylase determinations do not show a predominance of p-isoamylase except possibly for uremia and the rare tumors that secrete p-isoamylase.

6.3 OTHER LABORATORY TESTS

6.3.1 Miscellaneous

In acute pancreatitis, the white blood count is usually in the range of 9,000 to 18,000 but may be higher or lower.[70] Serum hemoglobin and hematocrit at first remain relatively normal, but may increase if pancreatic exudation into the retroperitoneal and peritoneal spaces causes a "chemical burn" and a substantial "third space loss." A hematocrit in excess of 50 is not unusual. If pancreatitis is associated with significant hemorrhage, hemoglobin and hematocrit decrease.

In 15%–25% of cases, there is a transient elevation in serum blood sugar caused at least in part by an increased secretion of glucagon by the pancreas.[71] Serum alkaline phosphatase, bilirubin, and SGOT are occasionally elevated either because of obstruction of the distal common bile duct by the edematous head of the pancreas,[72] or because of associated liver disease such as alcoholic hepatitis. If there is a significant disturbance of lipid metabolism, the serum is lactescent, and serum triglyceride level is increased.

6.3.2 Calcium

Serum calcium levels may decrease during acute pancreatitis. Hypocalcemia has been documented as early as the first day of hospitalization,[73] and frequently on the second to fifth day of illness.[63,70] In one report, the lowest level of serum calcium was recorded on the sixth day of illness,[74] but this is probably quite variable. Hypocalcemia may persist for several days and perhaps as long as 7 to 10 days.

The incidence of hypocalcemia during acute pancreatitis may be more common than is generally appreciated. In two recent studies, all 20 patients with moderate to severe acute pancreatitis were found to have ionized calcium and total calcium either lower than normal,[70,73] or in the low normal range.[73] In a third study, all 18 patients with hemorrhagic pancreatitis and one half of patients with severe edematous pancreatitis were demonstrated to have a decreased total serum calcium.[75] In general, the levels of serum calcium were lower in hemorrhagic than edematous pancreatitis.[75]

Some reduction in total serum calcium may occur on the basis of hypoalbuminemia. A decrease in ionized calcium requires a different explanation. During acute pancreatitis, there is deposition and sequestration of ionized calcium in areas of fat necrosis with formation of calcium complexes. Available evidence in man[74,76] and in the experimental animal[77] indicates that the amount of calcium deposited in areas of fat necrosis is substantial. If hypocalcemia were to take place on this basis alone, secretion of parathormone from the parathyroid gland should restore serum calcium completely to normal. The hypocalcemia of acute pancreatitis has been explained both on the basis of inadequate parathormine release,[70] and on the basis of refractoriness of the bone to adequate amounts of circulating parathormone.[73] It is not known at present which of these two effects is the more important, nor is the mediator of these effects understood. Serum magnesium levels were essentially normal in both reports.

A second explanation for hypocalcemia in pancreatitis relates specifically to a decrease in serum magnesium levels. There are multiple reasons for hypomagnesemia in acute pancreatitis.[79] Magnesium is deposited in areas of fat necrosis both in man[63] and in the experimental animal.[80] The use of alcohol may be associated with hypomagnesemia because of increased urinary loss of magnesium, poor dietary intake of magnesium, and diarrhea.[79,81,82] If serum magnesium levels are lower than normal, serum calcium cannot be restored to normal until magnesium is replaced.[78] The mechanism by which a decrease in serum magnesium prevents restoration of calcium level has not been fully elucidated. Two important physiologic effects would be that magnesium depletion either inhibits the synthesis of parathormone or renders bone refractory to its action.[83] One study has suggested the first mechanism[84]; another has suggested the second[78]; and a third suggests that both physiologic changes are important.[85]

A third explanation for hypocalcemia in pancreatitis is complex and probably not applicable. Serum glucagon levels are increased in acute pancreatitis.[70,71,73] Glucagon (and gastrin) stimulates calcitonin release. Calcitonin may contribute to hypocalcemia by inhibiting resorption of bone and thereby preventing the normalization of serum calcium. However, the amount of serum glucagon secreted in pancreatitis is probably not enough to influence serum calcitonin. Furthermore, serum gastrin levels are normal in acute pancreatitis.[71,73] Finally, a relationship has not been established between calcitonin levels and serum calcium levels in acute pancreatitis whether the serum calcitonin was normal,[73] slightly elevated,[70] or moderately elevated.[86]

6.3.3 Magnesium

There are at least three good reasons to measure serum magnesium as well as serum calcium several times during the course of acute pancreatitis: symptoms of hypomagnesemia may be suggestive of hypocalcemia such that the clinician expects clinical improvement with calcium replacement alone; serum magnesium may be reduced (as in cirrhosis) without an associated decrease in ionized calcium[87]; finally, if there is associated hypocalcemia, it cannot be corrected without first correcting hypomagnesemia. It may be of importance that serum magnesium may remain normal at a time that magnesium stores are depleted, as evidenced by a decreased magnesium content of skeletal muscle.[81,82,87] It is not known, however, whether a decrease in tissue magnesium influences ion-ized serum calcium when the serum magnesium is normal.

6.4 RADIOLOGIC DIAGNOSIS

6.4.1 Survey Film of the Abdomen

Many important radiologic features of pancreatitis are visible on plain roentgenogram of the abdomen. These features are caused for the most part by spread of pancreatic exudation along mesenteric planes.

The mesocolon of the transverse colon extends across the anterior surface of the pancreas throughout its length. Pancreatic exudation may spread to the lower border of the transverse colon within the mesocolon. With severe pancreatitis confined to the head of the pancreas, the exuda-tion may flow preferentially to the proximal transverse colon causing intense spasm with secondary dilatation of the ascending colon. This is one of the varieties of the "colon cut-off sign." A more uniform flow of exudation to the transverse colon may cause spasm and irregularity throughout the transverse colon (Figure 5). Alternatively, the flow of pancreatic exudation in the vicinity of the splenic flexure may become trapped in the phrenicocolic ligament causing spasm of the descending colon just below the splenic flexure with secondary dilatation of the entire transverse colon.[88,89] At times, the irritating effects of pancreatic exuda-tion on the transverse colon causes severe atony and dilatation rather than spasm.

The flow of pancreatic exudation down the length of the small bowel mesentery may cause an ileus of the duodenum, an ileus of one or more loops of jejunum ("sentinel loops"), or an ileus which may be restricted to the distal ileum and/or cecum[88,90] (Figure 6).

During pancreatitis, a marked phlegmon of the pancreas associated with significant exudation of fluid into the lesser sac displaces the stom-ach anteriorly. Marked anterior displacement of the stomach can be well visualized if an across-the-table view with the patient supine is taken after insertion of a nasogastric tube into the stomach. The course of the naso-gastric tube is well visualized and can be seen to be pushed far anteriorly. Exudation of fluid into the lesser sac also separates the contour of the stomach from the transverse colon on a conventional anterior–posterior view (Figure 5). In one recent report, there was at least a 3-cm separation of these contours in approximately 50% of patients.[91] In another report, while this finding was occasionally documented, the most common radio-

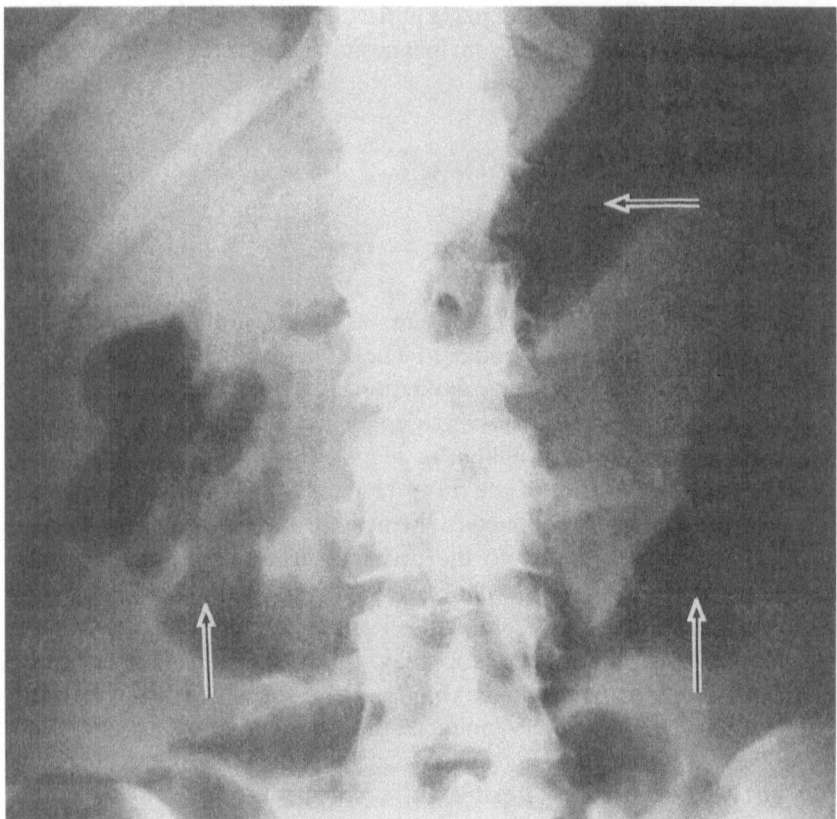

FIGURE 5 Plain Roentgenogram of the Abdomen in Acute Pancreatitis. A considerable amount
of air outlines both the stomach (horizontal arrow) and transverse colon (vertical arrows) in
an "air cast." The reason for this is that luminal structures bordering an inflammatory
process tend to develop an ileus. There is a gentle concavity of the greater curvature of the
stomach caused by the swollen pancreas. The contours of stomach and midtransverse
colon are separated by an inflammatory exudate.The haustral pattern of the transverse colon
is very irregular.

logic abnormality in pancreatitis involved the transverse colon, especially
spasm of the transverse colon and ileus of the transverse colon.[92]

A plain roentgenogram of the abdomen may reveal other important
abnormalities, including calcification of the pancreas (Figure 7), cholelithiasis, and a widening of the duodenal loop caused by marked edema of
the head of the pancreas. At times, the contiguously inflamed and
stretched duodenum becomes atonic and retains a column of air in the
form of an "air-cast" (Figure 8).

6.4.2 Chest Radiograph

A variety of radiologic abnormalities may be seen in acute pancreatitis. Diaphragms may be elevated and relatively fixed as a result of splinting. Platelike atalectasis may occur because of limited respiratory excursion. A pleural effusion may be visible at either base but more likely on the left side. There may be evidence of congestive heart failure or acute respiratory distress syndrome. On very rare occasions there is evidence of a pericardial effusion.

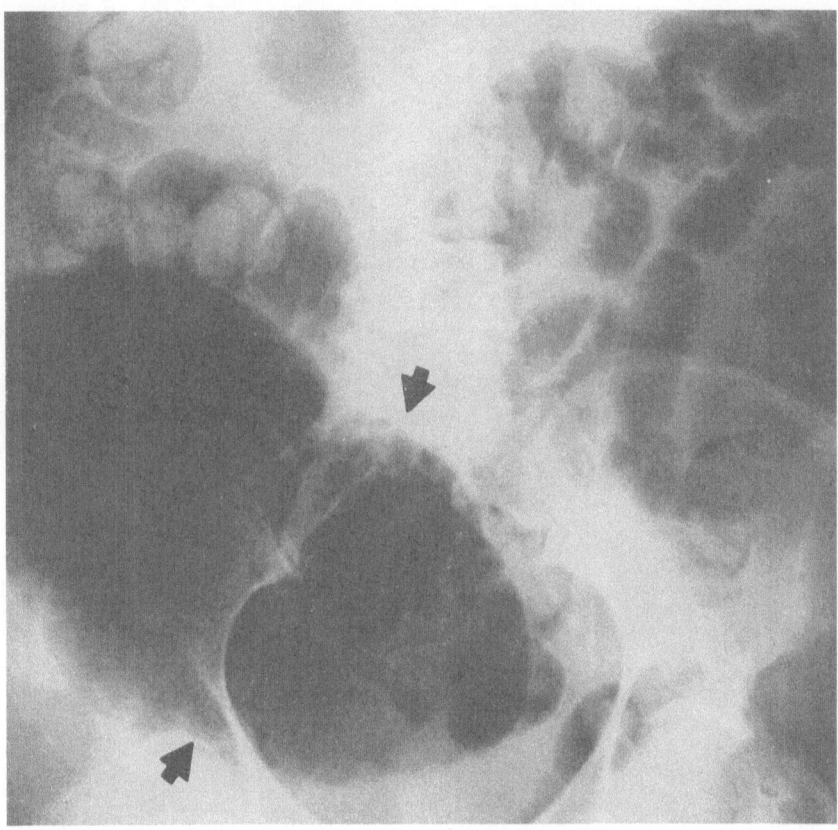

FIGURE 6 *Cecal Ileus in Acute Pancreatitis.* Extension of pancreatic exudation via the mesentery of the small intestine may cause a severe cecal ileus (arrows) that can be confused both clinically and radiologically with a volvulus of the cecum. A laparotomy disclosed severe hemorrhagic pancreatitis and a cecal ileus.

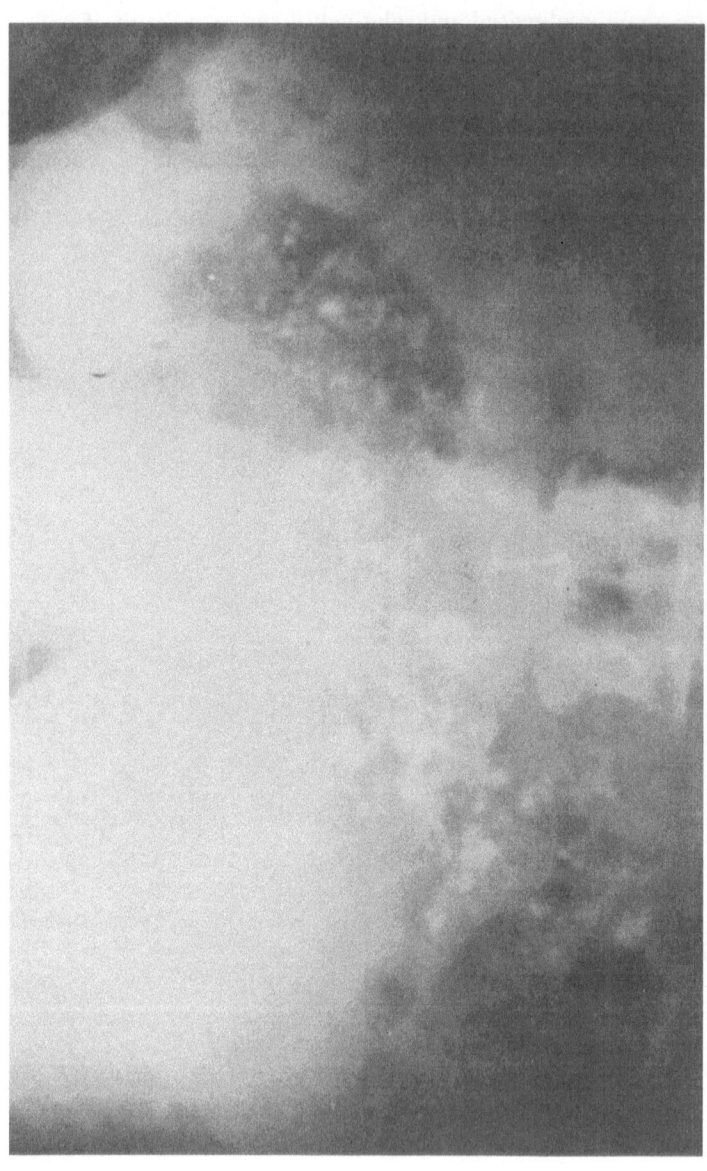

FIGURE 7 Pancreatic Calcification. Plain roentgenogram of the abdomen showing diffuse calcification of the pancreas during the first clinical episode of pancreatitis in a patient with at least 10 years of extensive alcoholic intake. The presence of calcification indicates severe chronic pancreatitis despite the absence of previous symptoms.

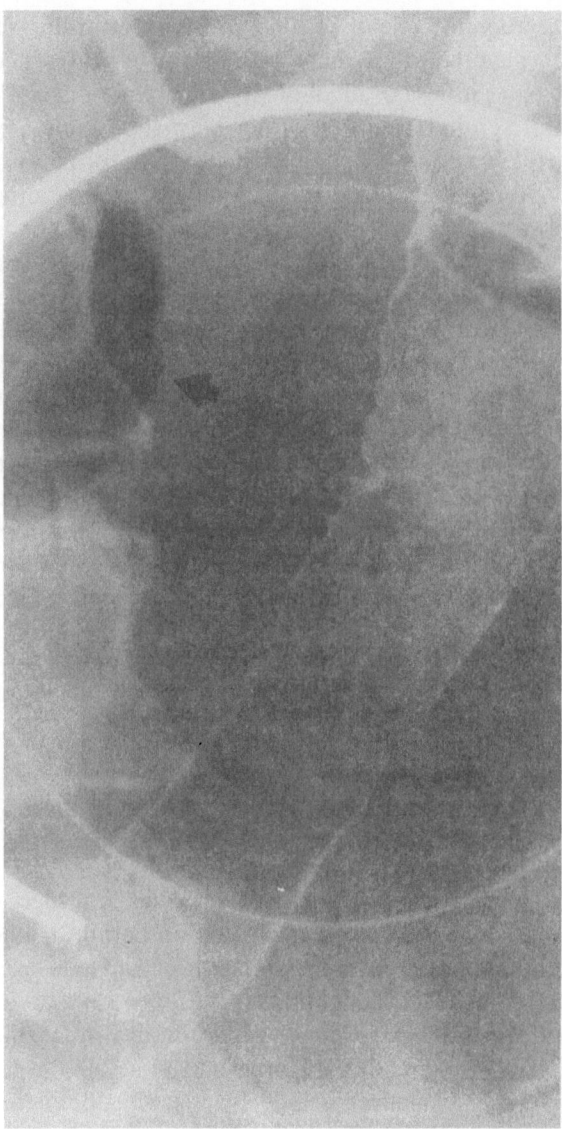

FIGURE 8 *Barium Enema in Acute Pancreatitis.* The haustral pattern of the transverse colon is absent, and tiny serrations are visible on the superior surface of the distal transverse colon. Note the "air-cast" in the upper left caused by a duodenal ileus (arrows). Note also that the nasogastric tube in the top center is curled and is probably ineffective in aspirating gastric juice. The barium enema was done prior to the gastrointestinal series (Figure 9) because of a clinical suspicion of mesenteric ischemia.

6.4.3 Cholecystographic Techniques

Cholecystographic techniques tend to be unrewarding early in the course of acute pancreatitis perhaps because of liver dysfunction associated with an acute illness or alcohol. If biliary tract disease is strongly suspected, and if serum bilirubin is either normal or minimally elevated, an intravenous cholangiogram may provide useful information. If visualization is not optimal, delayed films including a 24 hr radiograph may reveal the presence of calculi on upright compression spot films of the abdomen that were not visible at the time of the intravenous study.[93] Even if visualization appears reasonably adequate, an oral cholecystogram should be obtained during an asymptomatic interval in all patients whose pancreatitis has no clearly defined etiology. When performed several weeks after subsidence of symptoms, an oral cholecystogram not infrequently reveals the presence of tiny calculi in the gallbladder that were invisible on all cholecystographic studies performed during the illness. The optimal timing of oral cholecystography following pancreatitis remains controversial. In one recent report, oral cholecystography was almost uniformly successful in alcoholic pancreatitis when carried out in nonjaundiced patients shortly after resumption of food intake (approximately one week following hospitalization).[94] The resumption of food intake may cause contraction of the gallbladder and evacuation of thick bile thereby permitting contrast material to enter the gallbladder in quantity.

6.4.4 Barium Studies

Barium studies are occasionally helpful especially if there is diagnostic confusion. The major changes visualized on barium studies are displacement of a hollow viscus by an adjacent mass and mucosal abnormalities reflective of adjacent inflammation.

(a) *Upper Gastrointestinal Series.* A barium meal may show both of these effects in acute pancreatitis (Figure 9 and 10). Both the stomach and duodenum may be displaced anteriorly by a markedly edematous pancreas. The best way to demonstrate the draping of the posterior wall of the stomach over an edematous pancreas is an across-the-table view with the patient supine. Widening of the duodenal loop by an edematous head of the pancreas can be visualized radiologically by conventional oblique and anterior–posterior views after barium is permitted to opacify the duodenum. A variety of mucosal changes reflecting adjacent inflammation should be sought. Occasionally, the mucosal folds of the inner aspect of the duodenum are flattened and "pressed out" by an edematous head

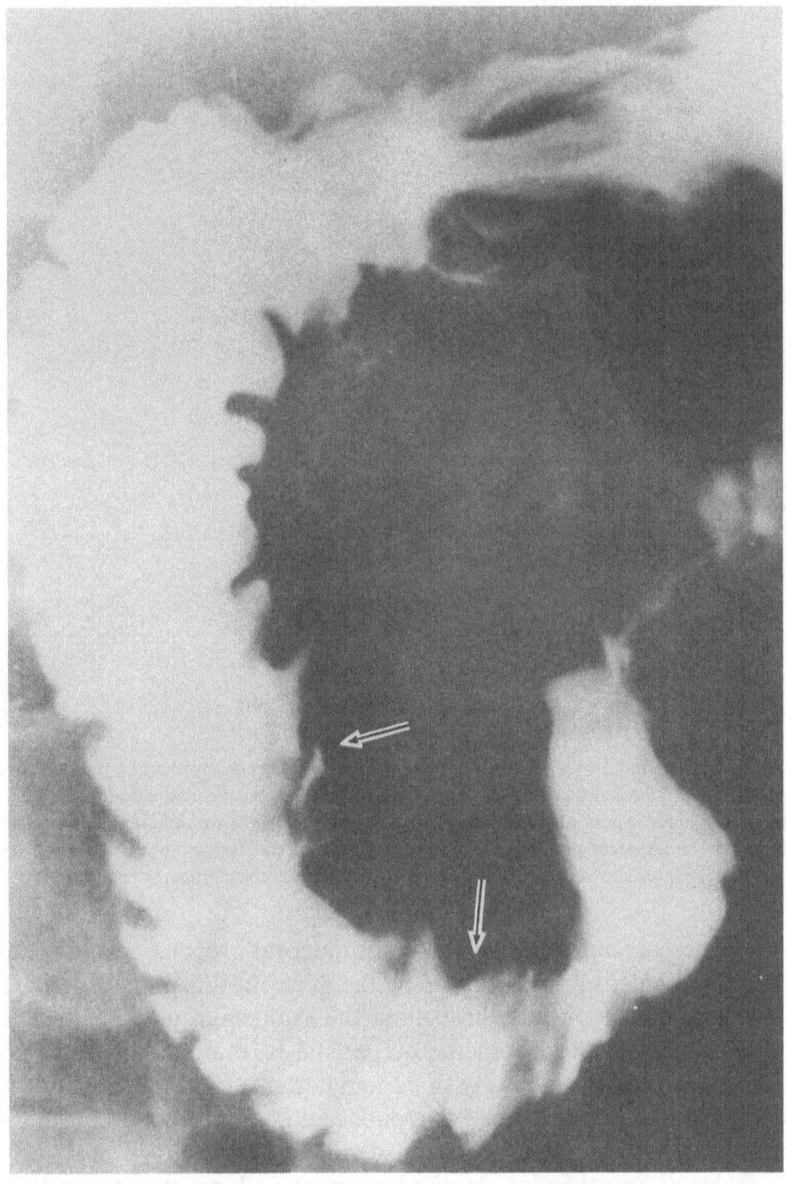

FIGURE 9 *Gastrointestinal Series in Acute Pancreatitis.* There are marked irregularities of the mucosal pattern on the inner aspect of the duodenum (arrows) and considerable spasm of the distal duodenum. The antrum and duodenal bulb are slightly stretched by the inflamed pancreas. Folds of the third portion of the duodenum are thickened and edematous. Note that the air in the duodenum in Figure 8 represented very accurately the configuration of the duodenum as outlined with barium.

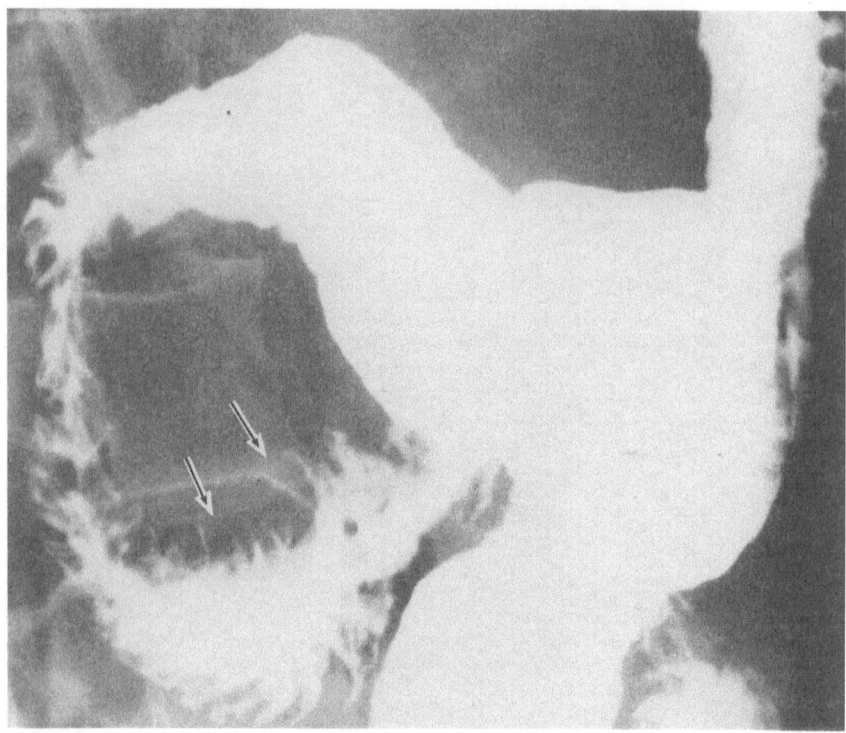

FIGURE 10 *Gastrointestinal Series in Acute Pancreatitis.* There is swelling of the head of the pancreas with encroachment of the undersurface of the antrum and duodenal bulb. The folds on the inner aspect of the duodenum are smoothed in the descending portion and are tethered to the adjacent pancreas in the third portion of the duodenum (arrows). GI series several weeks later showed complete resolution of these abnormalities.

of the pancreas; at other times, there is mucosal irregularity and pleating of duodenal mucosal folds caused by the adjacent inflammatory process. In general, mucosal folds throughout the duodenum may be thickened and edematous. If there is increased peristalsis, there may be poor coating of the duodenal mucosa with barium because of rapid transit of barium into the jejunum. If there is a duodenal ileus, the column of barium may maintain itself indefinitely in the duodenal loop.

(b) Small-Bowel Series. Marked pancreatic edema may cause depression of the ligament of Treitz such that its uppermost position is no longer on a horizontal line with the duodenal bulb. If there is an associated jejunal ileus, the column of barium may move very slowly resulting in marked fragmentation and flocculation of barium. If the differential diagnosis includes a perforation of a duodenal ulcer, a water-soluble material

such as Gastrografin should be utilized in place of barium. Excellent visualization of esophagus, stomach, and duodenum can usually be achieved before the Gastrografin becomes diluted with fluid in the small intestine giving rise to an amorphous hazy whitish opacification yielding no further diagnostic information. If a Gastrografin study does not reveal the correct diagnosis, delayed abdominal films should always be obtained. If the proper diagnosis is a perforation of a hollow viscus, Gastrografin may extravasate into the peritoneal cavity, even if this can not be seen radiologically. Once it is reabsorbed into the circulation from peritoneal surfaces, it is then excreted by the kidneys and opacifies the urinary bladder. Opacification of the urinary bladder on delayed films would be firm evidence for a perforation of a hollow viscus.

(c) *Barium Enema.* Barium enema is occasionally utilized especially if the differential diagnosis includes mesenteric vascular disease of the colon. In acute pancreatitis, there may be displacement of the transverse colon downward by pancreatic exudation or by a pancreatic pseudocyst (Figure 11). The mucosal folds may show spiculization because of the presence of the adjacent inflammatory mass (Figure 8). At times, major changes are visible on the inferior haustral margin of the transverse colon because pancreatic exudation tends to extend preferentially to this location. Under these circumstances, the inferior haustral pattern may be somewhat flattened or irregular.

A view of the transverse colon can also be achieved as a follow-up of an upper gastrointestinal series. Once the stomach and duodenum are properly visualized with barium, a second glass of barium can be utilized to visualize the small intestine in a conventional small bowel series. Late films of the colon can then be obtained once the barium traverses the transverse colon. Displacement of the transverse colon may be well visualized with this technique. If the changes are not diagnostic, air can be introduced per rectum in order to achieve distensibility of the transverse colon. The mixing of air per rectum with the advancing barium column frequently yields a most satisfactory air-contrast view of the colon that permits identification of abnormalities.

6.4.5 Angiography

Pancreatic angiography has limited application in the diagnosis and treatment of acute pancreatitis but at times is helpful in visualizing a complication of pancreatitis. One indication for angiography during acute pancreatitis is severe upper gastrointestinal bleeding. Possible angiographic findings are thrombosis of the splenic vein with esophagogastric varices or bleeding from a false aneurysm in a pseudocyst.

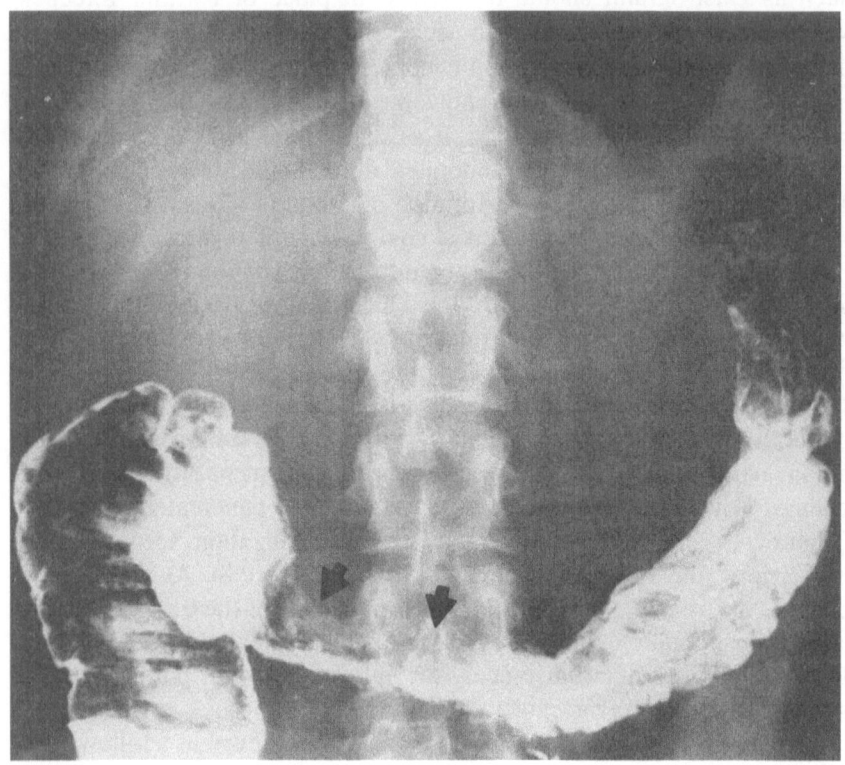

FIGURE 11 *Barium Enema in Acute Pancreatitis.* The transverse colon is displaced downward, and there is evidence of extrinsic compression (arrows). This barium enema was done
a few days after the plain film of Figure 5. Note how much information was secured on the
basis of the plain film.

Other angiographic findings are not visible unless the pancreatitis is
at least several years in duration.[95,96] These findings include a variety of
arterial abnormalities, distorted parenchymal accumulation of contrast
material, narrowing of splenic veins,[95] and aneurysms of the peripancreatic arteries.[96]

6.5 ULTRASONOGRAPHY

Gray-scale ultrasonic examination of the pancreas is an important
diagnostic procedure in severe pancreatitis. Normal measurements of the
pancreas based on large numbers of studies serve as a comparison for

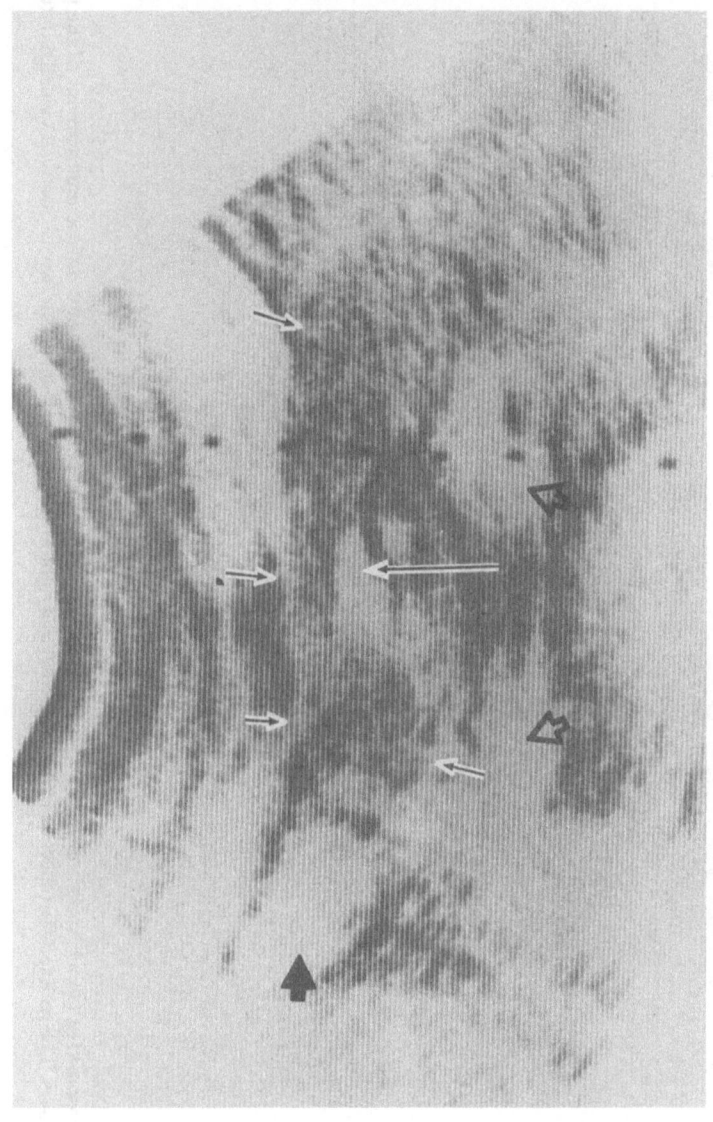

FIGURE 12 *Ultrasound of Upper Abdomen: Normal Pancreas.* Gray-scale transverse scan of upper abdomen shows a normal-sized pancreas outlined with four short vertical arrows. The gallbladder is visible at the left (short thick black arrow), the splenic vein is directly behind the pancreas (long vertical arrow), the superior mesenteric artery is unmarked but is just to the right of the long vertical arrow. The short thick clear arrow on the lower left marks the inferior vena cava; the short thick clear arrow on the lower right marks the aorta. The large clear area at the bottom in the center is the spine. (Courtesy of Dr. C. McArdle.)

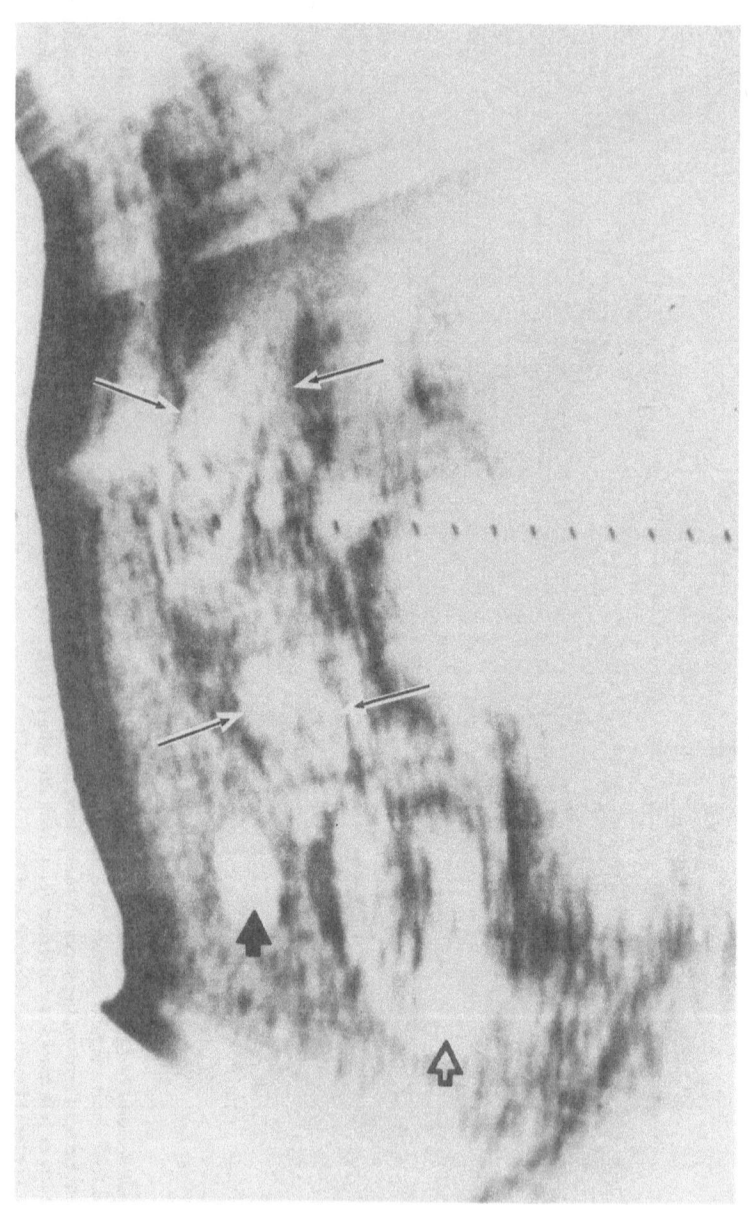

FIGURE 13 *Ultrasound of Upper Abdomen: Acute Pancreatitis.* Gray-scale transverse scan shows diffuse enlargement of the pancreas bordered by four long arrows. The gallbladder (short thick black arrow) and right kidney (short thick clear arrow) are well visualized. (Courtesy of Dr. P. McLellan.)

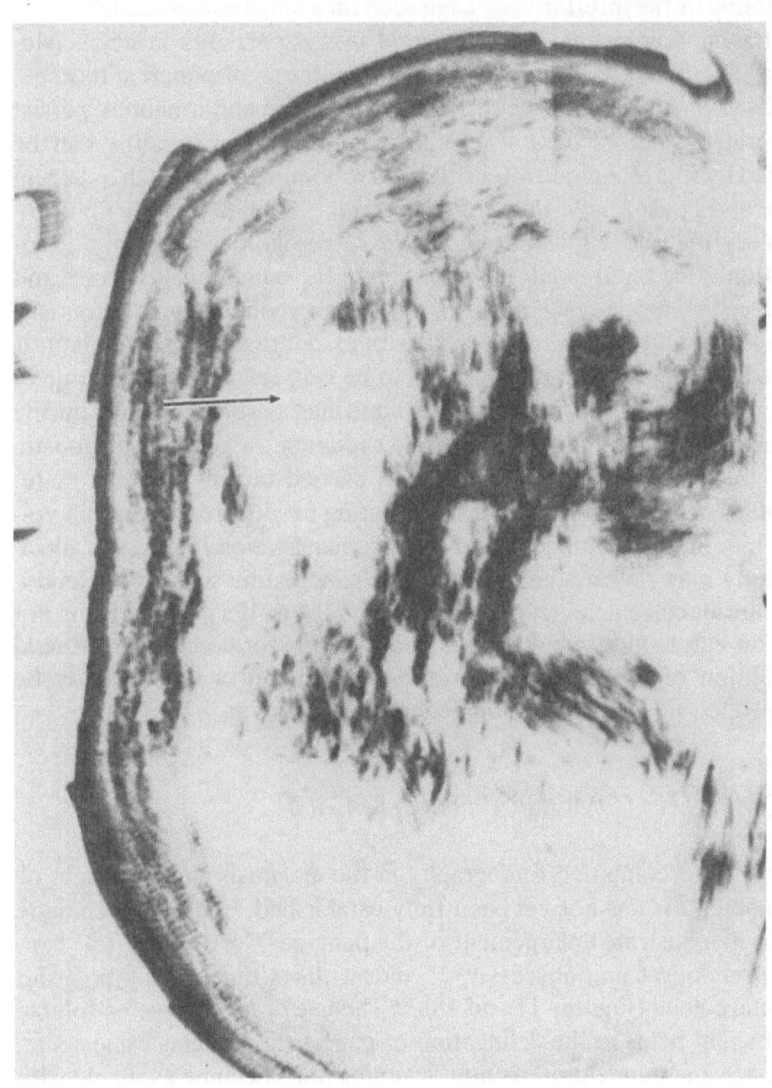

FIGURE 14 Ultrasound of Upper Abdomen: Pancreatic Pseudocyst. Gray-scale transverse scan reveals a large echo-free area that is diagnostic of a pancreatic pseudocyst (arrow). The liver at the left is essentially echo-free because the gain has been reduced considerably for technical reasons. (Courtesy of Dr. C. McArdle.)

abnormalities[97] (Figure 12). Severe pancreatic edema may be visible on the basis of an increased anterior–posterior diameter of the gland, loss of normal internal echos, and loss of the normal distinction between the pancreas and splenic vein[98] (Figure 13). On rare occasions, there may be compression of the inferior vena cava seen on a longitudinal scan.[99]

Ultrasonography may serve several useful purposes in acute pancreatitis. The first is to confirm a clinical impression of pancreatitis especially if the diagnosis is in doubt. Since ultrasonic abnormalities persist for several days to several weeks, a diagnosis of pancreatitis can be supported by this technique after other corroborating tests, such as serum amylase and lipase, have returned to normal.[98] Second, follow-up ultrasonic study may be a sensitive indicator of resolution of pancreatic inflammation. Third, ultrasonic examination of the common bile duct[100] and gallbladder[101,102] may reveal dilatation of the common bile duct secondary to obstruction and the presence of gallstones. Ultrasonic examination of the gallbladder in particular has proven to be very reliable and accurate in documenting cholelithiasis. This technique has particular value during pregnancy since there is no exposure to radiation. In general, diagnostic accuracy can be improved if the test is carried out in a fasting state. Gallbladder contraction associated with eating may decrease residual volume of bile in the gallbladder and impair visualization.[102] Finally, ultrasonic study may reveal a complication of pancreatitis such as a pseudocyst or intraductal calculi (Figures 14 and 15). Even if a pseudocyst is not visible, an early study would serve as a baseline for comparison should the condition of the patient deteriorate and should a repeat study be performed to rule out the development of a pseudocyst.

6.6 COMPUTED TOMOGRAPHY (C-T SCAN)

The role of computed tomography in the diagnosis and treatment of acute pancreatitis has not yet been fully established.[103,104] This technique is able to demonstrate enlargement of the pancreas[105,106] (Figure 16), pancreatic pseudocyst and abscess,[103–105] and at times ductal dilatation and intraductal calculi (Figures 17 and 18).[106] The use of an oral water-soluble contrast agent helps in the delineation of pancreatic margins by visualizing stomach and duodenum. As new scanning units become available with scan time less than 18 sec per section, visibility should improve.

C-T scan may detect a pancreatic pseudocyst that is not visible by diagnostic ultrasound,[106] but as a general screening test, diagnostic ultrasound is almost as accurate. The radiation exposure of C-T scan renders ultrasound more valuable during pregnancy.

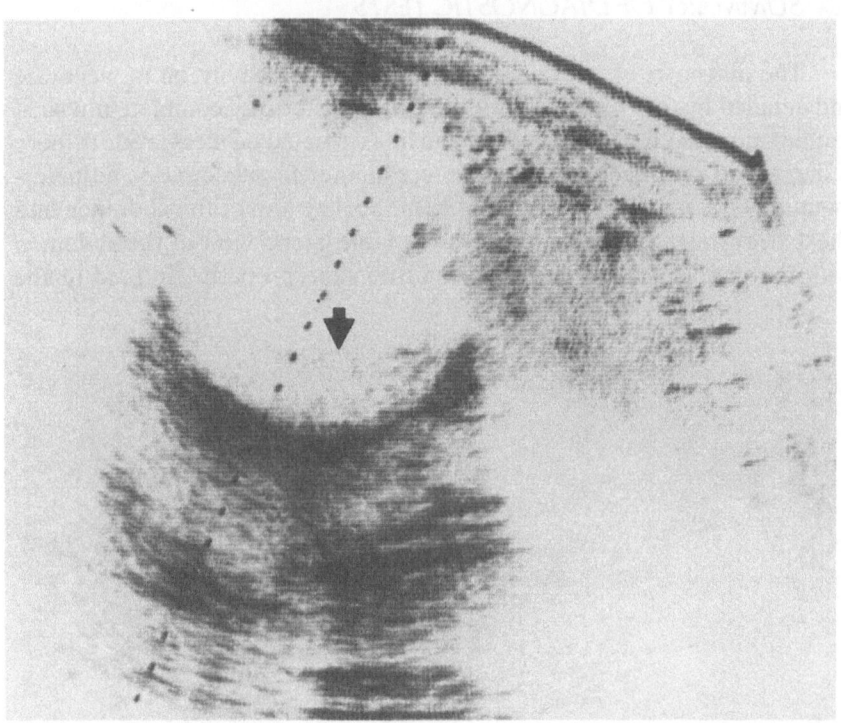

FIGURE 15 *Ultrasound of Upper Abdomen: Pancreatic Pseudocyst.* Gray-scale parasagittal longitudinal scan with the patient supine shows a large echo-free area indicative of a pseudo-cyst. The patient's head is to the left and feet to the right; the anterior abdomen is at the top and the spine at the bottom. Since the patient is supine, debris within the pseudocyst settles to the most dependent portion of the cyst (arrow). (Courtesy of Dr. C. McArdle.)

Computed tomography of the pancreas is recommended if unexplained abdominal pain suggests either pancreatitis or pancreatic carcinoma. This technique is also recommended in prolonged pancreatitis or severe recurrent pancreatitis if diagnostic ultrasound has failed to reveal a complication such as a pseudocyst or intraductal calculi causing ductal obstruction. The detection of carcinoma of the pancreas coexisting with chronic pancreatitis is very difficult.[103] On occasion, a carcinoma of the pancreas causing pancreatitis can be properly identified on C-T scan by the visualization of a large mass at the head of the pancreas and either ductal dilatation or a pseudocyst proximal to the mass.[105]

6.7 SUMMARY OF DIAGNOSTIC TESTS

The diagnosis of acute pancreatitis depends heavily on an accurate and detailed history coupled with the performance of a complete physical examination. Both serum amylase and lipase should be measured. If there is diagnostic confusion, an amylase–creatinine clearance ratio and determination of isoamylases may be of help. Survey film of the abdomen and chest x-ray are indicated. An across-the-table lateral view of the abdomen with the patient supine and a nasogastric tube properly situated in the

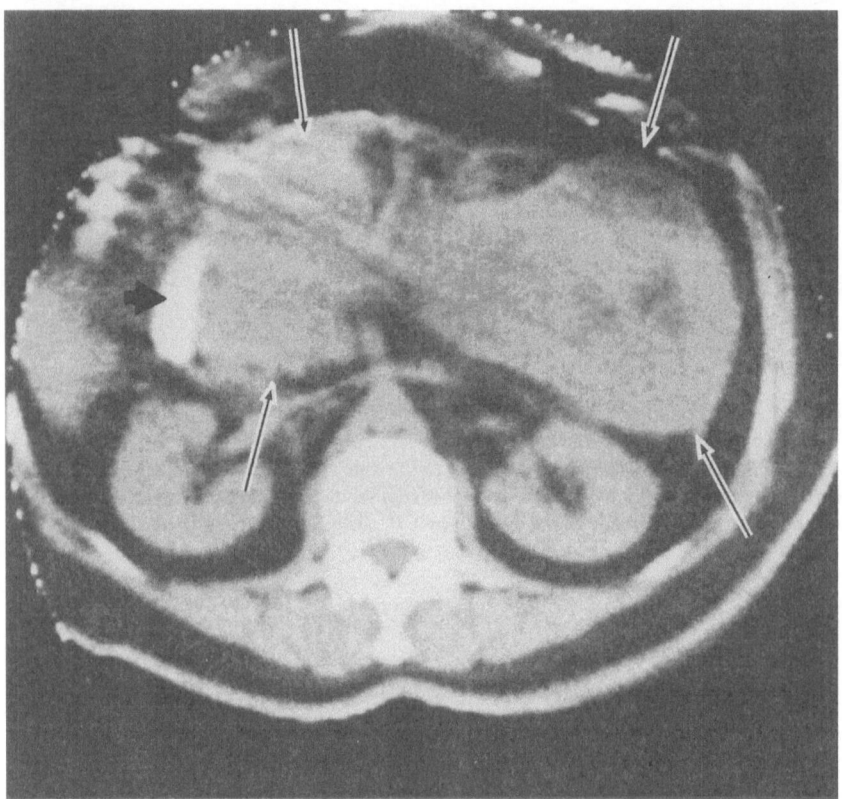

FIGURE 16 C-T Scan: Acute Pancreatitis. Transaxial section through upper abdomen with EMIC-T 5005 computed tomographic body scanner shows marked enlargement of the pancreas in acute pancreatitis (four vertical arrows). Gastrografin is visible in the descending duodenum (horizontal black arrow) and helps delineate the head of the pancreas. Note the marked encroachment of the pancreas anteriorly on the posterior wall of the stomach (top of figure). The two kidneys are alongside the vertebral body (bottom of figure). Scan time—eighteen seconds per section. (Courtesy of Dr. J. Ferrucci, Jr.)

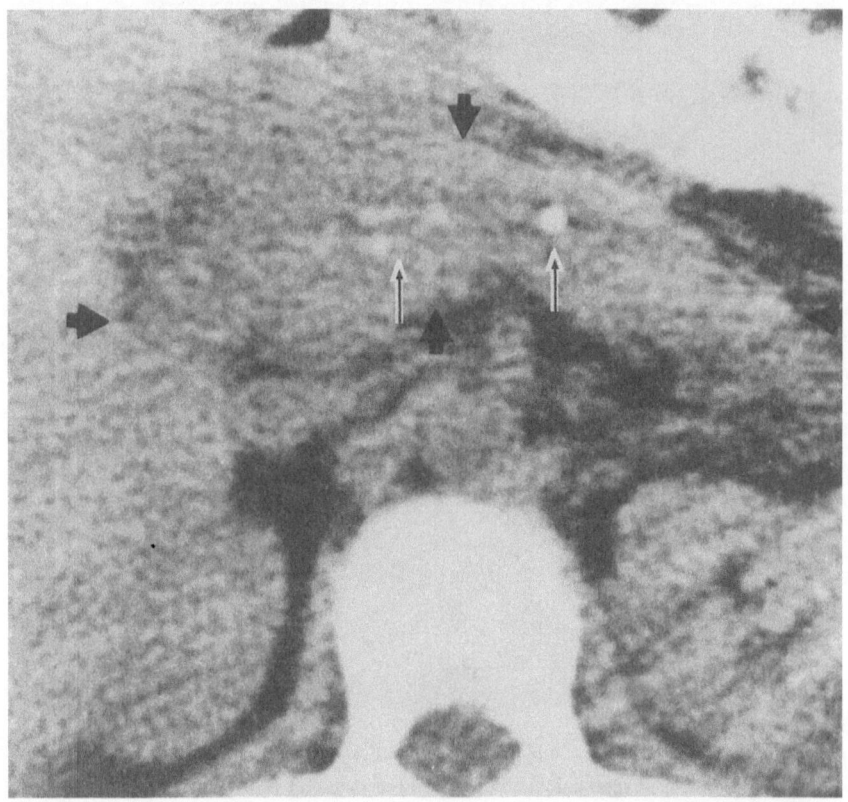

FIGURE 17 C-T Scan: Calcific Pancreatitis. Transaxial section through upper abdomen showing calcific densities in the body of the pancreas indicative of intraductal calculi (thin vertical
arrows). The pancreas is slightly enlarged (thick black arrows). (Courtesy of Dr. J. Ferrucci,
Jr.)

stomach may reveal anterior displacement of the stomach consistent with
a phlegmon of the pancreas. Ultrasonic study of the gallbladder, common
bile duct, and pancreas should be performed if equipment is available. If
an ultrasonic study is not done or is equivocal, there may be a role for
intravenous cholangiography in selected instances. Radiologic examination with Gastrografin is helpful if the differential diagnosis includes a
perforation of stomach or duodenum.

Serum calcium and magnesium should be measured on at least several occasions. Measurement of serum calcium should also be performed
after the patient has recovered completely in order to be sure that preexisting hypercalcemia did not decrease into a normal range during the
episode of pancreatitis.

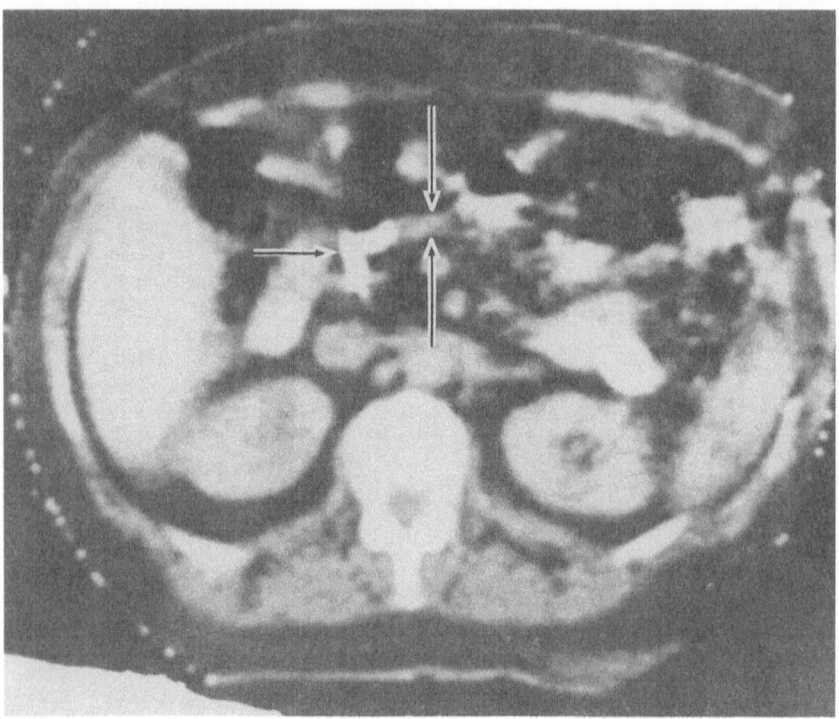

FIGURE 18 C-T Scan: Chronic Pancreatitis. Transaxial section through upper abdomen shows large dense L-shaped calcification at head of pancreas (horizontal arrow). The gland is markedly atrophic. The width of the pancreas is enclosed between the two vertical arrows and may represent a dilated pancreatic duct. Gastrografin is visible in the stomach (under the upper vertical arrow), in the descending duodenum (under the horizontal arrow), and in loops of jejunum (to the right of the lower vertical arrow). (Courtesy of Dr. J. Ferrucci, Jr.)

REFERENCES

1. Skude G: Sources of the serum isoamylases and their normal range of variation with age. *Scand J Gastroenterol* 10:577–584, 1975.
2. Warshaw AL, Lee K-H: Characteristic alterations of serum isoenzymes of amylase in diseases of liver, pancreas, salivary gland, lung, and genitalia. *J Surg Res* 22:362–369, 1977.
3. Shimamura J, Fridhandler L, Berk JE: Does human pancreas contain salivary-type isoamylase? *Gut* 16:1006–1009, 1975.
4. Warshaw AL, Lee L-H: The mechanism of increased renal clearance of amylase in acute pancreatitis. *Gastroenterology* 71:388–391, 1976.
5. Long WB, Grider JR Jr: Amylase isoenzyme clearances in normal subjects and in patients with acute pancreatitis. *Gastroenterology* 71:589–593, 1976.

6. Levitt MD, Ellis C, Engel RR: Isoelectric focusing studies of human serum and tissue isoamlases. *J Lab Clin Med* 90:141–152, 1977.
7. Duane WC, Frerichs R, Levitt MD: Distribution, turnover, and mechnism of renal excretion of amylase in the baboon. *J Clin Invest* 50:156–165, 1971.
8. Schonebeck J, Soderberg M: Serum amylase in renal failure. *Scand J Urol Nephrol* 5:257–262, 1971.
9. Blainey JD, Northam BE: Amylase excretion by the human kidney. *Clin Sci* 32:377–383, 1967.
10. Morton WJ, Tedesco FJ, Harter HR, et al: Serum amylase determinations and amylase to creatinine clearance ratios in patients with chronic renal insufficiency. *Gastroenterology* 71:594–598, 1976.
11. Levitt MD, Rapoport M, Cooperband SR: The renal clearance of amylase in renal insufficiency, acute pancreatitis, and macroamylasemia. *Ann Intern Med* 71:919–925, 1969.
12. Seward CW: Diagnosing pancreatitis the first day: a comparison of urinary amylase and serum enzymes in pancreatic dysfunction. *South Med J* 63:286–289, 1970.
13. Salt WB II, Schenker S: Amylase—its clinical significance. *Medicine* 55:269–289, 1976.
14. Levitt MD, Johnson SG, Ellis CJ, et al: Influence of amylase assay technique on renal clearance of amylase-creatinine ratio. *Gastroenterology* 72:1260–1263, 1977.
15. Lifton LJ, Slickers KA, Pragay DA, et al: Pancreatitis and lipase. *JAMA* 229:47–50, 1974.
16. Song H, Tietz NW, Tan C: Usefulness of serum lipase, esterase, and amylase estimation in the diagnosis of pancreatitis—a comparison. *Clin Chem* 16:264–268, 1970.
17. Albo R, Silen W, Goldman L: A clinical analysis of acute pancreatitis. *Arch Surg* 86:1032–1038, 1963.
18. Warshaw AL, Fuller AF Jr: Specificity of increased renal clearance of amylase in diagnosis of acute pancreatitis. *N Engl J Med* 292:325–328, 1975.
19. Sherr HP, Light RW, Merson MH, et al: Origin of pleural fluid amylase in esophageal rupture. *Ann Intern Med* 76:985–986, 1972.
20. Patt HH, Kramer SP, Woel G, et al: Serum lipase determination in acute pancreatitis. *Arch Surg* 92:718–723, 1966.
21. Warshaw AL, Bellini CA, Lee K-H; Electrophoretic identification of an isoenzyme of amylase which increases in serum in liver diseases. *Gastroenterology* 70:572–576, 1976.
22. MacGregor IL, Zakim D: A cause of hyperamylasemia associated with chronic liver disease. *Gastroenterology* 72:519–523, 1977.
23. Lehrner LM, Ward JC, Karn RC, et al: An elevation of the usefulness of amylase isozyme differentiation in patients with hyperamylasemia. *AJCP* 66:576–587, 1976.
24. Ammann RW, Berk E, Fridhandler L, et al: Hyperamylasemia with carcinoma of the lung. *Ann Int Med* 78:521–525, 1973.
25. Berk JE, Shimamura J, Fridhandler L: Hyperamylasemia associated with cancer. *Gastroenterology* 73:A-6/1029, 1977.
26. Kitamura T, Yoshioka K, Ehara M, et al: A study on the nature of macroamylase complex. *Gastroenterology* 73:46–51, 1977.
27. Levitt MD, Cooperband SR: Hyperamylasemia from the binding of serum amylase by an 11S IgA globulin. *N Engl J Med* 278:474–478, 1968.
28. Barrows D, Berk E, Fridhandler L: Macroamylasemia—survey of prevalance in a mixed population. *N Engl J Med* 286:1352, 1972.
29. Berk JE, Kizu H, Wilding P et al: Macroamylasemia: a newly recognized cause for elevated serum amylase activity. *N Engl J Med* 277:941–946, 1967.
30. Hedger RW, Hardison WGM: Transient macroamylasemia during an exacerbation of acute intermittent porphyria. *Gastroenterology* 60:903–908, 1971.

31. Berggren T and Levitt MD: An unusual form of macroamylasemia. *Gastroenterology* 67:149–154, 1974.

32. Pederson EB, Brock A, Kornerup HJ: Serum amylase activity and renal activity clearance in patient with severely impaired renal function and in patients treated with renal allotransplantation. *Scand J Clin Lab Invest* 36:137–140, 1976.

33. Warshaw AL, Feller ER, Lee K-H: On the cause of raised serum-amylase in diabetic ketoacidosis. *Lancet* 1:929–931, 1977.

34. Takagi H, Yasue M, Morimoto T, et al: Asymptomatic transient hyperamylasemia after a large intravenous dose of steroid hormone. *Am J Surg* 133:322–325, 1977.

35. Henn RM, Selcon S, Sturdevant RAL, et al: Experience with synthetic secretin in the treatment of duodenal ulcer. *Am J Dig Dis* 21:921–925, 1976.

36. Hanafy HM, Gursel EO, Veenema RJ: Increased serum amylase levels in prostatic disease. *Urology* 1:372–373, 1973.

37. Skude G, Wehlin L, Maruyama T, et al: Hyperamylaseamia after duodenoscopy and retrograde cholangiopancreatography. *Gut* 17:127–132, 1976.

38. Nardi GL: Remediable chronic pancreatitis. *Surg Clin North Am* 54:613–620, 1974.

39. Saxon EI, Hinkley WC, Vogel WC, et al: Comparative value of serum and urinary amylase in the diagnosis of acute pancreatitis. *Arch Intern Med* 99:607–621, 1957.

40. Johnson SG, Ellis CJ, Levitt MD: Mechanism of increased renal clearance of amylase/creatinine in acute pancreatitis. *N Engl J Med* 295:1214–1217, 1976.

41. Dreiling DA, Leichtling JJ, Janowitz HD: The amylase-creatinine clearance ratio. *Am J Gastroenterol* 61:290–296, 1974.

42. Murray WR, MacKay C: The amylase-creatinine clearance ratio in acute pancreatitis. *Br J Surg* 64:189–191, 1977.

43. Duane WC, Frerichs R, Levitt MD: Simultaneous study of the metabolic turnover and renal excretion of salivary amylase-^{125}I and pancreatic amylase-^{131}I in the baboon. *J Clin Invest* 51:1504–1513, 1972.

44. Noda A: Renal handling of amylase: evidence for reabsorption by stop-flow analysis. *Metabolism* 21:351–355, 1972.

45. Warshaw AL, Lesser RB: Amylase clearance in differentiating acute pancreatitis from peptic ulcer with hyperamylasemia. *Ann Surg* 181:314–316, 1975.

46. Lesser RB, Warshaw AL: Differentiation of pancreatitis from common bile duct obstruction with hyperamylasemia. *Gastroenterology* 68:636–641, 1975.

47. Berk JE, Fridhandler L, Montgomery K: Simulation of macroamylasemia by salivary-type ('S type') hyperamylasaemia. *Gut* 14:726–729, 1973.

48. Warshaw AL: The kidney and changes in amylase clearance. *Gastroenterology* 71:702–704, 1976.

49. Lesser PB, Warshaw AL: Diagnosis of pancreatitis masked by hyperlipemia. *Ann Intern Med* 82:795–798, 1975.

50. Warshaw AL, Bellini CA, Lesser PB: Inhibition of serum and urine amylase activity in pancreatitis with hyperlipemia. *Ann Surg* 182:72–75, 1975.

51. Donaldson LA, McIntosh W, Joffe SN: Amylase creatinine clearance ratio after biliary surgery. *Gut* 18:16–18, 1977.

52. Levine RI, Glauser FL, Berk JE: Enhancement of the amylase-creatinine clearance ratio in disorders other than acute pancreatitis. *N Engl J Med* 292:329–332, 1975.

53. Watkins PJ: The effect of ketone bodies on the determination of creatinine. *Clin Chim Acta* 18:191–196, 1967.

54. Sidi S, Warshaw AL, Banks PA: Amylase-creatinine clearance ratios and serum amylase isoenzymes in moderate renal insufficiency. *Gastroenterology* 74:1094, 1978.

55. Skude G: Human amylase isoenzymes. *Scand J Gastroenterol* 12 (supp 44):1–37, 1977.
56. Magid E, Horsing M, Rune SJ: On the qualification of isoamylases in serum and the diagnostic value of serum pancreatic type amylase in chronic pancreatitis. *Scand J Gastroenterol* 12:621–627, 1977.
57. Warshaw AL: Serum amylase isoenzyme profiles as a differential index in disease. *J Lab Clin Med* 90:1–3, 1977.
58. Fridhandler L, Berk JE, Montgomery K: Nature of isoamylases released, by acidification, from macroamylase complexes. *Clin Chem* 20:26–29, 1974.
59. Skude G, Eriksson S: Serum isoamylases in chronic pancreatitis. *Scand J Gastroenterol* 11:525–527, 1976.
60. Skude G, Ihse I: Isoamylases in pancreatic carcinoma and chronic relapsing pancreatitis. *Scand J Gastroenterol* 12:53–57, 1977.
61. Light RW, Ball WC Jr: Glucose and amylase in pleural effusions. *JAMA* 225:257–260, 1973.
62. Mitchell CE: Relapsing pancreatitis with recurrent pericardial and pleural effusions. *Ann Intern Med* 60:1047–1053, 1964.
63. Edmondson HA, Berne CJ, Homann RE Jr, et al: Calcium, potassium, magnesium and amylase disturbances in acute pancreatitis. *Am J Med* 12:34–42, 1952.
64. Finch WT, Sawyers JL, Schenker S: A prospective study to determine the efficacy of antibiotics in acute pancreatitis. *Ann Surg* 183:667–671, 1976.
65. Feller JH, Brown RA, Toussaint GPM, et al: Changing methods in the treatment of severe pancreatitis. *Am J Surg* 127:196–201, 1974.
66. Berk JE: Serum amylase and lipase. *JAMA* 199:134–138, 1967.
67. Greenberger NJ, Hatch FT, Drummey GD, et al: Pancreatitis and hyperlipemia. *Medicine* 45:161–174, 1966.
68. Mullin GT, Caperton EM, Crespin SR, et al: Arthritis and skin lesions resembling erythema nodosum in pancreatic disease. *Ann Intern Med* 68:75–87, 1968.
69. Sileo AV, Chawla SK, LoPresti PA: Pancreatic ascites: diagnostic importance of ascitic lipase. *Am J Dig Dis* 20:1110–1114, 1975.
70. Robertson GM Jr, Moore EW, Switz DM, et al: Inadequate parathyroid response in acute pancreatitis. *N Engl J Med* 294:512–516, 1976.
71. Donowitz M, Hendler R, Spiro HM, et al: Glucagon secretion in acute and chronic pancreatitis. *Ann Intern Med* 83:778–781, 1975.
72. Lukash WM, Bishop RP, Nielsen OF: Transaminase levels in acute pancreatitis and after secretin stimulation. *JAMA* 197:927–929, 1966.
73. Weir GC, Lesser PB, Drop LJ, et al: The hypocalcemia of acute pancreatitis. *Ann Intern Med* 83:185–189, 1975.
74. Edmondson HA, Berne CJ: Calcium changes in acute pancreatic necrosis. *Surg, Gynecol Obstet* 79:240–243, 1944.
75. Geokas MC, Rinderknecht H, Walberg CB, et al: Methemalbumin in the diagnosis of acute hemorrhagic pancreatitis. *Ann Intern Med* 81:483–486, 1974.
76. Edmondson HA, Fields IA: Relation of calcium and lipids to acute pancreatic necrosis. *Arch Intern Med* 69:177–190, 1942.
77. Storck G, Bjorntorp P: Chemical composition of fat necrosis in experimental pancreatitis in the rat. *Scand J Gastroenterol* 6:225–230. 1971.
78. Estep H, Shaw WA, Watlington C, et al: Hypocalcemia due to hypomagnesemia and reversible parathyroid hormone unresponsiveness. *J Clin Endocrinol* 29:842–848, 1969.
79. Hersh T, Siddique DA: Magnesium and the pancreas. *Am J Clin Nutr* 26:362–366, 1973.

80. Hernandez IA, Powers SR, Frawley TF: The role of the parathyroid glands in calcium and magnesium metabolism in acute hemorrhagic pancreatitis. *Surgery* 50:143–150, 1961.

81. Lim P, Jacob E: Magnesium status of alcoholic patients. *Metabolism* 21:1045–1051, 1972.

82. Lim P, Jacob E: Tissue magnesium level in chronic diarrhea. *Lab Clin Med* 80:313–321, 1972.

83. Muldowney FP, McKenna TJ, Kyle LH, et al: Parathormone-like effect of magnesium replenishment in steatorrhea. *N Engl J Med* 282:61–68, 1970.

84. Suh SM, Tashjian AH Jr, Matsuo N, et al: Pathogenesis of hypocalcemia in primary hypomagnesemia: normal end-organ responsiveness to parathyroid hormone, impaired parathyroid gland function. *J Clin Invest* 52:153–160, 1973.

85. Rude RK, Oldham SB, Singer FR: Functional hypoparathyroidism and parathyroid hormone end-organ resistance in human magnesium deficiency. *J Clin Endocrinol* 5:209–224, 1976.

86. Gillquist J, Larsson J, Sjodahl R: Serum calcitonin in acute pancreatitis in man. *Scand J Gastroenterol* 12:21–25, 1977.

87. Lim P, Jacob E: Magnesium deficiency in liver cirrhosis. *Q J Med* 41:291–300, 1972.

88. Meyers MA, Evans JA: Effects of pancreatitis on the small bowel and colon: spread along mesenteric planes. *Am J Roentgenol Radium Ther Nucl Med* 119:151–165, 1973.

89. Meyers MA: Roentgen significance of the phrenicocolic ligament. *Radiology* 95:539–545, 1970.

90. Meyers MA: The spread and localization of acute intraperitoneal effusions. *Radiology* 95:547–554, 1970.

91. Moreno G, Rivera HH: Evaluation of the gastrocolic space in 100 cases of acute pancreatitis. *Radiology* 118:535–538, 1976.

92. Miller IM, Irving MH: The value of the plain abdominal roentgenogram in the diagnosis of acute pancreatitis. *Am J Surg* 123:671–673, 1972.

93. Ounjian ZJ, Laing FC: Stratification in the gallbladder on intravenous cholangiography. *Radiology* 121:591–593, 1976.

94. Roller RJ, Mallory A, Caruthers SB Jr, et al: Oral cholecystography after alcoholic pancreatitis. *Gastroenterology* 73:218–220, 1977.

95. Reuter SR, Redman HC, Joseph RR: Angiographic findings in pancreatitis. *Am J Roentgenol* 107:56–64, 1969.

96. White AF, Baum S, Buranasiri S: Aneurysms secondary to pancreatitis. *Am J Roentgenol* 127:393–396, 1976.

97. Weill F, Schraub A, Eisenscher A, et al: Ultrasonography of the normal pancreas. *Radiology* 123:417–423, 1977.

98. Doust BD, Pearce JD: Gray-scale ultrasonic properties of the normal and inflamed pancreas. *Radiology* 120:653–657, 1976.

99. Walls WJ, Templeton AW: The ultrasonic demonstration of inferior vena caval compression: a guide to pancreatic head enlargement with emphasis on neoplasm. *Radiology* 123:165–167, 1977.

100. Goldberg BB: Ultrasonic cholangiography. *Radiology* 118:401–404, 1976.

101. Bartrum RJ Jr, Crow HC, Foote SR: Ultrasonic and radiographic cholecystography. *N Engl J Med* 296:538–541, 1977.

102. Lawson TL: Gray scale cholecystosonography. *Radiology* 122:247–251, 1977.

103. Wittenberg J, Ferrucci JT, Jr: Computed body tomography. *Gastroenterology* 74:287–293, 1978.

104. Abrams HL, McNeil BJ: Medical implications of computed tomography ("Cat scanning"). *N Engl J Med* 298:310–318, 1978.
105. Stanley RJ, Sagel SS, Levitt RG: Computed tomographic evaluation of the pancreas. *Radiology* 124:715–722, 1977.
106. Haaga JR, Alfidi RJ, Havrilla TR, et al: Definitive role of C-T scanning of the pancreas: the second year's experience. *Radiology* 124:723–730, 1977.

7

Differential Diagnosis of Acute Pancreatitis

7.1 ACUTE PANCREATITIS VS. OTHER INTRAABDOMINAL DISORDERS

7.1.1 Perforation of Duodenal Ulcer

Abdominal pain caused by a perforated gastric or duodenal ulcer usually increases to maximum intensity extremely quickly; in pancreatitis, the rate of increase is usually not as rapid. After perforation of an ulcer, abdominal tenderness and guarding is usually prompt and generalized, and the patient remains immobile in bed since motion tends to increase the severity of discomfort; in pancreatitis, abdominal guarding and tenderness are usually restricted to the upper abdomen, and the patient may adjust his position at least a little seeking a more comfortable position.

A film of the abdomen and a chest x-ray should be obtained with the patient standing in order to visualize the accumulation of air under the diaphragm. Alternatively, a left lateral decubitus film of the abdomen can be obtained after the patient has lain in this position for at least 10 min. This interval of time permits air to collect along the right gutter of the abdomen.

A duodenal ulcer that penetrates posteriorly into the pancreas may create a focal form of pancreatitis that produces severe abdominal and back pain. Under these circumstances, epigastric tenderness may be minimal or moderate rather than severe. A gastrointestinal series (using Gastrografin if a perforation is strongly suspected) will disclose the presence of severe ulcer disease and should be utilized early if the differential diagnosis is unclear.

7.1.2 Biliary Tract Disease

In acute cholecystitis, pain is usually maximal in the right upper quadrant or epigastrium, and frequently radiates to the right infrascapular area. A tender gallbladder may be palpable. There may be tenderness and guarding in the right upper quadrant but usually not generalized in the upper abdomen. Chills and fever may indicate ascending cholangitis.

In biliary colic, pain is usually present in the right upper quadrant or epigastrium and on rare occasions is substernal or confined to the back. The pain is characteristically steady and may be quite severe. Right upper quadrant tenderness is usually less pronounced than in the case of acute cholecystitis. Chills and fever may indicate ascending cholangitis. If there is obstruction of the common bile duct, the patient may be jaundiced.

7.1.3 Mesenteric Vascular Disease

In mesenteric vascular occlusion, pain may increase very promptly and mimic a perforated ulcer. Abdominal pain and tenderness tend to be diffuse but guarding is minimal for a prolonged interval of time. Mesenteric vascular disease should be strongly suspected in an older patient who looks acutely ill and has severe abdominal pain, especially if abdominal findings are equivocal.

7.1.4 Miscellaneous Conditions

A dissecting or expanding abdominal aneurysm may cause severe abdominal and back pain and simulate acute pancreatitis. A pulsating mass may be present in the region of the umbilicus. If this diagnosis is suspected, additional x-rays should be obtained including a lateral view of the abdomen utilizing lumbosacral technique. Abdominal ultrasound is extremely helpful in confirming a diagnosis of abdominal aneurysm.

It is extremely important to rule out pelvic disease, particularly ectopic pregnancy or ruptured ovarian cyst. A careful gynecologic and obstetric history must be obtained. Rectal and pelvic examinations must always be performed on a female patient with abdominal pain.

Occasionally left renal colic may cause pain that simulates acute pancreatitis. Usually this type of pain is more lateral, localizes in the flank rather than in the abdomen, and tends to radiate in the left lower quadrant and inner thigh. Hematuria can usually be documented. An intravenous pyelogram is helpful in ruling out this possibility.

Acute myocardial infarction occasionally causes severe pain in the lower xiphoid and high epigastric regions. An electrocardiogram should therefore be obtained on all patients with upper abdominal symptoms.

Other important intraabdominal conditions such as appendicitis, diverticulitis, and small-bowel obstruction should be considered and usually can be distinguished from pancreatitis. It should be borne in mind that on occasion a patient with pancreatitis has pain that is confined to the lower abdomen.

A variety of unusual illnesses may create a confusing picture of severe abdominal pain. These illnesses include lead poisoning, acute intermittent porphyria, familial Mediterranean fever, abdominal migraine, Henoch's purpura, and sickle cell crisis.

7.2 EDEMATOUS VS. HEMORRHAGIC PANCREATITIS

One might anticipate that a patient who appears seriously ill probably has hemorrhagic rather than edematous pancreatitis. However, hypovolemic shock may occur as a result of either edematous or hemorrhagic pancreatitis if intravenous fluid replacement does not adequately compensate for a substantial third space loss.

The precise level of serum amylase is not an indicator of the severity of the illness. Very high levels often occur in relatively mild edematous pancreatitis, and slight elevations may occur in both hemorrhagic pancreatitis and mild edematous pancreatitis.

There are only a few tests to help in this differentiation. A low serum calcium is indicative of a severe episode of acute pancreatitis associated with necrosis. In one study, the serum calcium level in hemorrhagic pancreatitis was uniformly depressed (the majority were less than 8 mg%, with some much lower), whereas in severe acute edematous pancreatitis most of the calcium levels were higher than 8 mg%, with none below 7.2 mg%.[1]

A decrease in serum hemoglobin or hematocrit not associated with an obvious source such as gastrointestinal bleeding or hemolysis is evidence for hemorrhagic pancreatitis. In edematous pancreatitis, the serum hematocrit usually increases because of a loss of fluid associated with a chemical burn.

Hemorrhagic pancreatitis can be confirmed by diagnostic paracentesis. If there is substantial hemorrhage, ascitic fluid resembles beef-broth or prune juice in appearance. The ascitic fluid is an exudate with a protein level usually in excess of 3 gm%. If diagnostic paracentesis reveals a more cloudy brown fluid and especially if it contains bacteria, food particles, or bile, a perforation of a hollow viscus is the correct diagnosis even if the ascitic fluid amylase is elevated.

In hemorrhagic pancreatitis, pancreatic proteolytic enzymes convert hemoglobin to hematin which then binds with albumin to form methemalbumin. Since normal levels have been recorded among patients with hemorrhagic pancreatitis and increased levels among patients with gastrointestinal bleeding and soft tissue trauma, the diagnostic specificity of this test has frequently has been questioned.[2] More recently, measurement of serum methemalbumin has reliably distinguished edematous pancreatitis from hemorrhagic pancreatitis,[1] and hemorrhagic pancreatitis from other serious intraabdominal diseases.[3] Measurement of levels in ascitic fluid and pleural effusion were also diagnostic in hemorrhagic pancreatitis.[1]

7.3 PANCREATITIS SECONDARY TO BILIARY TRACT DISEASE VS. ALCOHOLIC PANCREATITIS

Pancreatitis associated with biliary tract disease occurs predominantly in women (roughly 3:1) in the age group generally from 30 to 40; alcoholic pancreatitis takes place predominantly in men (3:1) with an average age in the late 30s.[4-6] In pancreatitis associated with biliary tract disease, serum amylase, bilirubin, and alkaline phosphatase tend to be higher than in alcoholic pancreatitis.[4]

Occasionally, a patient with known alcoholic pancreatitis and cholelithiasis develops a flare-up of pancreatitis, and it may be extremely difficult to determine whether the symptoms are caused by alcohol or biliary tract disease. From a clinical standpoint, the development of chills, fever, and jaundice is suggestive of the latter. A variety of diagnostic procedures help in the distinction, including intravenous cholangiogram, "skinny needle" transhepatic cholangiography, or endoscopic retrograde cholangiopancreatography (ERCP). Examination of the stool for the passage of gallstones is extremely important in this clinical setting.[5] The recovery of gallstones strongly supports the formulation that cholecystectomy should be performed. If gallstones cannot be recovered in the stool or visualized in the common bile duct, the cholelithiasis is probably asymptomatic, and cholecystectomy will not prevent further episodes of pancreatitis.

REFERENCES

1. Geokas MC, Rinderknecht H, Walberg CB, et al: Methemalbumin in the diagnosis of acute hemorrhagic pancreatitis. *Ann Intern Med* 81:483–486, 1974.

2. Battersby C, Green MK: The surgical significance of methaemalbuminaemia. *Gut* 12: 995–1000, 1971.
3. Kelly TR, Klein RL, Porquez JM, et al: Methemalbumin in acute pancreatitis. *Ann Surg* 175:15–18, 1972.
4. Paloyan D, Simonowitz D: Diagnostic considerations in acute alcoholic and gallstone pancreatitis. *Am J Surg* 132:329–331, 1976.
5. Acosta JM, Ledesma CL: Gallstone migration as a cause of acute pancreatitis. *N Engl J Med* 290:484–487, 1974.
6. Kelly TR: Gallstone pancreatitis. *Arch Surg* 109:294–297, 1974.

8

Treatment of Acute Pancreatitis

8.1 MEDICAL TREATMENT

8.1.1 General Treatment of Acute Pancreatitis

(a) *Putting the Gland to Rest.* A fundamental principle in the treatment of acute pancreatitis is the prevention of pancreatic secretion. This approach is based on the concept that the secretion of an enzyme-rich juice may intensify the inflammation and increase symptomatology especially if there is significant ductal obstruction.

The easiest way to eliminate pancreatic secretion is to maintain the patient in a fasting state and aspirate gastric acid via an indwelling nasogastric tube. The importance of this strategy can be best appreciated by a review of the mechanisms of stimulation of pancreatic secretion that are outlined in Chapter 1. The proper placement of the nasogastric tube in the stomach is critical to prevent acid from reaching the duodenum and stimulating both secretin and cholecystokinin-pancreozymin (CCK-PZ). The optimal position of the tube is along the greater curvature of the body of the stomach and not in the antrum. The reason for this is that gastric acid tends to puddle in the fundus and body with the patient in the conventional supine position in bed. If the tube is advanced into the antrum (an anterior structure) gastric juice sequestered in the posterior fundus of the stomach would not be aspirated. Should the patient then change position (such as turn to the right or stand up) a considerable amount of acid might then enter the antrum and disappear into the duodenum before it could be aspirated. Similarly, if the nasogastric tube is curled back on itself, quantitative evacuation of gastric acid may not occur. The best way to ensure proper localization of the nasogastric tube is to utilize a radiopaque tube and position the tube with fluoroscopic control or with the help of a plain roentgenogram of the abdomen.

Once the tube has been properly positioned, efforts must be made to prevent occlusion of its apertures by tenacious material or by the agglutination of rugal folds. Two methods can be utilized to ensure patency. The first is the use of a nasogastric sump tube which has an inlet for air that prevents mucosal folds from occluding the apertures. The other is to instill 20 to 30 ml of fluid every 2 hr via the nasogastric tube to displace tenacious material or agglutinated folds. In either situation, the clinician should gently hand-aspirate the nasogastric tube periodically in order to be absolutely sure that total recovery of gastric juice is being achieved.

The care of the nasogastric tube extends also to management of the suction apparatus. The patient can participate considerably in his own care by noting whether the machine is actually on (as evidenced by a flashing red light), whether it is providing proper suction (as evidenced by an increasing volume in the receptacle), and by making sure that the nasogastric tube is aspirated by hand at frequent intervals. Each time the nasogastric tube is disconnected from the machine, a gurgling sound indicating suction should be heard. If the noise of suction is not clearly audible, there is a malfunction which is preventing proper aspiration of gastric juice.

These small details, such as proper localization of the nasogastric tube in the stomach, maneuvers to ensure patency of the nasogastric tube, and assurance that the aspirating machinery is providing proper suction are all very important in preventing acid from stimulating pancreatic secretion. The pH of the gastric aspirate should be checked at regular intervals. If the pH is extremely low (such as 1 or 2) and the volume of gastric juice is considerable, it is likely that at least some acid (and perhaps a large quantity) will escape into the duodenum despite all the above efforts. Under these circumstances, an antacid can be instilled every 1 to 2 hr via the nasogastric tube in order to maintain an intragastric pH greater than 5. One method of administering an antacid is to instill a quantity of liquid antacid (such as 30 to 60 cc), disconnect the suction apparatus for $1/2$ hr, reconnect it for another $1/2$ hr, and then check the pH of the gastric aspirate. Increments of antacid should be added on an hourly basis as above until the pH is maintained without difficulty at a level of 5 or higher. In time, the schedule can be altered such that testing of the pH takes place every 2 hr, and a quantity of antacid is administered on an every 2-hr basis sufficient to keep the gastric aspirate at a pH greater than 5 each 2 hr. This approach is not necessary if gastric acid is being readily removed and the patient is making a rapid recovery. The instillation of antacids via the nasogastric tube has the disadvantage of complicating the bedside management of the patient by the nursing service. Antacids also tend to render nasogastric tubes relatively ineffective because of their tenacious consistency following contact with gastric juice.

A reasonable alternative to the use of antacids when there is marked hypersecretion of acid is the use of Cimetidine, an H-2 receptor antagonist that markedly inhibits gastric acid secretion.[1-3] Basal acid secretion has been found to be inhibited by 95% for at least 5 hr by 300 mg of Cimetidine.[3] Cimetidine can be administered intravenously in a dosage of 300 mg every 6 hr if renal function is normal.[4] Since the drug half-life is prolonged in renal insufficiency, the dosage should be decreased to 300 mg every 8 hr in moderate renal failue and to 300 mg every 12 hr in severe renal failure.[4] Thus far, Cimetidine has been proven to be safe in therapeutic dosages for periods of 6 to 8 weeks.[5]

Other measures to reduce the secretion of acid and also reduce pancreatic flow include anticholinergic agents, acetazolamide,[6,7] antidiuretic hormone,[8] and glucagon.[9,10] Anticholinergic agents are capable of decreasing basal secretion of both acid and pancreatic juice. This group of medications has important side effects including urinary retention, tachycardia, increase in abdominal ileus, and excessive dryness of the mouth. If the nasogastric tube is functioning properly, the usefulness of this type of medication is probably marginal. Since there are no well-controlled clinical trials affirming the efficacy of anticholingergic agents, it is my practice not to use them. Acetazolamide has been utilized on occasion in acute pancreatitis,[11] but there are no controlled clinical trials that substantiate its value. Vasopressin has been used in experimental pancreatitis with some benefit, but has not been utilized in clinical trials in man.[12]

There has been considerable speculation that the administration of glucagon would be of benefit either because of a diminution of pancreatic secretion or improvement in mesenteric blood flow. Unless glucagon is shown to improve morbidity or survival in properly controlled clinical trials, it should not be administered in acute pancreatitis. Thus far, in randomized trials in experimental pancreatitis[13] and pancreatitis in man,[14] glucagon therapy did not diminish mortality.

In summary, a properly functioning nasogastric tube is the best method of allowing the pancreas to rest. A second benefit of this approach is that it prevents swallowed air from reaching the small intestine and intensifying an ileus. If clinical improvement is slow and there is marked hypersecretion of acid, either Cimetidine should be administered intravenously or antacid therapy started in order to diminish acid delivery into the duodenum. The suggestion has recently been made that mild to moderate alcoholic pancreatitis is not favorably influenced by the use of nasogastric suction.[15] A reasonable approach is to utilize the nasogastric tube and be prepared to remove it if there is rapid clinical improvement.

(b) Fluid and Electrolyte Replacement. Twenty to thirty percent of the normal circulating blood volume may be sequestered in the form of a "third-space" loss as a consequence of extensive pancreatic exudation and a "chemical burn" of the retroperitoneum and peritoneum. Additional sources of fluid loss include vomiting, nasogastric aspiration, as well as sensible and insensible loss. Should significant retroperitoneal bleeding occur, hypovolemia is even more pronounced. If the systemic circulation is not adequately maintained, the microcirculation of the pancreas does not receive an adequate flow of blood. Numerous experimental studies have ascertained that adequate circulation in the pancreas is essential in preventing a fatal outcome (see Chapter 3). The use of intravenous fluids that include colloid (such as albumin) is helpful in maintaining an adequate blood volume and in protecting the microcirculation of the pancreas. An effort should be made to maintain a serum albumin greater than 3 gm% by administration of albumin-containing preparations. Experimentally, a variety of agents including plasma, dextran, and heparin have been utilized in an effort to improve survival, but widespread clinical trials in man have not taken place.[16]

The measurements that are important is assessing adequacy of circulation include pulse, blood pressure, hourly urine output, hematocrit every 6 hr at first, electrolytes, BUN, and creatinine. A central venous pressure line should be inserted if the patient is seriously ill in order to monitor the volume of intravascular space relative to the ability of the heart to tolerate additional intravenous fluids. A metabolic flow sheet is indispensable in assessing the needs of the patient. Measurements that are important (at times hour by hour, at times each nursing shift, and certainly on a daily basis) include weight, urine output and urine specific gravity, nasogastric output and electrolyte content, amount of intravenous fluids and electrolyte content, measurement of vital signs and central venous pressure, and measurement of serum electrolytes, calcium, magnesium, BUN, creatinine, blood sugar, and CBC. If the patient is unable to void, a urinary catheter should be inserted. Intravenous fluids should include copious amounts of saline or half-strength saline, potassium replacement, a colloid such as albumin, whole blood or packed red blood cells if the hematocrit falls, and in general sufficient fluid replacement to maintain a urinary output of at least 50 cc/hr.

If there is clinical or laboratory evidence of hypocalcemia, 10 cc of 10% calcium gluconate can be slowly infused intravenously over a period of 6–8 hr either on a daily basis or more frequently if needed. Calcium deficiency can be suspected either from carpopedal spasm, a positive

Trousseau test, or a positive Shvostek test. A simple bedside test is simply to tap lightly on the bridge of the nose and observe whether the frontalis muscle undergoes spasm. If there is magnesium deficiency, parenteral magnesium sulfate is required. It should be remembered that serum calcium is not likely to return to normal until serum magnesium levels are first restored to normal.

The administration of a multivitamin preparation intravenously would be of importance especially in a patient with malnutrition. Parenteral thiamine should always be administered for several days in a patient with alcoholism.

(c) Pain. Before the administration of medication to relieve abdominal pain, the clinician must be assured that the pain is caused by either pancreatic inflammation or pancreatic exudation into the peritoneal cavity resulting in peritonitis, and not gastric dilatation, small bowel ileus, or urinary retention. Gastric dilatation and an ileus can be helped considerably by a nasogastric tube that functions properly. If an ileus is severe, an attempt can be made to decompress the small intestine by advancing a long tube. Urinary retention is managed by either standing to void or catheterization.

Abdominal pain secondary to pancreatitis may be managed by the use of meperidine (Demerol) in a dosage of 50 to 100 mg intramuscularly every 4 to 6 hr. The physician should remain alert to the amount of medication that is required and the indications for its use rather than permitting the injections on a "prn" basis. The use of morphine is generally not recommended because of its presumed greater tendency to promote spasm of the sphincter of Oddi.

An intensification of pain during the course of acute pancreatitis may herald an important complication such as a pancreatic pseudocyst. The physician must remain alert to various causes of pain and not order medication indiscriminately.

(d) Infection. The value of antibiotics remains controversial. There is general agreement that when pancreatitis is associated with biliary tract disease, bile is likely to be infected with bacteria (usually a gram-negative organism), and antibiotic therapy is recommended. An antibiotic agent that is frequently utilized is Ampicillin in a dosage of 1 gm every 4 hr intravenously. In the presence of gram-negative septicemia, Gentamicin would be the drug of first choice,[17] in a dosage of 1.5 mg/kg IM every 8 hr if renal function is normal.

The value of antibiotic coverage in alcoholic pancreatitis is unproved. Thus far, in controlled studies of patients with relatively mild alcoholic pancreatitis, the use of Ampicillin did not improve the clinical course.[18-20] In addition, a retrospective analysis has shown that the prophylactic use of antibiotics in pancreatitis of diverse etiologies did not reduce the incidence of infectious complications.[21]

Despite this evidence that prophylactic use of an antibiotic is not helpful, faced with a severe case of hemorrhagic pancreatitis, the physician may feel compelled to use an antibiotic in the hope that secondary infection in bloody necrotic material can be minimized. At present, there is no evidence that this approach protects against the development of a pancreatic abscess. Indeed, the physician may be lulled into a false sense of security so that he becomes less perceptive to the early signs of an abscess.

The discovery that pancreatic juice may contain bacteria during pancreatitis is of interest, but the clinical importance of bacteria within pancreatic juice is not clear.[22]

(e) Removal of Activated Pancreatic Enzymes. Trasylol is a polypeptide which inhibits trypsin and kallikrein. Theoretically, a proteinase inhibitor would be valuable in treating acute pancreatitis since activated pancreatic enzymes play an important role in the pathophysiology. Many studies have found this agent ineffective,[16] perhaps because it does not inhibit elastase or phospholipase-A. A more recent controlled study has reawakened interest in this preparation by showing a reduction in mortality in an older age group.[23] Unfortunately, an even more recent randomized double-blind trial has failed to confirm the usefulness of trasylol in reducing mortality.[14] In any case, trasylol is at present not available in the United States.

(f) Treatment of Metabolic Complications. Hyperglycemia may occur early in acute pancreatitis because of release of glucagon from α cells.[24] Increased levels of pancreatic glucagon may recede promptly. For this reason, the diabetes associated with acute pancreatitis may be extremely brittle, and insulin should be administered with extreme caution. Mild hyperglycemia should be noted but not treated with insulin. The appearance of modest amounts of sugar in the urine (1 to 2+) should also be noted but not treated. Insulin should be reserved for diabetic ketoacidosis or for impressive elevations in blood sugar associated with significant glycosuria (3 to 4+).

Evidence of hypocalcemia and hypomagnesemia should be sought on the first day of clinical illness and for several days thereafter.

Patients with alcoholic pancreatitis should be observed closely for early signs of alcohol withdrawal. Parenteral vitamins should be utilized including Thiamine.

(g) Respiratory and Cardiac Care. Acute pancreatitis may be associated with a decrease in respiratory reserve. Measurement of pulmonary function including arterial pH, pO_2, and pCO_2 are helpful in monitoring the respiratory status. Oxygen should be administered as needed by face mask or nasal catheter. Pulmonary infection should be treated promptly with antibiotics. Chest physiotherapy is of great help in encouraging deep breathing and full aeration of lungs. A decreasing pulmonary reserve associated with physical exhaustion may necessitate a tracheostomy with assisted ventilation. Acute respiratory distress syndrome associated with acute pancreatitis and other cardiopulmonary complications of pancreatitis are discussed in the next chapter. Evidence of congestive heart failure requires parenteral digitalization and at times the use of diuretic agents.

(h) Miscellaneous. Varities of medications have been thought to be beneficial in the treatment of acute pancreatitis. There is no evidence that adrenal corticosteroid agents are helpful unless there is coexisting adrenal insufficiency. The use of insulin has been suggested for relief of pain. The mechanism may be inhibition of fat necrosis.[25]

Peritoneal lavage to remove activated enzymes and other toxic materials from the peritoneal cavity has been utilized on numerous occasions,[26-29] but controlled clinical studies to confirm the efficacy of this maneuver are lacking.

Consideration has been given to the possibility that circulating endotoxins play a role in some of the serious complications of acute pancreatitis.[30] Endotoxins would presumably gain access to the circulation following inflammation of the transverse colon by pancreatic exudation. Controlled data are lacking on this point. If circulating endotoxins are important, sterilization of the bowel by the administration of Kanamycin either by mouth or in the form of an enema could be beneficial.

8.1.2 Treatment of Severe Protracted Pancreatitis

The persistence of fever, tachycardia, abdominal tenderness and pain, and elevated serum amylase requires the clinician to reevaluate all important information. This reassessment includes a review of the medical history of the patient, a thorough physical examination, a review of all laboratory tests, careful inspection of both the medication Kardex and the metabolic flow sheet, and reappraisal of therapeutic strategy. The clinician may find to his dismay that the patient is receiving an excessive amount of medication for pain for inappropriate reasons, such as discomfort from an ileus. The metabolic flow sheet may document that fluid replacement has been woefully inadequate and that uncorrected hypovolemia has led to splanchnic vasoconstriction which in turn has decreased perfusion through the microcirculation of the pancreas and increased pancreatic hypoxia (both of which increase pancreatic inflammation and contribute to pancreatic necrosis). The proper position of the nasogastric tube, its patency, and adequacy of suction must all be confirmed. The tube may be found to be hopelessly coiled and ineffective in preventing acid from reaching the duodenum and stimulating pancreatic secretion.

The major possibilities that may be uncovered from this detailed analysis are the following. First, the original diagnosis was incorrect, and the patient is suffering from a serious intraabdominal disease masquerading as pancreatitis. Second, the diagnosis of pancreatitis was correct but additional efforts must be made for proper treatment. Third, a major complication of pancreatitis has occurred (such as pancreatic pseudocyst). From a diagnostic standpoint, another chest x-ray, a new series of plain roentgenogram and upright films of the abdomen, and a repeat ultrasound study of the pancreas and gallbladder should be obtained. If liver function tests are reasonably normal and obstruction in the biliary tract is strongly suspected, an intravenous cholangiogram may be attempted. If there is a possibility of ischemic disease of the colon, a barium enema should be administered (possibly with Gastrografin if perforation is strongly suspected). If other important diagnoses have not been excluded such as severe duodenal ulcer disease or ischemic disease of the small intestine, a barium meal study and small bowel series should be obtained. If the barium enema was not obtained prior to the gastrointestinal series, late films should be obtained in order to visualize barium in the transverse and descending colon. Air can then be instilled via the rectum to obtain an air contrast study which may reveal evidence of ischemic disease or stenosis. When Gastrografin rather than barium is utilized for either a gastrointestinal series or barium enema because of a possibility of perforation, a plain film of the abdomen should be taken several hours after the completion of the examination unless the study yielded diagnostic information. The reason for the late film is the fact that if a perforation is present and a small quantity of Gastrografin extravasated into the peritoneal cavity, this material is then reabsorbed into the systemic circulation and excreted by the kidneys. Visualization of kidneys, ureters, or urinary bladder would be confirmatory evidence of a perforation.

If the prevailing clinical impression is severe protracted pancreatitis, there are at least three areas of therapy that must be reinforced. First, efforts must be redoubled to prevent acid from reaching the duodenum. Once it has been ascertained that the nasogastric tube is functioning properly, consideration may be given to instilling liquid antacid through the nasogastric tube at frequent enough intervals to maintain the intragastric pH above 5. Alternatively, if there is marked hypersecretion of acid and major difficulty in neutralizing intragastric pH, consideration can be given to the use of Cimetidine intravenously.

A second area of improved therapy relates specifically to the fluid needs of the patient. Sufficient fluid and colloid must be administered intravenously to protect the microcirculation of the pancreas. Measurement of central venous pressure and urinary output are helpful in gauging adequacy of replacement. Sufficient amounts of albumin should be administered to maintain a serum level in excess of 3 gm%. Blood must be administered either in the form of whole blood or packed red blood cells to maintain a hematocrit at 30 or higher.

A third area focuses on nutritional needs of the patient. Standard intravenous fluids contain insufficient calories and are lacking in protein. Even if 10% dextrose is mixed with an equal quantity of 8.5% freamine such that each liter contains 5% dextrose and 4.25% freamine (plus electrolytes and vitamins as needed), the protein and calorie needs of the patient suffering from an intensely catabolic illness such as pancreatitis will probably not be met. In other illnesses, supplemental intravenous therapy with a 10% soybean oil emulsion (Intralipid 10%) has been well tolerated and has established itself as an effective source of calories,[33] but there is reluctance in utilizing this preparation in the treatment of pancreatitis because of a concern that serum lipid levels may increase and cause additional damage to the pancreas. A valuable alternative to satisfy the nutritional needs of the patient is the use of total parenteral nutrition.[26,31,34-36] By this technique, 2,000 to 3,000 calories can be administered each day in the form of hypertonic glucose and either amino acids or protein hydrolysates for several weeks to several months if needed.[36] The side-effects and morbidity of total parenteral nutrition must be understood in advance, and the technique should be supervised by an experienced team. It is not known at present to what extent nutritional support via total parenteral nutrition has a beneficial influence on the natural history of pancreatitis or its complications,[36] but at the very least it can sustain the nutritional needs of the patient and provide the proper nutriments to heal inflammation. Total parenteral nutrition does not increase pancreatic secretion.[32] Total parenteral nutrition decreases basal serum gastrin levels in the dog.[37] Since gastrin is a trophic hormone for acinar tissue of the pancreas,[38,39] a reduction in serum gastrin level during total parenteral nutrition might be beneficial if a decrease in pancreatic weight means a decrease in enzyme synthesis and secretion. Since intravenous infusion of amino acids stimulates acid secretion,[40,41] additional efforts may be required to prevent acid from reaching the duodenum in quantity during this therapy. The two choices are the use of Cimetidine intravenously or the use of liquid antacids orally.

The use of an elemental diet in the treatment of pancreatitis will be discussed in succeeding sections.

8.1.3 Treatment of Subsiding Acute Pancreatitis

Once there has been definite clinical improvement, consideration is given to removal of the nasogastric tube. The timing of this step depends to a large extent on the following guidelines: stabilization of vital signs; marked subsidence of abdominal discomfort and tenderness; improvement of appetite and disappearance of nausea; marked reduction in serum amylase but not necessarily to a normal serum amylase level; and absence of complications such as pseudocyst. Once the nasogastric tube has been removed, a liquid antacid should be administered every 2 hr by day and every 4 hr by night to maintain an intragastric pH at a near-neutral level. After 24 to 72 hr of antacid therapy (depending on the severity of the pancreatitis and the clinical response), consideration can be given to offering food in small amounts. It should be emphasized that this interval is a critical one for a smooth convalescence, and that an inappropriately large meal may cause a clinical setback. It is for this reason that a cautious dietary approach is desirable, starting with small portions of foods that are primarily carbohydrate, four to six times each day. Items such as water, jello, and toast with clear jelly are usually well tolerated. Liquid antacids should be continued indefinitely. The patient must understand this protocol so that he will not be tempted if a magnificent tray of food reaches his bedside by accident. After several more days, again depending on the severity of the initial episode and the pace of clinical improvement, additional foods can be provided, such as thin cooked cereal, skim milk, baked potato, and vanilla cookies. As additional food is cautiously added, the basic principle of small feedings with emphasis on carbohydrates should continue to be observed. The reader is encouraged to review the basic physiology of the pancreas in Chaper 1 in order to help him in the formulation of a rational dietary program which provides calories without excessive stimulation of the pancreas.

The use of an elemental diet (otherwise known as a chemically defined diet)[42] has gained popularity. These preparations provide most of their calories in the form of carbohydrates and some from a source of protein. A few contain fat.[42] An important consideration in their use is the ability to stimulate pancreatic secretion. Experimentation in animals suggests that an elemental diet given by mouth stimulates pancreatic volume and enzymes, that when introduced directly into the duodenum it produces a brisk enzyme but not volume response, and that when introduced into the jejunum causes only a minimal enzyme response.[32,43,44] However, an elemental diet taken orally stimulates less pancreatic volume than a standard diet.[45] It would appear on the basis of this information that an elemental diet given by mouth stimulates both volume and enzyme output by the usual physiologic mechanisms but probably less than a standard diet; when introduced directly into the small intestine, an elemental diet stimulates CCK-PZ but not secretin. Intrajejunal elemental feedings have been safely instituted among patients with relatively severe pancreatitis, suggesting that stimulation of pancreatic enzyme secretion by CCK-PZ has limited if any injurious capability unless coupled with stimulation of a brisk volume output in response to secretin.[26,31,46] The use of an elemental diet by mouth has also been well tolerated by patients with severe pro-tracted pancreatitis at a time when a regular house diet caused significant symptoms.[34] An elemental diet by mouth can be considered in the early dietary program of a patient with subsiding pancreatitis especially if the clinical course was protracted and difficult. It is not known at present which of the many preparations are best tolerated clinically. It is possible that preparations either lacking a source of fat or containing fat in the form of medium-chain triglycerides stimulates less enzyme output than those with a source of dietary fat. The composition of protein (whether in the form of amino acids or oligopeptides) may also influence enzyme output.

If there is marked secretion of gastric acid which was difficult to control during the acute phase of the illness, and especially if there is coexisting duodenal ulcer disease, antacid therapy should be continued for several weeks. The use of a 30-ml dose of liquid Maalox 1 and 3 hr after mealtime markedly decreases the postprandial delivery of acid into the duodenum.[2] Alternatively, the administration of Cimetidine before mealtimes reduces the postprandial delivery of acid into the duodenum to the same degree.[1,2] It would be reasonable to use either approach.

During the recovery phase of a particularly serious episode of pan-creatitis, both antacids and Cimetidine can be utilized. One might also combine Cimetidine in a dosage of 300 mg with the anticholinergic Pro-pantheline in a dosage of 15 mg before each meal now that it has been determined that the suppression of acid secretion in response to food is more complete when both drugs are utilized than with either alone.[47]

The continuation of smoking may be of benefit for pancreatitis (by decreasing basal flow of pancreatic juice) but may be injurious to coexist-ing ulcer disease (by permitting the maintenance of an acid pH in the proximal duodenum).[48]

The results of therapy may differ depending on etiology. In pancrea-titis caused by gallstones, most patients are clinically improved in 3 to 5 days and may be ready for discharge by 7 days unless there is a serious complication such as a pseudocyst or abscess. In alcoholic pancreatitis, the clinical course is usually more variable, ranging from a very mild episode with substantial improvement within a few days to a more protracted course that requires several weeks of intensive treatment. In general, a full 7- to 10-day course of hospitalization is advised for the proper treatment of alcoholic pancreatitis in order to ensure full resolution of the acute inflammatory process and early recognition of a complication. Serum amylase levels should be normal at the time of discharge. A persistingly elevated serum amylase level indicates either unresolved acute inflammation or the development of a serious complication such as a pseudocyst. Since the clinical course of alcoholic pancreatitis may differ considerably from pancreatitis in association with gallstones, published results of therapy are difficult to appraise unless the etiologies are clearly identified.

8.2 SURGICAL TREATMENT

8.2.1 Urgent Indications

There are several urgent indications for surgery during acute pancreatitis. First, pancreatic trauma caused by either blunt trauma or a penetrating wound to the abdomen requires an exploratory laparotomy. Discussion of the surgical approach to pancreatic trauma is covered in Chapter 2.

Second, biliary tract sepsis and especially sepsis associated with deepening jaundice requires urgent surgical treatment even if there is a clinical suspicion of coexisting pancreatitis. This approach is strongly recommended because gram-negative septicemia is often fatal without proper surgical drainage, the coexisting pancreatitis may be either extremely mild or not even visible at the time of surgery, and finally because the postoperative course of patients with coexisting pancreatitis who are operated on for biliary tract disease and jaundice has been extremely favorable.[49-51] On the other hand, it should be clearly understood that alcoholic pancreatitis associated with jaundice is usually not treated surgically, first because there are many causes of jaundice unrelated to obstruction in the common bile duct, and second because there is an excessively high surgical mortality if the patient has alcoholic hepatitis.

A third indication for surgery is uncertainty of diagnosis. Diseases that may masquerade as acute pancreatitis include gangrene of an afferent loop causing a closed-loop obstruction (even long after the original gastric surgery), mesenteric infarction, and perforated duodenal ulcer. While the level of serum amylase does not distinguish pancreatitis from a surgical crisis, serum amylase values above 1,000 are not infrequently recorded in surgical emergencies.

Fourth, laparotomy is required if there is serious progressive clinical deterioration of the patient even when the diagnosis of pancreatitis appears secure. At times a disease masquerading as pancreatitis is discovered, or a specific complication of pancreatitis is found and lends itself to specific therapy (such as drainage of a pseudocyst externally). At other times, the surgeon discovers severe necrotizing hemorrhagic pancreatitis, and has three basic therapeutic choices.[31] The first is to attempt a major pancreatic resection and possibly even a near total pancreatectomy.[52] The second is to provide adequate drainage,[53] and possibly proceed with a trial of peritoneal dialysis. The third approach is to perform a gastrostomy (to aspirate acid and decrease ileus), a jejunostomy (for the purpose of feeding), a decompressing cholecystostomy (if there is evidence of biliary tract obstruction or impending obstruction), and drainage of the peritoneal cavity and retroperitoneal spaces.[31,54,55] While there are proponents for each of these techniques, there is not as yet a properly controlled clinical trial which compares these surgical alternatives and contrasts them with a medical form of treatment. In one small trial comparing the triple-ostomy approach with a nonoperative approach, there were no deaths in either group and the surgical group developed a variety of severe complications.[56]

If a surgical approach is required, postoperative nutritional support can be facilitated (and apparently without exacerbation of pancreatitis) by intrajejunal feeding of an elemental diet.[26,31,46] A simplified surgical technique for insertion of a feeding catheter into the jejunum using a needle has been described.[57]

Specific complications of pancreatitis that require surgical therapy are described in Chapter 9. These include pancreatic abscess (which should be drained surgically as promptly as the diagnosis is made), pancreatic pseudocyst (which usually resolves spontaneously but at times requires drainage), and a variety of complications including massive gastrointestinal bleeding, infarction of loops of jejunum, and perforation of the colon or small intestine.

8.2.2 Semiurgent or Elective Surgery

There is general agreement that cholecystectomy (and, if indicated, common bile duct exploration as well) should be performed if acute pancreatitis is caused by biliary tract disease. If the patient is seriously ill with increasing jaundice and sepsis, corrective surgery should be performed promptly as described in the previous section. When this is done, there is an acceptably low morbidity and mortality.[50,58] If there is no urgent indication to operate, a traditional approach has been to delay surgery on the biliary tract for at least 4 to 6 weeks to allow subsidence of pancreatitis. There are, however, several compelling reasons to consider an earlier surgical approach. First, some cases of biliary tract disease associated with an elevation in serum amylase are accompanied by only minimal pancreatitis or none at all.[59] Second, if symptoms of acute pancreatitis subside and serum amylase returns to normal during the initial hospitalization, biliary tract surgery can be carried out within 12 days of onset of pancreatitis without major risk of postoperative complications or postoperative pancreatitis.[50,58] Also, among patients who have required surgery on a semiurgent basis within 20 days of initial hospitalization for pancreatitis associated with biliary tract disease and jaundice, mortality has been found to be negligible and the incidence of postoperative pancreatitis very low.[51] Finally, if corrective surgery is deferred, there is a likelihood that a majority of patients will experience a second episode of pancreatitis within 30 days of the initial attack.[50] In the light of these observations, it appears reasonable to consider corrective surgery on the biliary tract during the initial hospitalization once the patient's condition has fully stabilized and associated pancreatitis has resolved completely.

If a diagnosis of hyperparathyroidism is substantiated, surgical exploration of the parathyroid glands is indicated. Diagnosis of hyperparathyroidism should be strongly suspected if hypercalcemia is documented during an episode of pancreatitis or if serum calcium is found to be elevated following subsidence of an episode of pancreatitis.

Recurrent episodes of acute pancreatitis of obscure etiology in time require a careful surgical approach. This topic is considered in a subsequent section.

8.2.3 Surgical Treatment of Recurrent Pancreatitis

Recurrent pancreatitis of unknown etiology poses a difficult dilemma for the clinician. Additional medical efforts include measurements of serum calcium and triglyceride, an evaluation of drug history, and attempts to visualize the gallbladder and common bile duct by oral cholecystography and IV cholangiography. If the cause of recurrent pancreatitis cannot be elucidated by usual means, endoscopic retrograde cholangiopancreatography (ERCP) should be performed in an effort to find abnormalities of the common bile duct, gallbladder, or pancreatic duct. Abnormalities of importance that may be discovered include biliary calculi not visualized by other techniques, stenosis of the sphincter of Oddi, stenosis of the pancreatic duct, marked ductal dilatation associated with sludge (Figure 19), and pancreatic pseudocyst not visualized by ultrasonic examination (Figure 20).

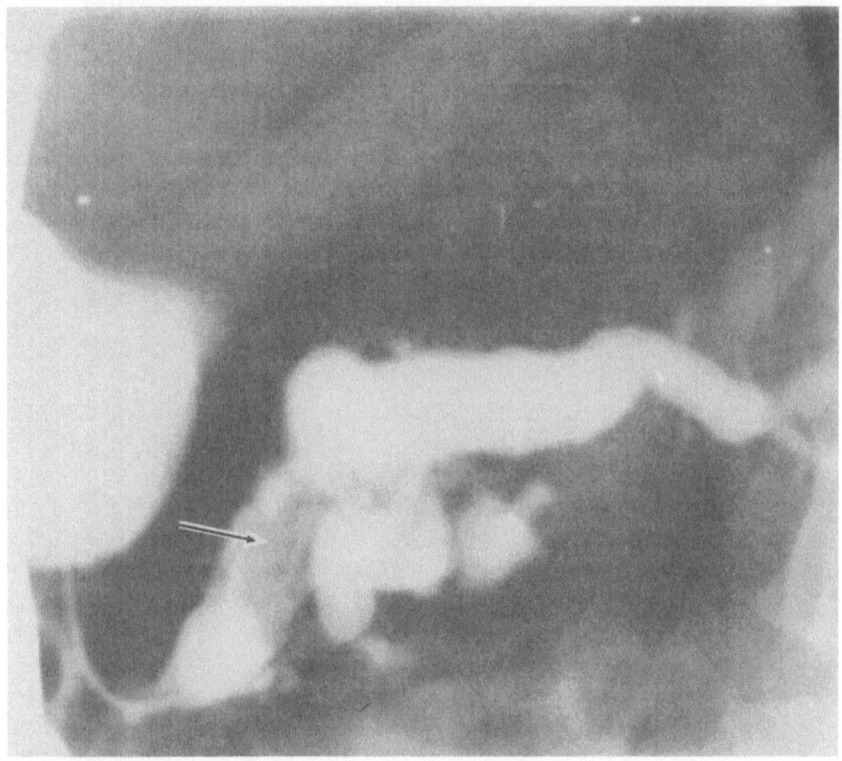

FIGURE 19 ERCP: Pancreatic Ductal Dilatation. ERCP shows greatly dilated pancreatic duct and its major branches. There is amorphous material within the duct lumen (arrow). The cannula is seen extending from the endoscope at the far left, entering the pancreatic duct in the lower left, and passing through the amorphous material to the right of the arrow. At surgery, a chronically inflamed fibrotic pancreas with dilated ducts was visualized. Following a lateral pancreaticojejunostomy, there was complete relief of pain. (Courtesy of Dr. R. Norton.)

Stenosis of the sphincter of Oddi is an intriguing problem. Some patients show no evidence of associated biliary tract disease and the cause of the stenosis is unknown. Other patients have already undergone cholecystectomy for cholelithiasis or are found to have cholelithiasis, and may have developed fibrotic and inflammatory changes of the sphincter as a result of the passage of gallstones or gravel.[60–62] These changes in the sphincter cause narrowing and inadequate drainage of the common bile duct and at times the pancreatic duct as well. An elevated pressure in the common bile duct may be documented on manometric studies at the time of surgery. Clinically, there are recurrent episodes of abdominal pain

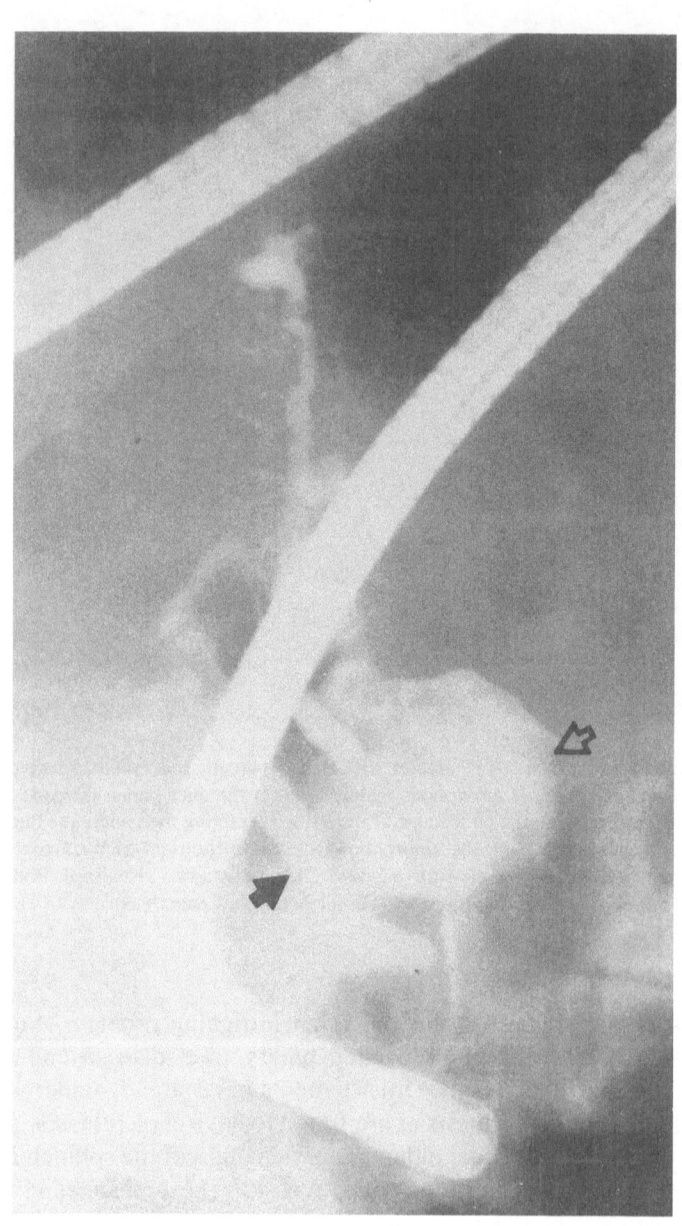

FIGURE 20 ERCP: Pancreatic Pseudocyst. ERCP visualizes a large slightly irregular pancreatic pseudocyst at the head of the pancreas (clear arrow). Secondary pancreatic ducts are dilated and shortened in the body and tail of the pancreas. The common bile duct is also visualized (black arrow). (Courtesy of Dr. R. Norton.)

associated with elevation of serum amylase. ERCP occasionally shows abnormalities including delayed emptying of contrast material from the common bile duct,[63] stenosis of the orifice of the pancreatic duct, or dilatation of the pancreatic duct,[61,64] but may be entirely normal.[61] Morphine-prostigmine test has produced chemical abnormalities in at least some patients with this condition.[61,64] Unfortunately, in many patients all the diagnostic studies are normal and the characteristic changes of the sphincter of Oddi are only discovered at the time of surgical exploration. Surgical correction of the stenotic sphincter of Oddi requires a sphincteroplasty, and will be discussed in a subsequent paragraph.

A standard surgical approach for recurrent pancreatitis of uncertain etiology starts with a cholecystectomy. At times, when the gallbladder is open, very tiny stones are discovered that were not visible by any preoperative technique.[65] If intraductal stones are also visualized by cystic duct cholangiogram, exploration of the common bile duct is then undertaken. Once it has been ascertained that there is normal flow of cholangiographic material into the duodenum without visualization of retained stones, the operation is usually then terminated. At other times, no gallstones are found in the gallbladder or common bile duct, but manometric studies reveal an elevated pressure in the common bile duct. Under these circumstances, a sphincteroplasty of the sphincter of Oddi is then performed. A more difficult decision awaits the surgeon if no calculi are discovered and if manometric studies are completely normal. Some surgeons would terminate the operation at this point having performed only a cholecystectomy. Others would proceed with a sphincteroplasty apparently not trusting the validity of manometric studies in an anesthetized patient, and in addition would inspect the orifice of the pancreatic duct to be sure that it is fully patent.

The technique of sphincteroplasty has been well described.[60,62,66] The distal common bile duct is opened, and the mucosa of the common bile duct is sutured to the mucosa of the duodenum. The opening of the main pancreatic duct also requires a sphincteroplasty if there is narrowing of this orifice.[60] A more vigorous surgical approach to provide adequate egress of pancreatic fluid is actual excision of the common wall of the terminal bile duct and duct of Wirsung.[67] Once proper drainage has been achieved with sphincteroplasty of the sphincter of Oddi and either sphincteroplasty or septectomy of the orifice of the pancreatic duct, the operation has been completed. The decision as to the patency of the orifice of the pancreatic duct is based partly on close inspection at the time of surgery, partly on evidence secured by preoperative ERCP, and at times by pancreatic ductography performed at the time of surgery.

Among reported series of patients with histologic verification of sphincter of Oddi stenosis, surgical benefit has been reported in the majority. It has been emphasized that this approach is not helpful for patients with alcoholic pancreatitis.[60] In general, a longer period of observation will be required to analyze the results of surgery in this syndrome.

Recurrent pancreatitis of uncertain etiology may have causes other than undocumented biliary tract disease or sphincter of Oddi stenosis. These involve structural abnormalities of the common bile duct, duodenum, and pancreatic duct, and have been described in Chapter 2. An interesting but rare cause of recurrent pancreatitis is pancreas divisum, in which the main pancreatic duct of Wirsung drains only a small portion of the pancreas (the ventral bud), whereas the accessory duct of Santorini drains the major portion of the adult pancreas (the dorsal bud). In one series, among 33 patients that were demonstrated by ERCP to have pancreas division, 15 experienced pancreatitis (usually of the dorsal bud).[68] This anatomic variation was suggested at ERCP by the small amount of dye that was required to opacify acinar tissus via the main duct and by the copious amount of pancreatic secretion that gushed from the accessory duct following the administration of intravenous secretin.

8.2.4 Surgical Treatment of Severe Protracted Pancreatitis

A surgical approach may be required if pancreatitis persists for an indefinite period despite all efforts of medical management including the use of total parenteral nutrition. A reasonable course would be to continue medical management for 4 to 6 weeks unless there is evidence of clinical deterioration. Prior to laparotomy, all clinical information should be reviewed by the entire staff of physician (including medical staff, surgeons, and radiologists) to be sure there is no misunderstanding or confusion about the available data. A final ultrasonic study or a C-T scan may be of help by revealing a surgically correctable problem such as a pseudocyst or pancreatic ductal dilatation secondary to stone or stricture.

The surgeon may be greatly helped by a preoperative mapping out of the ductal anatomy with the technique of ERCP. If the patient is critically or seriously ill such as with severe intractable pain, marked peritoneal guarding, and other evidence of severe pancreatitis, ERCP should generally be avoided for fear of causing further deterioration. However, for a patient who is chronically but not seriously ill and especially if it is a patient who experiences recurrent pain with each attempt to eat during convalescence, the technique of ERCP can generally be performed safely and yield valuable information.[34]

The preoperative or intraoperative discovery of a pancreatic pseudocyst or ductal stenosis facilitates surgical correction, as outlined in Chapters 9 and 15. If neither is identified, the choice of an operation is more difficult. Devitalized tissue can be removed, retroperitoneal and peritoneal drainage secured, gastrostomy performed for aspiration of acid, and jejunostomy performed to provide postoperative feeding. The advantages of a feeding jejunostomy have been outlined in a previous section.

REFERENCES

1. Longstreth GF, Go VLW, Malagelada J–R: Postprandial gastric, pancreatic, and biliary response to histamine H_2–Receptor antagonist in active duodenal ulcer. *Gastroenterology* 72:9–13, 1977.
2. Deering TB, Malagelada J–R: Comparison of an H_2–Receptor antagonist and a neutralizing antacid on postprandial acid delivery into the duodenum in patients with duodenal ulcer. *Gastroenterology* 73:11–14, 1977.
3. Richardson CT: Effect of H_2–Receptor antagonist on gastric acid secretion and serum gastrin concentration. *Gastroenterology* 74:366–370, 1978.
4. Ma KW, Brown DC, Masler DS, et al: Effects of renal failure on blood levels of Cimetidine. *Gastroenterology* 74:473–477, 1978.
5. Kruss DM, Littman A: Safety of Cimetidine. *Gastroenterology* 74:478–483, 1978.
6. Banks PA, Sum PT: Mode of action of acetazolamide on pancreatic exocrine secretion. *Arch Surg* 102:505–508, 1971.
7. Dyck WP, Hightower NC, Janowitz HD: Efect of acetazolamide on human pancreatic secretion. *Gastroenterology* 62:547–552, 1972.
8. Banks PA, Rudick J, Dreiling DA, et al: Effect of antidiuretic hormone on pancreatic exocrine secretion. *Am J Physiol* 215:361–365, 1968.
9. Dyck WP, Texter EC Jr, Lasater JM, et al: Influence of glucagon on pancreatic exocrine secretion in man. *Gastroenterology* 58:532–538, 1970.
10. Konturek SJ, Biermat J, Kwiecien N, et al: Effect of glucagon on meal-induced gastric secretion in man. *Gastroenterology* 68:448–454, 1975.
11. Anderon MC, Copass MK: Use of carbonic anhydrase inhibitor in the treatment of pancreatitis. *Am J Dig Dis*, 11:367–376, 1966.
12. Pissiotis CA, Condon RE, Nyhus LM: Effect of vasopressin on pancreatic blood flow in acute hemorrhagic pancreatitis. *Am J Surg* 123:203–208, 1972.
13. Condon RE, Woods JH, Poulin TL, et al: Experimental pancreatitis treated with glucagon or lactated ringer solution. *Arch Surg* 109:154–158, 1974.
14. Welbourn RB, Armitage P, Gilmore OJA, et al: Death from acute pancreatitis. *Lancet* 2:632–635, 1977.
15. Levant JA, Secrist DM, Resin H, et al: Nasogastric suction in the treatment of alcoholic pancreatitis. *JAMA* 229:51–52, 1974.
16. Banks PA: Acute pancreatitis. *Gastroenterology* 61:382–397, 1971.
17. The choice of antimicrobial drugs. *The Medical Letter* 20:1–8, January 13, 1978.
18. Howes R, Zuidema GD, Cameron JL: Evaluation of prophylactic antibiotics in acute pancreatitis. *J Surg Res* 18:197–200, 1975.
19. Craig RM, Dorday E, Myles L: The use of ampicillin in acute pancreatitis. *Ann Int Med* 83:831–832, 1975.
20. Finch WT, Sawyers JL, Schenker S: A prospective study to determine the efficacy of antibiotics in acute pancreatitis. *Ann Surg* 183:667–671, 1976.

21. Kodesch R, DuPont HL: Infectious complications of acute pancreatitis. *Surg Gynecol Obstet* 136:763–768, 1973.

22. Gregg JA: Detection of bacterial infection of the pancreatic ducts in patients with pancreatitis and pancreatic cancer during endoscopic cannulation of the pancreatic duct. *Gastroenterology* 73:1005–1007, 1977.

23. Trapnell JE, Rigby CC, Talbot Ch, et al: A controlled trial of Trasylol in the treatment of acute pancreatitis. *Br J Surg* 61:177–182, 1974.

24. Donowitz M. Kerstein MD, Spiro HM: Pancreatic ascites. *Medicine* 53:183–195, 1974.

25. Svensson J–O: Role of intravenously infused insulin in treatment of acute pancreatitis. *Scand J Gastroenterol* 10:487–490, 1975.

26. Feller JH, Brown RA, Toussaint GPM, et al: Changing methods in the treatment of severe pancreatitis. *Am J Surg* 127:196–201, 1974.

27. Paoloyan D, Skinner DB: Clinical significance of pancreatic ascites. *Am J Surg* 132:114–117, 1976.

28. Gjessing J: Renal failure in acute pancreatitis. *Brit Med J* 4:359–360, 1972.

29. Hartong WA, Skibbe RM and Greenberger NJ: Spontaneous Pseudocystogastrostomy associated with pancreatitis. *Arch Intern Med* 136:1287–1289, 1976.

30. Fine J: Acute pancreatitis. *Lancet* 1:1092, 1975.

31. White TT, Heimbach DM: Sequestrectomy and hyperalimentation in the treatment of hemorrhagic pancreatitis. *Am J Surg* 132:270–275, 1976.

32. Kelly GA, Nahrwold DL: Pancreatic secretion in response to an elemental diet and intravenous hyperalimentation. *Surg Gynecol Obstet* 143:87–91, 1976.

33. Hansen LM, Hardie WR, Hidalgo J: Fat emulsion for intravenous administration. *Ann Surg* 184:80–88, 1976.

34. Blackburn GL, Williams LF, Bistrian ER, et al: New approaches to management of severe acute pancreatitis. *Am J Surg* 131:114–124, 1976.

35. Law DH: Total parenteral nutrition. *N Engl Med* 297:1104–1107, 1977.

36. Goodgame JT, Fischer JE: Parenteral nutrition in the treatment of acute pancreatitis. *Ann Surg* 186:651-658, 1977.

37. Thor PJ, Copeland EM, Dudrick SJ, et al: Effect of long-term parenteral feeding on gastric secretion in dogs. *Am J Physiol* 232:E39–E43, 1977.

38. Johnson LR: The trophic action of gastrointestinal hormones. *Gastroenterology* 70:278–288, 1976.

39. Johnson LR, Lichtenberger LM, Copeland EM, et al: Action of gastrin on gastrointestinal structure and function. *Gastroenterology* 68:1184–1192, 1975.

40. Landor JH, Ipapo VS: Gastric secretory effect of amino acids given enterally parenterally in dogs. *Gastroenterology* 73:781–784, 1977.

41. Isenberg JI, Maxwell V: Intravenous infusion of amino acids stimulates gastric acid secretion in man. *N Engl J Med* 298:27–29, 1978.

42. Young EA, Heuler N, Russell P, et al: Comparative nutritional analysis of chemically defined diets. *Gastroenterology* 69:1338–1345, 1975.

43. Wolfe BM, Keltner RM, Kaminske DL: The effect of an intraduodenal elemental diet on pancreatic secretion. *Surg Gynecol Obstet* 140:241–245, 1975.

44. Ragins H, Levensen SM, Signer R, et al: Intrajejunal administration of an elemental diet at neutral pH avoids pancreatic stimulation. *Am J Surg* 126:606–614, 1973.

45. McArdle AH, Echave W, Brown RA, et al: Effects of elemental diet on pancreatic secretion. *Am J Surg* 128:690–692, 1974.

46. Voitk A, Brown RA, Echave V, et al: Use of an elemental diet in the treatment of complicated pancreatitis. *Am J Surg* 125:223–227, 1973.

47. Feldman M, Richardson CT, Peterson WL, et al: Effect of low-dose Propantheline on food-stimulated gastric acid secretion. *N Engl J Med* 297:1427–1430, 1977.

48. Murphy SNS, Dinoso VP Jr, Clearfield HR, et al: Simultaneous measurement of basal pancreatic, gastric acid secretion, plasma gastrin, and secretin during smoking. *Gastroenterology* 73:758–761, 1977.
49. Cohen R, Priestley JT, Gross JB: Abdominal surgery in the presence of acute pancreatitis. *Mayo Clin Proc* 44:309–317, 1969.
50. Paloyan D, Simonowitz D, Skinner DB: The timing of biliary tract operations in patients with pancreatitis associated with gallstones. *Surg Gynecol Obstet* 141:737–739, 1975.
51. Acosta MA, Ledesma CL: Gallstone migration as a cause of acute pancreatitis. *N Engl J Med* 290:484–487, 1974.
52. Norton L, Eiseman B: Near total pancreatectomy for hemorrhagic pancreatitis. *Am J Surg* 127:191–195, 1974.
53. Jordon GL Jr, Spjut HJ: Hemorrhagic pancreatitis. *Arch Surg* 104:489–493, 1972.
54. Lawson DW, Daggett WM, Civetta JM, et al: Surgical treatment of acute necrotizing pancreatitis. *Ann Surg* 172:605–617, 1970.
55. Warshaw AL, Imbembo AL, Civetta JM, et al: Surgical intervention in acute necrotizing pancreatitis. *Am J Surg* 127:484–491, 1974.
56. Ranson JHC, Rifkind KM, Roses DF, et al: Prognostic signs and the role of operative management in acute pancreatitis. *Surg Gynecol Obstet* 139:69–81, 1974.
57. Delany HM, Carnevale N, Garvey JW, et al: Postoperative nutritional support using needle catheter feeding jejunostomy. *Ann Surg* 186:165–170, 1977.
58. Kelly TR: Gallstone pancreatitis. *Arch Surg* 109:294–297, 1974.
59. Dixon JA, Hillam JD: Surgical treatment of biliary tract disease associated with acute pancreatitis. *Am J Surg* 120:371–375, 1970.
60. White TT: Indications for sphincteroplasty as opposed to choledochoduodenostomy. *Am J Surg* 126:165–170, 1973.
61. Raskin JB, Kaplan S, Kafka E: Ampullary stenosis: clinical presentation, diagnosis and management. *Gastroenterology* 72:1116, 1977.
62. Jones SA, Smith LL, Gregory G: Sphincteroplasty for recurrent pancreatitis. *Ann Surg* 147: 180–190, 1958.
63. Belsito AA, Marta JB, Cramer GG, et al: Measurement of biliary tract size and drainage time. *Radiology* 122:65–69, 1977.
64. Gregg JA, Taddeo AE, Milano AF, et al: Duodenoscopy and endoscopic pancreatography in patients with positive morphine prostigmine tests. *Am J Surg* 134:318–321, 1977.
65. Freund H, Pfeffermann R, Durst AL, et al: Gallstone pancreatitis. *Arch Surg* 111:1106–1107, 1976.
66. Partington PF: Twenty-three years of experience with spincterotomy and sphincteroplasty for stenosis of the sphincter of Oddi. *Surg Gynecol Obstet* 145:161–168, 1977.
67. Moody FG, Berenson MM and McCloskey D: Transampullary septectomy for postcholecystectomy pain. *Ann Surg* 186:415–423, 1977.
68. Gregg JA: Pancreas divisum: its association with pancreatitis. *Am J Surg* 134:539–543, 1977.

9

Complications of Acute Pancreatitis

A complication of acute pancreatitis may occur during the first clinical episode or during a subsequent episode. It may occur whether the pancreas was previously normal (as in biliary tract disease) or already chronically inflamed (as in alcoholic pancreatitis). For the purposes of this chapter, the term acute pancreatitis refers to an episode of painful pancreatitis whether the pancreas was previously normal or not. Complications that relate specifically to chronic pancreatitis will be discussed in Chapter 16.

9.1 EARLY COMPLICATIONS

9.1.1 Shock

In either edematous or hemorrhagic pancreatitis, leakage of pancreatic exudate into retroperitoneal and peritoneal spaces may severely reduce intravascular volume and lead to systemic hypotension and shock. Vasoactive polypeptides released by the pancreas may contribute to this process. Once systemic hypotension occurs, splanchnic vasoconstriction develops as a compensatory mechanism. This effect may devastate the pancreas by reducing its supply of arterial blood and increasing pancreatic hypoxia. Owing to mechanisms outlined in Chapter 3, this combination provides a milieu that intensifies pancreatic inflammation and leads to pancreatic necrosis and hemorrhage. The process becomes self-perpetuating because of additional fluid losses that intensify systemic hypotension. Pancreatic ischemia must be prevented by providing sufficient amounts of intravenous fluids and colloids to counteract systemic hypotension and splanchnic vasoconstriction.

9.1.2 Renal Abnormalities

Pancreatic inflammatory exudate can burrow into the left kidney producing a mass lesion on intravenous pyelogram, causing hematuria.[1] A pancreatic pseudocyst may also erode the left kidney and displace it from its usual location[1] (Figure 21).

The kidney is vulnerable to hypotension, which may lead to acute tubular necrosis. A syndrome of acute renal failure has also been documented in the absence of demonstrable hypotension.[2,3] The explanation that has usually been offered is that an episode of transient hypotension

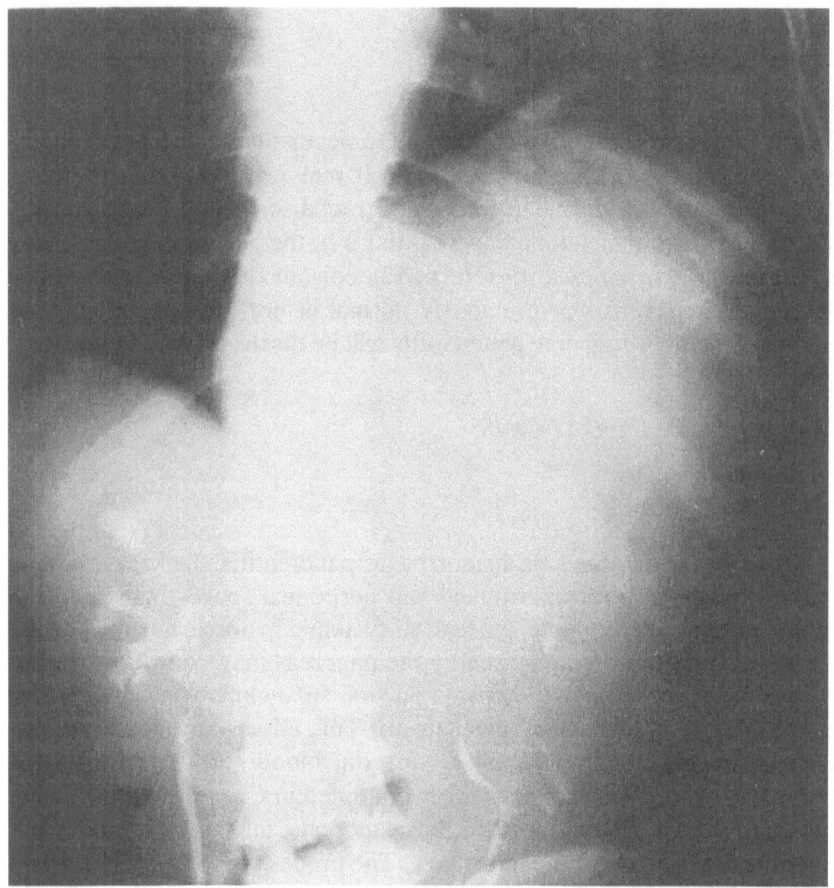

FIGURE 21 Intravenous Pyelogram in Pancreatitis: Pseudocyst. There is a large mass in the left upper quadrant of the abdomen displacing the left kidney downward and medially. At surgery, a large pseudocyst was identified and drained internally.

was not detected. Alternative explanations have also been offered. One is that elevated levels of trypsin activate the coagulation mechanism resulting in the deposition of fibrin in glomeruli.[4] Another is that in acute pancreatitis, there is release of a circulating vasopressor that increases total peripheral resistance (causing systemic hypertension) and renal vascular resistance (causing a decrease in renal plasma flow and glomerular filtration).[5] Transient systemic hypertension has been noted by other authors during the course of acute pancreatitis,[6] and the concept of a vasopressor is an attractive one.

In acute renal failure associated with pancreatitis, peritoneal dialysis[2,3] and hemodialysis[3] have been used with success.

9.1.3 Splenic Abnormalities

The spleen is rarely palpable in acute pancreatitis.[7] A palpable spleen or a mass in the left upper quadrant should raise the question of a complication of pancreatitis involving the spleen[8-11] One possibility is dissection of a pancreatic pseudocyst into the hilus of the spleen causing one or more of the following abnormalities: rupture of the spleen, splenic infarction, splenic artery hemorrhage, and splenic vein thrombosis.[9,12-14] Another possibility is splenic vein thrombosis secondary to either chronic pancreatitis or an acute exacerbation of pancreatitis.[8,10,11] A third possibility is that an inflammatory mass from the tail of the pancreas has extended into the hilum of the spleen causing a large hematoma.[12,15]

Splenic involvement in pancreatitis can be documented by a liver–spleen scan, by abdominal ultrasound, or by selective celiac arteriogram.[9] The treatment of choice for bleeding esophagogastric varices secondary to splenic vein thrombosis is splenectomy.[8,10,11] Treatment of choice for a pseudocyst of the tail of the pancreas extending into the spleen is distal pancreatectomy and splenectomy.[9]

9.1.4 Gastrointestinal Bleeding

Gastrointestinal bleeding may occur through a variety of mechanisms in acute pancreatitis. A full differential diagnosis should include alcoholic gastritis, mucosal tear of the esophagogastric junction caused by retching or vomiting (Mallory–Weiss syndrome), active duodenal ulcer, or active gastric ulcer.

In addition, there are sources of bleeding that are specifically related to pancreatitis. One is diffuse mucosal bleeding of the duodenum caused by contiguous inflammation from the head of the pancreas. Another is esophageal or gastric varices secondary to splenic vein thrombosis.[8,10,11] Varices not associated with bleeding do not require therapy; the treatment of choice for variceal bleeding caused by splenic vein thrombosis is a splenectomy.[8,10,11] Gastrointestinal bleeding may occur in association with a pancreatic pseudocyst or abscess should either rupture into a hollow viscus such as stomach, duodenum, or transverse colon. Occasionally, an arterial aneurysm in association with chronic pancreatitis erodes directly into the pancreatic duct causing a brisk flow of blood into the duodenum.[16]

Diagnostic evaluation of gastrointestinal bleeding during acute pancreatitis usually includes panendoscopy and at times arteriography.

9.1.5 Liver

Varieties of biochemical and morphologic abnormalities of the liver have been reported in pancreatitis.[17] Some relate specifically to the toxic effect of alcohol on the liver such as steatosis and alcoholic hepatitis.

An interesting question that has yet to be completely resolved is whether alcoholic cirrhosis is likely to occur in a patient with clinically significant (i.e., painful) alcoholic pancreatitis. There is general agreement that abnormalities of the liver including alcoholic fatty liver and alcoholic hepatitis may occur in alcoholic pancreatitis, but until recently the reported incidence of coexisting cirrhosis has been extremely low (2%,[18] 5%,[19] and 8%[20] in three reports around the world). In support of this nonassociation is the infrequency of bleeding from esophageal varices in alcoholic pancreatitis unless there is coexisting splenic vein thrombosis. Nonetheless, several recent studies have suggested that patients with clinically significant alcoholic pancreatitis may have a substantially higher incidence of coexisting alcoholic cirrhosis than was formerly appreciated.[21,22] Accordingly, the possibility of either alcoholic hepatitis or cirrhosis should be kept in mind before planning an operation on the pancreas in alcoholic pancreatitis since surgery may be more hazardous if there is serious liver disease.

Jaundice may develop during the course of acute pancreatitis for a variety of reasons. These include alcoholic hepatitis, cirrhosis with activation of liver disease, viral hepatitis, and drug hepatitis. Viral agents may cause both hepatitis and pancreatitis. A pancreatic abscess is not infrequently associated with jaundice.[23,24] Other causes are common bile duct obstruction and hemolysis of blood in the peritoneal cavity or retroperitoneum.

9.1.6 Common Bile Duct Obstruction

Obstruction of the common bile duct may occur on the basis of gallstones,[25-27] a pancreatic pseudocyst of the head of the pancreas,[26-32] a carcinoma of the head of the pancreas,[25-27] acute inflammation of the head of the pancreas in the form of a phlegmon,[25,26,30,31,33] or chronic inflammation of the head of the pancreas.[18,26,30,33-40]

The presence of gallstones in the common bile duct may be associated with jaundice and sepsis, or simply an elevation of serum alkaline phosphatase and possibly SGOT and SGPT. A pancreatic pseudocyst obstructing the common bile duct usually causes jaundice and abdominal pain, but occasionally is painless and not even associated with an elevation of serum amylase or lipase. A carcinoma obstructing the distal common bile duct usually causes jaundice having developed as a complication of chronic pancreatitis or as an unrelated coincidence. Compression of the distal common bile duct during acute pancreatitis occasionally causes jaundice but at other times is asymptomatic and causes no liver dysfunction whatsoever. Since the distal common bile duct is embedded in the posterior portion of the head of the pancreas, it is vulnerable to circumferential compression by the inflamed pancreas. With subsidence of pancreatitis, jaundice and other abnormalities of liver function usually resolve, and patency of the distal common bile duct is restored.

Obstruction of the distal common bile duct by a cicatrix of chronic pancreatitis is an important entity (Figure 22). Almost all patients have chronic alcoholic pancreatitis severe enough to cause calcific pancreatitis. Clinical symptomatology has been variable, but most patients have had abdominal discomfort either continuously or intermittently; most have been jaundiced, and some have had evidence of ascending cholangitis. In the context of alcoholic pancreatitis, these symptoms should not be misinterpreted as another bout of pancreatitis or alcoholic hepatitis. There are a few laboratory clues. Almost all patients have a marked elevation of alkaline phosphatase; some have had an elevation of SGOT higher than customary for alcoholic hepatitis. Levels of bilirubin have varied from normal to moderately elevated. Serum amylase and lipase may be either increased or normal. A plain roentgenogram of the abdomen frequently shows calcification of the pancreas but need not. This diagnosis can be confirmed by additional radiologic studies. An oral cholecystogram may be entirely normal, but occasionally sufficient contrast material enters the common bile duct to reveal ductal dilatation. An intravenous cholangiogram should be performed if liver function tests are not severely deranged. A dilated common bile duct that tapers smoothly to a zone of

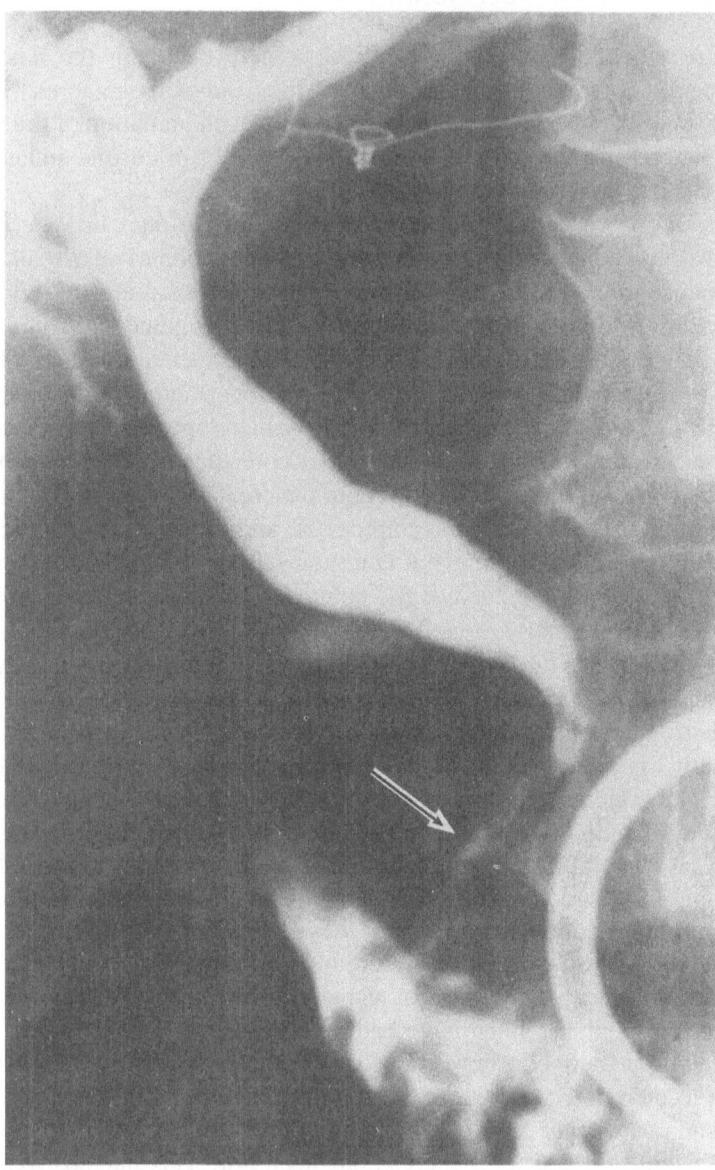

FIGURE 22 *Operative Cholangiogram in Chronic Pancreatitis.* There is marked tapering of distal common bile duct (arrow) with proximal dilation in a patient with severe chronic pancreatitis secondary to alcohol. The narrowing is secondary to entrapment of the distal common bile duct within the fibrotic head of the pancreas. Major symptoms were recurrent chills and fever. Following choledochojejunostomy, the patient has remained well aside from an episode of alcoholic hepatitis.

marked narrowing is the characteristic finding of a long ductal stricture within the substance of the pancreas. Other techniques that may be required to define this entity are ERCP, "skinny needle" transhepatic cholangiography, and ultrasonography. During ERCP, multiple views of the common bile duct must be obtained with the patient rotated in a variety of positions and the endoscope withdrawn from the duodenum to be sure that the endoscope has not caused distortion of the distal common bile duct in the form of temporary narrowing.[41] The importance of extrahepatic obstruction is the threat of ascending cholangitis and secondary biliary cirrhosis. Treatment of choice is a surgical bypass usually by anastomosing the dilated common bile duct to the duodenum or a loop of jejunum. Occasionally, biochemical and structural abnormalities recede during recovery from an exacerbation of pancreatitis. It is for this reason that surgery can usually be delayed for a few weeks unless there is increasing jaundice, sepsis, evidence of biliary cirrhosis on liver biopsy, or intractable pain.

9.1.7 Fat Necrosis

Fat necrosis may occur in a wide variety of tissues. These include retroperitoneal tissue, peritoneal tissue including the mesentery, mediastinum, pleura, pericardium, subcutaneous tissue, and bone.[42-49] Fat necrosis in the mesentery may be severe enough to cause small-bowel obstruction.[43] At least 20 patients have been reported with subcutaneous fat necrosis. This sign appears to carry a grave prognosis in that approximately half of the patients did not survive.[42] The lesions are circumscribed tender red nodules adherent to the skin but movable over deeper structures. They are most commonly located in the region of the ankles, fingers, knees, and elbows.[44] On occasion the lesions are more diffuse.[45] The differential diagnosis includes erythema nodosum and Weber–Christian disease (nodular nonsuppurative panniculitis). The histologic appearance of subcutaneous fat necrosis is characterized by necrotic ghostlike fat cells and a diffuse inflammatory infiltration. The foci may be fluctuant and drain through the skin. Amylase has been recovered from the fluctuant material.[42,43]

The cause of fat necrosis is unclear. A frequent suggestion is that lipase liberated into the blood stream during the course of pancreatitis is responsible. An alternative suggestion is that immunologic mechanisms play a role when subcutaneous fat necrosis occurs in association with arthritis and at times pleuritis and pericarditis.[42] Among 20 patients with subcutaneous fat necrosis, arthritis was demonstrated in 10 (usually involving ankles, knees, wrists, or elbows),[42] and only 4 of these 10 patients survived.

There have been 8 reports of intramedullary fat necrosis[46-49] during pancreatitis. Painful osteolytic lesions and chronic intramedullary calcification have been reported. One patient required total pancreatectomy because of progressive bone destruction.[46]

Subcutaneous fat necrosis has been reported in pancreatitis of various etiologies including alcohol, trauma, and biliary tract disease. This complication appears to herald a very serious prognosis.

9.1.8 Respiratory Complications

A variety of respiratory complications may occur during acute pancreatitis, including pleural effusions, atelectasis caused by splinting of the diaphragm, pneumonia, pulmonary emboli, and pulmonary edema.

Pleural effusions are generally attributed to passage of pancreatic exudate via lymphatic channels into the chest or extravasation of exudate through the diaphragm. At times, a pancreatic pseudocyst or pancreatic abscess creates a fistula into the pleural space.[50-52] Pleural effusions may be either bilateral or unilateral; if unilateral, either on the right or left side.[53] At times, the pleural fluid is hemorrhagic. Levels of amylase and lipase in pleural fluid are invariably higher than in serum. The effusion may be large but more often is moderate to small. A constricting pleuritis requiring surgical decortication for proper expansion has been reported.[53]

Clinical and radiologic evidence of pulmonary edema may occur within several days of the onset of acute pancreatitis. One mechanism that has been accepted is left ventricular failure causing congestive heart failure as in an older population with coronary artery disease.[54] Under these circumstances, pulmonary congestion is a transudate, and cardiac enlargement would be expected. Possible contributing factors include excessive intravenous fluid replacement, toxic effects of pancreatic enzymes on the myocardium, and alcoholic cardiomyopathy.

Some patients, however, have not fit a classic description for congestive heart failure. The measurements of central venous pressure, pulmonary artery pressure, pulmonary capillary wedge pressure, and pulmonary vascular resistance have substantiated the fact that hydrostatic pressure was not increased but that the alveolar–capillary membrane was disrupted causing the leakage of protein-rich fluid into the pulmonary interstitium.[55,56] An early clue was the development of diffuse pulmonary infiltrates and progressive hypoxemia in severe pancreatitis requiring massive fluid replacement and characterized by marked hypocalcemia.[55] This sequence of events is generally called the adult respiratory distress syndrome.[57] The cause of the lung damage leading to exudation of fluid and impaired gas exchange is not clearly understood. Possibilities include circulating free fatty acids, activated phospholipase-A, vasoactive substances, or circulating endotoxins. Phospholipase-A is known to disrupt phospholipids and may injure the lung by altering lecithin (which is a normal component of surfactant).[58]

On admission, basic laboratory data including chest x-rays and measurement of arterial blood gases usually do not predict that a serious complication such as adult respiratory distress syndrome may develop.[55] Some degree of arterial hypoxia occurs not infrequently during the first 48 hr in most cases of acute pancreatitis,[59,60] but usually resolves on simple nasal oxygen and chest physiotherapy without causing either clinical or radiologic evidence of respiratory difficulty. Extreme arterial hypoxia tends to correlate with a more severe form of pancreatitis, but even mild pancreatitis may on occasion cause severe hypoxia. Since hypoxia on occasion progresses to a serious form of respiratory insufficiency, measurement of serial blood gases is recommended every 12 hr for the first 2 to 3 days of hospitalization until there is evidence of an uneventful convalescence.

Treatment of pulmonary complications incudes oxygen by nasal catheter or face mask, aspiration of pleural fluid if there is respiratory embarrasssment, chest physiotherapy, and treatment of pneumonia. If pulmonary edema occurs on the basis of congestive heart failure, there is ample justification for the use of diuretic therapy and parenteral digitalization. If pulmonary edema occurs on the basis of an acute respiratory distress syndrome, there are several therapeutic choices. One is to provide endotracheal intubation and assisted ventilation with positive end-expiratory pressure (PEEP).[55] A second choice is to administer salt-poor albumin and diuretic therapy.[59] Since Furosamide (Lasix) increases pancreatic secretion (see Chapter 2), perhaps a different diuretic should be chosen in acute pancreatitis. If pulmonary function deteriorates and there is an increase in respiratory rate associated with fatigue, tracheostomy and assisted ventilation is essential.

9.1.9 Cardiac Complications

A variety of electrocardiographic changes may occur in acute pancreatitis. There may be evidence of electrolyte disturbance such as hypocalcemia or hyperkalemia. An alcoholic cardiomyopathy may induce changes of myocarditis. On rare occasions, there are electrocardiographic changes consistent with an acute myocardial infarction,[54,61] but no confirmation of this event at autopsy. Severe ischemic changes have been documented on the basis of a rapid ectopic tachycardia possibly associated with hypotension.[62]

Occasionally, a significant pericardial effusion results in cardiac tamponade.[53] The possibility of congestive heart failure leading to pulmonary edema has been discussed in the previous section.

9.1.10 Coagulation Abnormalities

Coagulation changes have been documented during acute pancreatitis. While the mechanism or mechanisms are not clearly defined, release of trypsin into the blood stream is thought to be one possible cause.[63-65] This enzyme could then cause severe coagulation abnormalities leading to disseminated intravascular coagulation and the development of microthrombi in various organs. In one study, the early alterations in coagulation factors involve an increase in fibrinogen, fibrinogen-fibrin-related antigen, and prothrombin time.[63]

9.2 LATE COMPLICATIONS

9.2.1 Colon

During acute pancreatitis, there may be spasm of the transverse colon caused by passage of pancreatic exudation from the anterior surface of the pancreas via the two leaves of the transverse mesocolon to the transverse colon (Figure 5). In addition to spasm, there may be evidence of inflammatory changes involving part or all of the transverse colon, and occasionally gaseous distention.[66] As the pancreatitis subsides, there usually is complete resolution of changes involving the transverse colon. Sometimes a portion of the colon remains narrowed, usually the area of the splenic flexure,[66] but occasionally the right colon or hepatic flexure.[67,68] Even in instances of severe stenosis, there is usually no clinical sign or symptom of obstruction. If an abdominal mass develops, or if there are guaiac positive stools, a barium enema should be done and may show a stenotic lesion that is often misinterpreted as a carcinoma of the colon.[66,69,70] At surgery, a large mass may be seen enveloping the tail of the pancreas, omentum, splenic flexure, and occasionally the stomach and the spleen. There is usually evidence of fat necrosis in and around the zone of stricture. This appearance has led to the belief that the cause of the stricture was an intense local reaction to the extravasation of pancreatic exudate through the transverse mesocolon. There is also the possibility that local ischemia and not pericolic inflammation plays a role.[71]

Since at least some strictures tend to resolve in time, the radiologic distinction from carcinoma is essential. A barium enema using air contrast technique may be of help in differentiating destruction of mucosa by carcinoma from pericolonic inflammation.[71] The use of parenteral glucagon to achieve distention of the colon may also be helpful in making this distinction. I have some hesitancy in recommending colonoscopy in an acute inflammatory process involving the colon.

A much more serious complication is fistulization into the colon. A fistula may occur in any portion of the transverse, ascending, or descending colon; most have occurred in the region of the splenic flexure. A fistula usually occurs when a pancreatic pseudocyst or pancreatic abscess erodes into a portion of the colon.[72,73] Occasionally, severe pericolic inflammation alone causes a perforation.[74] The development of a fistula appears to depend on a variety of factors including pressure from a contiguous mass, bacteria in an abscess, infarction of local vessels by fat necrosis, and possibly enzymatic activity. The most important symptoms of a fistula into the colon are massive gastrointestinal bleeding and evidence of severe sepsis.[72-74] Massive gastrointestinal bleeding in association with severe pancreatitis and an abdominal mass should alert the clinician to the possibility of this complication. At surgery, a large mass is usually encountered with an intense inflammatory reaction agglutinating all tissues in the vicinity. The surgical approach involves a proximal colostomy, drainage of pseudocyst or abscess, and ligation of bleeding vessels. A fistula may penetrate not only the colon but also the small intestine or stomach. On rare occasions, many weeks or even months after successful surgical drainage of a pancreatic abscess, a fistula burrows from colon to abdominal wall if there is residual suppuration adjacent to the colon.

9.2.2 Small Intestine

Pancreatic exudation may extravasate through the mesentery of the small intestine causing an ileus of the small intestine (sentinal loops). At times, the ileus is confined to the distal small bowel or cecum and may resemble a cecal volvulus (Figure 6). In general, sentinal loops disappear with clinical improvement.

Occasionally, there is substantial fat necrosis in the mesentery of the small intestine causing small-bowel obstruction.[43,75,76] Severe fat necrosis leading to thrombosis of arteries and veins may result in infarction of the small intestine.[75-77] The symptoms that suggest this serious complication include a prolonged ileus, persisting partial small-bowel obstruction, and local peritoneal signs.[76-77] The important clinical point to be reemphasized is that medication for pain must not be given until the clinician is fully satisfied he is not camouflaging an important complication of pancreatitis.

A pancreatic pseudocyst or abscess may erode into a loop of small intestine causing massive gastrointestinal bleeding or sepsis (Figure 23).

Pancreatic exudation in the root of the mesentery may cause obstruction of the duodenum in the form of a superior mesenteric artery syndrome.[78] This complication should resolve with subsidence of pancreatitis. In addition to an organic obstruction such as this, a profound duodenal ileus may occur which is clearly visible on the flat plate of the abdomen by virtue of the fact that the entire duodenal segment is outlined with air in the form of an "air cast" (Figure 8). Severe duodenal obstruction may occur in chronic pancreatitis. This will be discussed in Chapter 16.

9.2.3 Pancreatic Pseudocyst

(a) Definition and Pathophysiology. A pancreatic pseudocyst is a collection of enzyme-rich pancreatic fluid containing variable amounts of tissue debris and blood. It occurs on the basis of autodigestion and liquefaction of pancreatic tissue during severe pancreatitis associated with necrosis and perhaps hemorrhage. Adjacent structures tend to contain this amorphous collection of fluid reasonably well. The interface between the collection and neighboring structures is at first composed of fibrinous material and granulation tissue which in time develops into a relatively sturdy "capsule" that appears to resist rupture reasonably well.[79] It should be emphasized that a pseudocyst is not a true cyst in that it is lined by inflammatory tissue and not epithelium.

A pseudocyst appears to have no particular predilection for the head, body, or tail of the pancreas.[80,81] Several pseudocysts may be present simultaneously.[80] The size of a pseudocyst is variable. Expansion of a cyst implies that a duct or ductule is continuing to elaborate pancreatic fluid that "feeds" the cyst. Expansion also appears to depend on pancreatic ductal obstruction such that the pseudocyst cannot empty itself properly into the larger pancreatic ducts. Partial or total obstruction of the main pancreatic duct in association with a pseudocyst has been demonstrated on numerous occasions.[82-85] Retrograde filling of a pseudocyst by ERCP further substantiates a continuity between the pancreatic ductal system and the cyst,[81,83-85] and suggests that spontaneous decompression of a pancreatic pseudocyst depends to a large extent on resolution of ductal obstruction. An alternative explanation for expansion of a pseudocyst is that tissue debris within the cyst is osmotically active and encourages insorption of interstitial fluid through the capsule. If this explanation

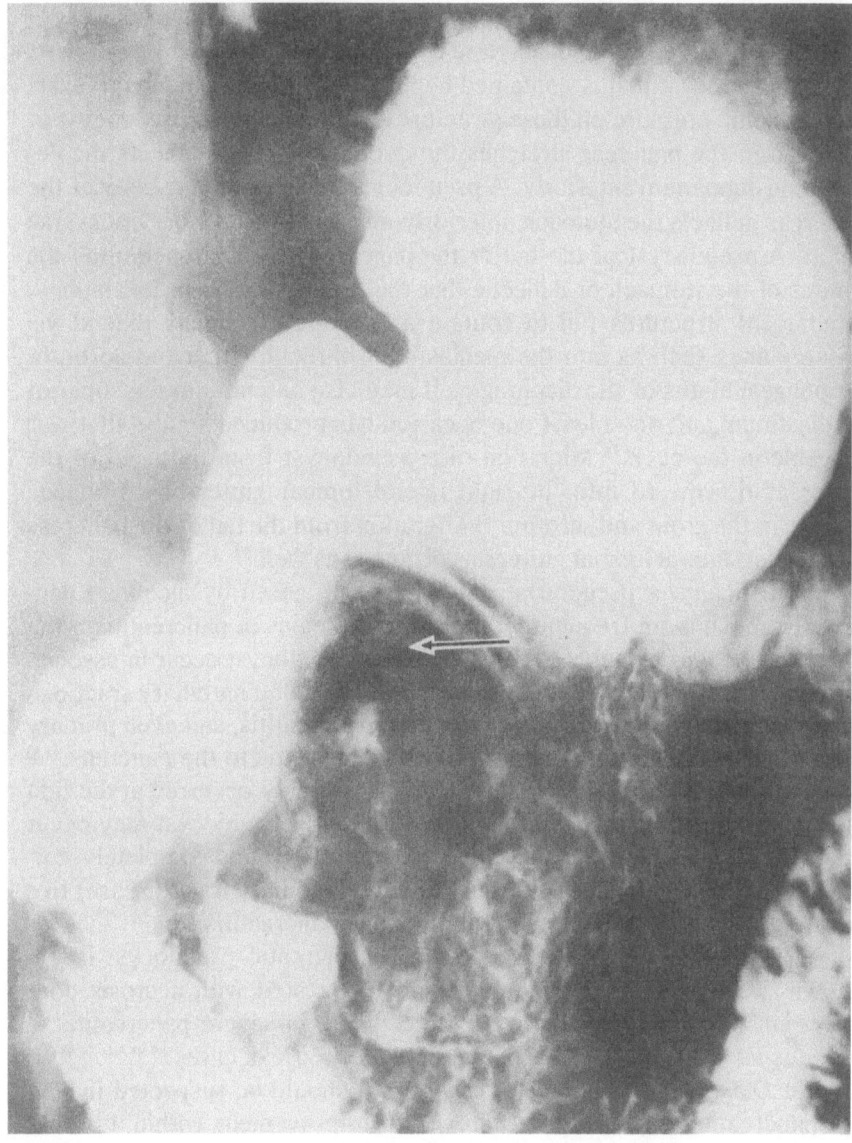

FIGURE 23 *Gastrointestinal Series Showing Pancreatic Abscess.* The greater curvature of the antrum is displaced superiorly. Amorphous bubbles of air are visible just below this deflection (arrow) as well as barium that has extravasated from the third portion of the duodenum into the pancreatic bed. A duodenal diverticulum is visible on the inner aspect of the descending duodenum. Several days after surgical drainage of this abscess, the patient underwent a fatal massive exsanguination from erosion of the abscess into a major duodenal vessel. The etiology of the pancreatitis was biliary tract disease.

were correct, the largest pseudocyst would contain fluid with relatively low concentrations of amylase (due to dilution), yet even large pseudocysts tend to have very high amylase concentrations.

A pseudocyst that is contained by adjacent structures tends to exert at least some pressure on these structures. For example, a pseudocyst of the head of the pancreas stretches the duodenal loop or deflects the descending duodenum anteriorly. A pseudocyst arising from the body of the pancreas deflects the stomach anteriorly and may depress the transverse colon. A pseudocyst of the tail of the pancreas may encroach upon the fundus of the stomach or deflect either the splenic flexure or left kidney. If adjacent structures fail to contain a pseudocyst, it may extend via tissue planes such as into the mediastinum through either the aortic or esophageal hiatus of the diaphragm. It may also extend into the superior mediastinum and on at least one occasion has produced a mass that was palpable in the neck.[86] Migration of a pseudocyst from the head of the pancreas downward into the right lateral lumbar gutter has produced masses in the groin and scrotum.[87] Migration from the tail of the pancreas into the left lateral lumbar gutter has occurred as well.[87]

Statistically, a pseudocyst appears to be caused by alcoholic pancreatitis much more frequently than other etiologies of pancreatitis.[80,88–91] Nonetheless, individual cases of pancreatic pseudocyst occur in association with most etiologies of acute pancreatitis including biliary tract disease, traumatic pancreatitis, postoperative pancreatitis, and even primary carcinoma of the pancreas and carcinoma metastatic to the pancreas.[92,93] Since a substrate of chronic pancreatitis has already occurred at the first episode of alcoholic pancreatitis, it is clear that a pseudocyst may occur at any stage in the natural history of pancreatitis from a completely normal pancreas (as in pancreatitis associated with biliary tract disease) to a severely damaged pancreas (such as alcoholic pancreatitis).

(b) Incidence. The true incidence of pancreatic pseudocyst is unknown. Mild edematous pancreatitis not associated with necrosis does not result in a pseudocyst. On the other hand, in severe pancreatitis, a pseudocyst has been reported in approximately 50% of cases.[89,91,94]

(c) Diagnosis. A pancreatic pseudocyst should be suspected in severe pancreatitis especially if there is no improvement within 1 week. Approximately 80% of cysts are associated with at least some abdominal discomfort, nausea, and vomiting. Temperature may be either normal or elevated. White blood count is usually at least slightly elevated. An abdominal mass is appreciated in only 30% to 40% of patients. It is important to remember that a tender abdominal mass may be caused by a phlegmon of the pancreas rather than a pseudocyst. A phlegmon represents marked tissue inflammation and bears no relationship to a pseudocyst.[87,95]

Serum amylase is increased in 50% to 85% but by no means in all cases.[80,81,88-91] There may be abnormalities of liver function tests but there is no pattern that is diagnostic of a pseudocyst. Hypocalcemia may occur if the pancreatitis is severe.

A plain film of the abdomen may show separation of the contour of the stomach from that of the transverse colon indicative of a mass in the lesser sac (either a phlegmon or pseudocyst). A gastrointestinal series may show an indentation in any portion of the stomach from the high fundic area to the pylorus (Figure 24). A lateral view may show the

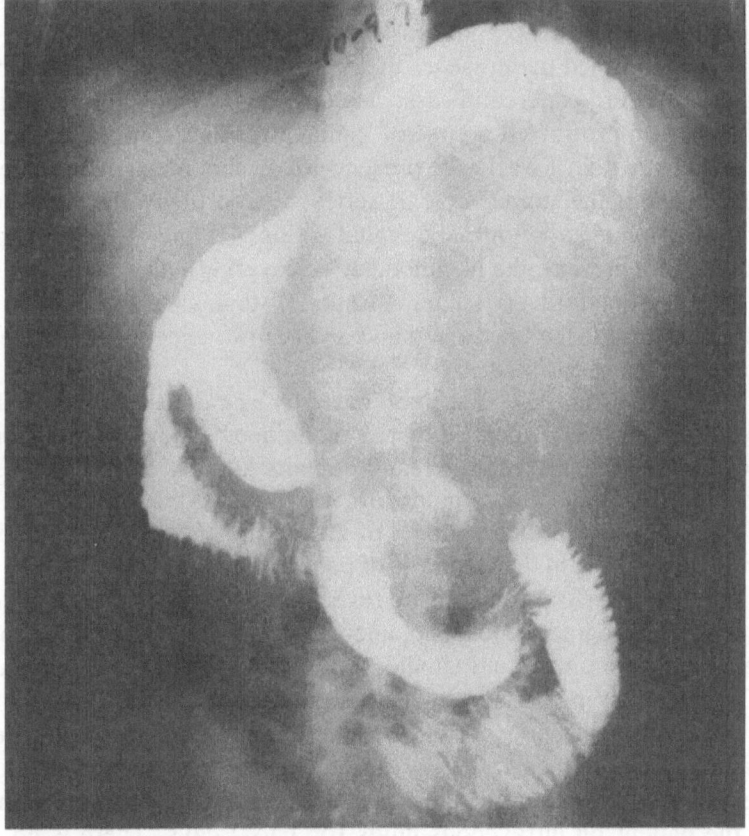

FIGURE 24 *Gastrointestinal Series Showing Pancreatic Pseudocyst.* A very large pancreatic pseudocyst displaces and indents the greater curvature of the stomach to the right, and depresses the ligament of Treitz. There is marked thickening of the folds of the descending duodenum. After cystgastrostomy, the patient continued to have episodes of pancreatitis thought attributable to alcohol. Several intravenous cholangiograms were normal. When an oral cholecystogram was finally performed during an asymptomatic interval, extensive cholelithiasis was demonstrated. (Courtesy of Dr. R. Langevin.)

presence of a very large mass posterior to the stomach. An even better view to confirm the draping of the posterior wall of the stomach over a retrogastric mass is an ''across-the-table'' lateral view with the patient in the supine position. Unfortunately, from a diagnostic standpoint, a large phlegmon of the pancreas may produce a radiologic picture identical to a pseudocyst (Figure 25). A barium enema examination may show extrinsic compression on the transverse colon if the pseudocyst impinges on this area. An intravenous pyelogram may show depression and medial displacement of the left kidney in the presence of a large pseudocyst of the tail of the pancreas (Figure 21). Chest x-ray has revealed a pleural effusion in approximately 20% of cases reported.

Diagnostic ultrasound is at present the most reliable diagnostic test in identifying a pancreatic pseudocyst (Figures 14 and 15). In one study, this technique confirmed the presence of a pseudocyst in approximately 50% of cases of severe pancreatitis associated with at least one of the following features: a protracted course of pancreatitis that showed no sign of improvement within 1 week; the presence of an abdominal mass; anterior displacement of the stomach on GI series; a persistingly elevated serum amylase; or evidence of intraabdominal sepsis.[89] If one or more of these features is not present, the likelihood of discovering a pancreatic pseudocyst by ultrasound is very small. Additional studies have confirmed the accuracy of diagnostic ultrasound and a very low incidence of false positive and false negative studies.[81,85,89,91,96,97]

The usefulness of a C-T scan is limited by lack of general availability. A pseudocyst is well visualized by this technique.[92] The demonstration of a pseudocyst and marked pancreatic ductal dilatation on C-T scan suggests the possibility of a carcinoma of the head of the pancreas as the etiology.[92] In general, the reliability of ultrasound has thus far minimized the role of C-T scan in the diagnosis of pancreatic pseudocyst.

If diagnostic ultrasound fails to reveal a pseudocyst, the technique of endoscopic retrograde cholangiopancreatography may reveal its presence. Diagnostic ultrasound should be the first step because it is safer. ERCP cautiously performed by skilled endoscopists is also safe but on rare occasions a pseudocyst can be converted into an abscess. Whenever a pseudocyst is demonstrated by this technique, the patient should be observed very closely in the hospital. A reasonable approach is to maintain the patient on intravenous fluids for 1 to 2 days. There is no firm consensus about the need for prophylactic antibiotic therapy.

Arteriography may reveal stretching and draping of pancreatic vessels around a pseudocyst. This radiologic technique has generally been replaced by diagnostic ultrasound for the diagnosis of a pancreatic pseudocyst.

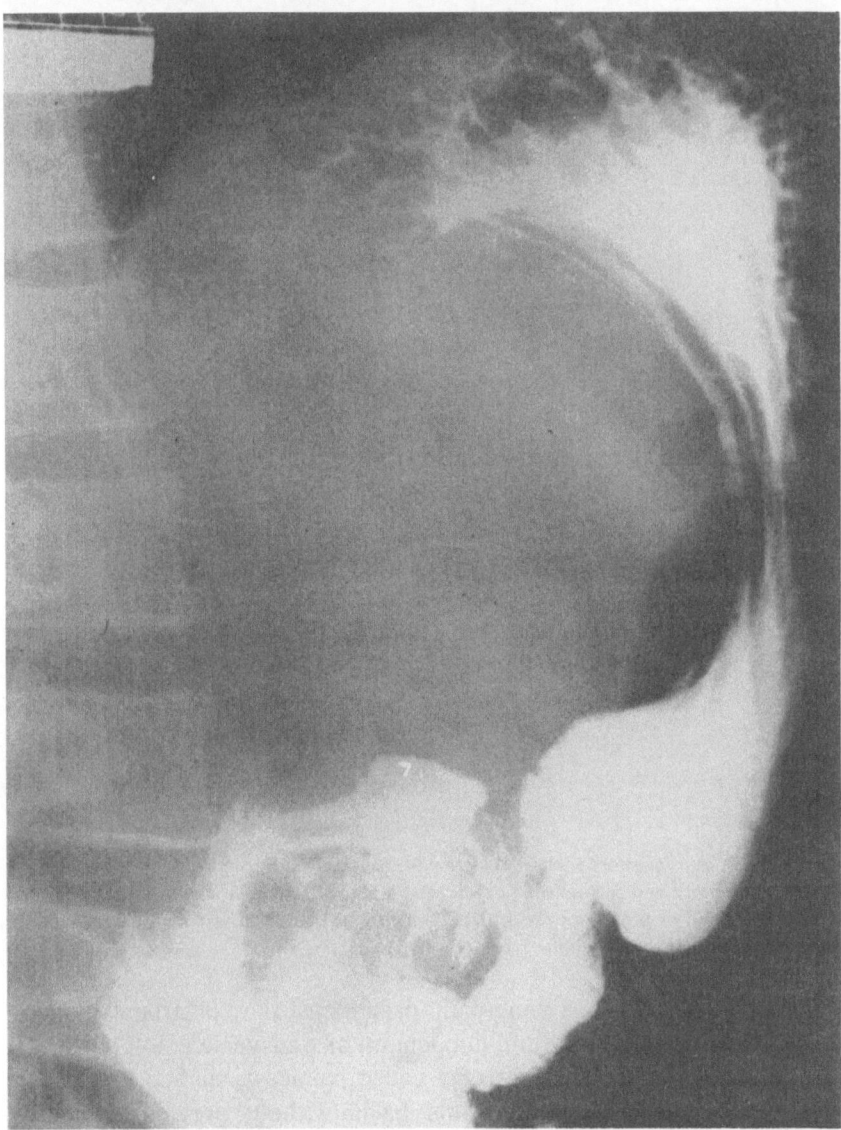

FIGURE 25A *Gastrointestinal Series in Pancreatitis.* There is marked anterior displacement of the posterior wall of the stomach by a retrogastric mass. This could be either a phlegmon or a pseudocyst.

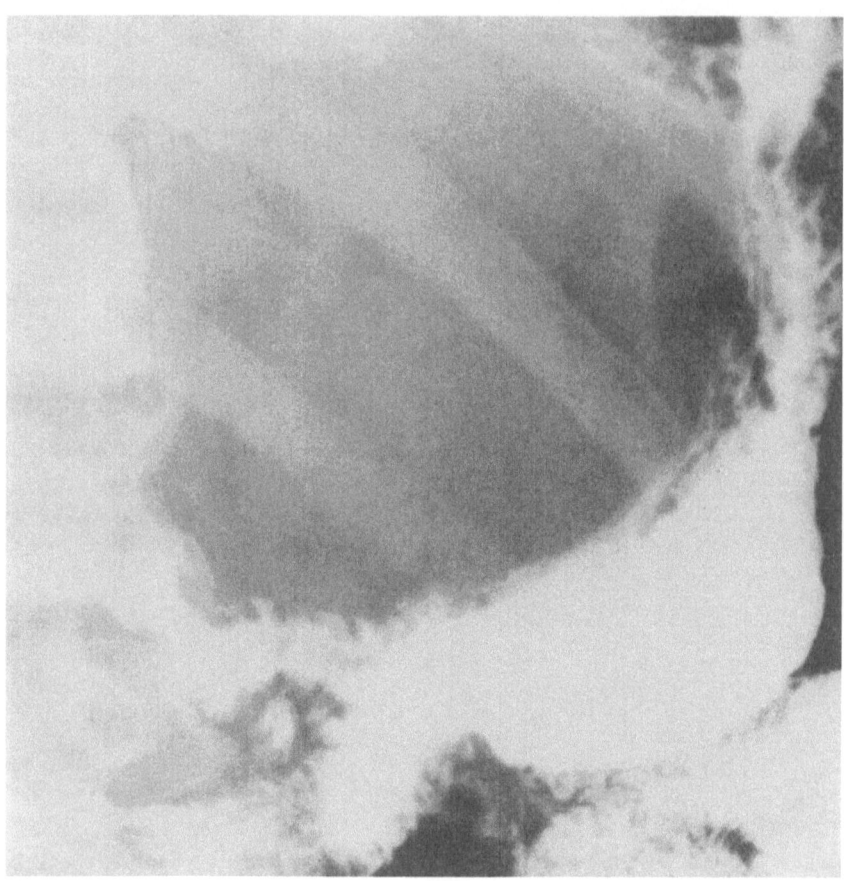

FIGURE 25B Gastrointestinal Series in Pancreatitis. There is marked extrinsic compression of the lesser curvature and antrum of the stomach by a large retrogastric mass. This could be either a phlegmon or a pseudocyst. In A, at surgery, a phlegmon was identified. In B, at surgery, a pseudocyst was identified.

(d) Complications. A pancreatic pseudocyst may obstruct a contiguous structure such as antrum, duodenum, or transverse colon. Obstruction of the common bile duct may cause painless jaundice.[26–29,31,32] On occasion, jaundice occurs on this basis without previous signs or symtpoms of pancreatitis.[32]

A much more serious complication is rupture of a pseudocyst into the peritoneal cavity.[29] Marked expansion of a pseudocyst and severe abdominal pain may herald this complication. (An alternative explanation for rapid expansion would be bleeding into a pseudocyst.) Treatment for rupture into the peritoneal cavity is surgical. Mortality owing to this complication is generally greater than 50%.

Alternatively, a pseudocyst may rupture into an adjacent structure such as the colon,[98-100] duodenum,[29,100] stomach,[100,101] esophagus,[100] or common bile duct.[102] Rupture of a pseudocyst into an adjacent hollow viscus can be suspected clinically by the disappearance of an abdominal mass, relief of abdominal pain, and development of gastrointestinal bleeding. Repeat diagnostic ultrasound study showing disappearance of a cystic mass confirms this clinical impression. If the cyst decompresses without massive bleeding or uncontrollable sepsis, surgical treatment may be unnecessary. If bleeding is brisk or sepsis occurs, prompt surgical intervention is usually necessary.

A pancreatic pseudocyst that invades the spleen may cause either rupture of the spleen or brisk bleeding from the splenic artery.[9,14,99] A splenic complication is suggested by a palpable mass in the left upper quadrant of the abdomen, abdominal pain, and pain referred to the left shoulder if there is diaphragmatic irritation caused by subcapsular hematoma or splenic rupture. This clinical impression can be substantiated by arteriography or by a liver–spleen scan.

A pseudocyst may rupture through the diaphragm causing a left pleural effusion,[103,104] and may subsequently erode from the pleural space into a bronchus causing a cyst-bronchial fistula.[29] Rupture through the diaphragm may also involve the pericardium.[29] Alternatively, a pseudocyst may first enter the mediastinum via the aortic or esophageal hiatus of the diaphragm,[105-107] and then rupture into the esophagus,[100] or more commonly into the pleura on either side causing a pleural effusion.[29,51,52,105,106] In most instances, abdominal symptoms are minimal. The most characteristic symptoms are shortness of breath and cough.[52] Pleural effusions caused by pancreatic pseudocysts are usually large, recur rapidly after thoracentesis, and require intensive medical management and if need be surgical intervention to resect or drain the pseudocyst.[52]

Hemorrhage associated with a pseudocyst may be a very serious complication. It can occur as a result of contiguous inflammation of an adjacent structure such as stomach, duodenum, or transverse colon resulting in mucosal oozing of blood. A pseudocyst may cause thrombosis of the splenic or portal vein resulting in portal hypertension and bleeding varices. Fistulization of a pseudocyst into an adjacent structure such as colon,[98] stomach,[101] and common bile duct[102] can cause bleeding that may become severe. Occasionally, bleeding occurs from the cyst itself. At times, the pseudocyst fills with blood from diffuse oozing from the capsule. At other times, the cyst encompasses a major artery which then becomes part of the cyst wall. With weakening of this artery, a false aneurysm may develop. A major bleed may be heralded by a rapidly expanding abdominal mass, a bruit over the mass, increasing abdominal pain, and a decrease in the hematocrit.[29,108] The vessel that is most commonly involved is the splenic artery, but the gastroduodenal artery or any blood vessel in the vicinity of a pseudocyst may also cause brisk bleeding,[109,110] even the abdominal aorta itself.[111] If the serum amylase is elevated, one should suspect that an aneurysm of the aorta was caused by a pancreatic pseudocyst.[111] At times, bleeding from a pseudocyst gushes from the main pancreatic duct into the duodenum.[112] It should be noted that bleeding via the pancreatic duct may occur not only on the basis of a pancreatic pseudocyst but also on the basis of erosion of a splenic aneurysm into the substance of the pancreas and then into the pancreatic duct.[16] At times, the etiology of a splenic artery aneurysm is chronic pancreatitis.[16]

In summary, massive bleeding as a complication of pancreatic pseudocyst may occur via the common bile duct, pancreatic duct, or an adjacent hollow viscus. It may take place in the peritoneal cavity or retroperitoneal space in association with rupture of a false aneurysm. The cyst itself may fill with blood and expand rapidly. Massive bleeding by any of these mechanisms is usually an indication for urgent surgery. Preoperative evaluation is helped enormously by arteriography and at times by endoscopy.

A pancreatic pseudocyst that becomes secondarily infected in essence becomes a pancreatic abscess. A pseudocyst that perforates into an adjacent hollow viscus such as the transverse colon may become secondarily infected and become a septic focus.

A pancreatic pseudocyst may cause chronic pancreatic ascites especially in a cachectic patient without overt signs or symptoms of acute pancreatitis or pseudocyst. These last two complications will be discussed in detail in subsequent sections.

(e) Medical Treatment of Pancreatic Pseudocyst. Evidence is accumulating that most pancreatic pseudocysts that occur during the course of acute pancreatitis resolve spontaneously.[89,91,96,113] Resolution appears to correlate with subsidence of acute inflammation. The important link may be resolution of ductal obstruction such that a pseudocyst then empties its contents via pancreatic ducts into the duodenum. Once a pancreatic pseudocyst has been documented, vigorous medical treatment should be undertaken in accordance with the basic principles outlined in Chapter 8 on treatment of acute pancreatitis. These efforts usually include the use of a nasogastric tube to aspirate acid, careful attention to fluid and electrolyte needs of the patient with emphasis on administration of colloid for hypoalbuminemia and blood for anemia, and maintenance of the nutritional needs of the patient with total parenteral nutrition. Liquid antacids can be administered via the nasogastric tube in order to neutralize gastric contents fully. If there is marked hypersecretion of acid that cannot be successfully neutralized, consideration can be given to the use of Cimetidine parenterally. The availability of total parenteral nutrition permits medical surveillance and therapy for an indefinite period of time if there is no urgent indication for surgery.

Resolution of the pseudocyst can be monitored by periodic ultrasonic examinations. Once there has been substantial improvement, the nasogastric tube can be discontinued and antacid therapy continued by mouth. Use of an elemental diet, small frequent feedings, emphasis on foods that are primarily carbohydrate, and other dietary considerations are identical to measures that are utilized in the recovery phase of acute pancreatitis.

Recently, there have been several reports of successful puncture and aspiration of pancreatic pseudocysts by introduction of a thin needle through the abdominal wall with the help of ultrasonic guidance.[84,85,114] The safety record has been impressive as well as ease of cyst puncture. It appears not to matter whether the needle tracks through the stomach or intestine, but each author has expressed caution lest the needle penetrate the liver. On occasion, evacuation of the cyst via a needle has apparently decompressed the cyst permanently. However, in most instances the cyst has reappeared in a matter of only a few weeks. If cyst puncture has value, it may be to decompress a rapidly expanding cyst in a patient who is too ill or debilitated to undergo emergency surgery. Presumably, with the availability of total parenteral nutrition, a surgical delay of even a few weeks would be of great nutritional value. More extensive investigation into this approach is required in order to establish its usefulness.

(f) Surgical Treatment. There are several indications for urgent surgical treatment. One is secondary infection of a pseudocyst such that it becomes a pancreatic abscess. Another indication is massive bleeding whether it be within the cyst itself, within the gastrointestinal tract as a result of a fistulous communication, or within the retroperitoneum or peritoneum as a result of leakage from the pseudocyst. A third indication is either frank perforation of the cyst into the peritoneal cavity or imminent perforation as suggested by rapid enlargement of the cyst.

There are other indications that can be classified either semiurgent or elective. These include compression of the common bile duct by a pseudocyst of the head of the pancreas, chronic pancreatic ascites caused by a leaking pseudocyst, and fistulous communication of a pseudocyst to the pleural space causing chronic respiratory symptoms.

The preferred surgical treatment of a pancreatic pseudocyst is anastomosis of the cyst to an adjacent hollow viscus.[81] A cyst of the head of the pancreas is often anastomosed to the duodenum, and a cyst of the body of the pancreas is anastomosed to the posterior wall of the stomach.

A cyst of the tail of the pancreas at times is decompressed by using a loop of jejunum with a Roux-en-Y anastomosis. If a pseudocyst of the tail of the pancreas involves the spleen, a splenectomy must be done in order to avoid postoperative complications such as hemorrhage from the spleen or from varices caused by splenic vein thrombosis.[115] Under these circumstances, the preferred surgical approach is distal pancreatectomy (including the pseudocyst) and splenectomy.[9]

An important technical detail in the anastomosis of the pseudocyst to the posterior wall of the stomach is first to aspirate the retrogastric mass by inserting a needle through the posterior wall of the stomach prior to actually incising the posterior wall with a scalpel. This detail is important because on rare occasions an aneurysm of a vessel (such as splenic artery) masquerades both clinically and by ultrasonic examination as a pseudocyst, and under these circumstances the aspirate is arterial blood rather than the expected cloudy or brownish enzyme-rich pancreatic fluid.

Following the anastomosis of a pseudocyst to the stomach, the cyst usually shrinks very rapidly and may be totally invisible several weeks later on a gastrointestinal series and diagnostic ultrasound.[96] A complication of cystgastrostomy is bleeding from the anastomotic site possibly as a result of erosive effects of gastric acid. The recurrence rate after an anastomotic procedure is approximately 5% and at times is related to additional bouts of pancreatitis.[89] Another reason for recurrent pseudocyst would be persisting ductal stenosis after surgical decompression of the initial pseudocyst.

An alternative to internal anastomosis is external drainage with creation of a pancreatic fistula to the skin. Although closure of the fistula has occurred with the use of an elemental diet,[116] the possibility of a persistingly draining fistula to the skin makes this a much less desirable alternative. External drainage is therefore reserved for the rare situation in which the capsule of the pseudocyst has not matured sufficiently to permit an anastomosis with an adjacent structure. It has been assumed that maturation of the capsule requires at least 6 weeks from the onset of the pseudocyst. Since a 6-week waiting period in the absence of complications is desirable in order to determine whether a pseudocyst will resolve medically, this interval is acceptable. It is reassuring that even if surgery is required on an urgent basis within the 6-week period, there is a possibility that the wall of the cyst will have already matured sufficiently to accommodate internal drainage.[90] Additional experience with diagnostic ultrasound will probably define more precisely the period of time that is required for maturation of a pseudocyst.

With a recurrence rate of approximately 4% to 5%[89] and an overall surgical mortality of 11%,[88] the seriousness of this complication is readily apparent.

Other techniques for the management of pancreatic pseudocyst have been advocated but not yet fully tested. One is the surgical evacuation of a cyst followed by corrosion with 20% sodium hydroxide.[117] It would be of interest to determine whether aspiration followed by corrosion could be achieved following puncture of a pseudocyst through the abdominal wall. A second experimental approach is the purposeful reduction of blood pressure with the use of intravenous trimethaphan (Arfonad) in order to stop bleeding associated with a pseudocyst.[81,118] The safety and usefulness of this approach will require considerable study.

(g) Prognosis. The overall mortality of a pancreatic pseudocyst is approximately 14%[90] with a surgical mortality of 11%.[88] Since the majority of pseudocysts occur in alcoholic pancreatitis, the general health of many patients is marginal, especially if there is coexisting alcoholic hepatitis which by itself increases surgical mortality. Some complications of a pseudocyst are associated with a mortality of at least 50%: sepsis, free perforation into the peritoneal cavity, and major bleeding either into the cyst, the peritoneal cavity, or into a hollow viscus.

A particularly difficult problem is the treatment of an asymptomatic pancreatic pseudocyst that does not resolve during the initial 6 weeks of observation. Evidence is accumulating that a pseudocyst can usually be followed safely during an initial 6-week period as long as a specific complication does not occur. However, the natural history of a pseudocyst is capricious, and the threat of a complication may be serious enough to warrant surgical drainage of most pancreatic pseudocysts that do not resolve on medical treatment within 6 weeks. It remains to be shown whether the use of diagnostic ultrasound or other techniques will improve our understanding of the natural history of pancreatic pseudocysts so that patients who are at greatest risk of developing a serious complication can be selected for surgery either urgently during the first 6 weeks or electively beyond this interval.

9.2.4 Pancreatic Abscess

(a) Definition and Pathophysiology. A pancreatic abscess is a collection of purulent and necrotic pancreatic tissue. It occurs if an episode of pancreatitis is severe enough to cause parenchymal necrosis, and if devitalized pancreatic and retroperitoneal tissue become secondarily infected. Usually, there are multiple foci of infected necrotic debris rather than a recognizable discrete abscess cavity that can be easily drained surgically.

On rare occasions, a pancreatic abscess is caused by secondary infection of a pseudocyst. In these circumstances, the surgical drainage can be accomplished much more easily.

The manner in which necrotic pancreatic tissue becomes secondarily infected is not entirely clear. Possible routes of infection include lymphatic pathways, the bloodstream, and even the swallowing of organisms that normally reside in the oral cavity.[119] The most likely pathway is migration of bacteria from the transverse colon to the nearby pancreatic bed. This pathway seems logical because the pancreatic inflammatory response may bathe the transverse colon. The organisms that most commonly cause a pancreatic abscess are either *E. coli* or a combination of coliform bacteria.[23,24,120-122]

Most pancreatic abscesses develop in the lesser sac after this space fills with pancreatic exudation and tissue debris. From this location an abscess may extend to both subphrenic areas (particularly on the left) causing secondary abscesses. It may also tract down behind either the ascending or descending colon (or both) and culminate as a pelvic abscess. It may follow the mesentery of the small intestine and cause secondary abscesses, or fistulize into the stomach, small intestine, or colon. At times, a pancreatic abscess fistulizes through the diaphragm causing a severe mediastinal infection. It is important to emphasize that aside from the relatively uncommon solitary infected pseudocyst, a pancreatic abscess tends to be a multilocular spreading infection.

(b) Etiology and Incidence. A pancreatic abscess may develop in pancreatitis of various etiologies including biliary tract disease, alcohol, and postoperative pancreatitis. Most cases have been reported in association with alcohol. An abscess may occur during the first clinical episode of pancreatitis or during a recurrence.

The incidence of pancreatic abscess is estimated to be 3% to 4% of all cases of pancreatitis.[121-123] Since this complication occurs only in a milieu of pancreatic necrosis, it would not be expected to follow an episode of edematous pancreatitis.

(c) Clinical Diagnosis. A pancreatic abscess generally is recognized 2 to 4 weeks after an episode of severe pancreatitis.[24] The most common sequence is subsidence of acute pancreatitis and then the development of fever and increasing abdominal tenderness and pain.[24,120,121,124] Less commonly a pancreatic abscess develops without a recognizable lull. The clinical features have been well described.[23,24,95,119,123-125] Almost all patients are febrile, either low-grade in the range of 100–101°F, frequently 102–103°F, and on occasion 104–105°F associated with shaking chills. If a patient with a suspected pancreatic abscess remains afebrile, a look at the medication list may reveal that an antipyretic medication such as aspirin

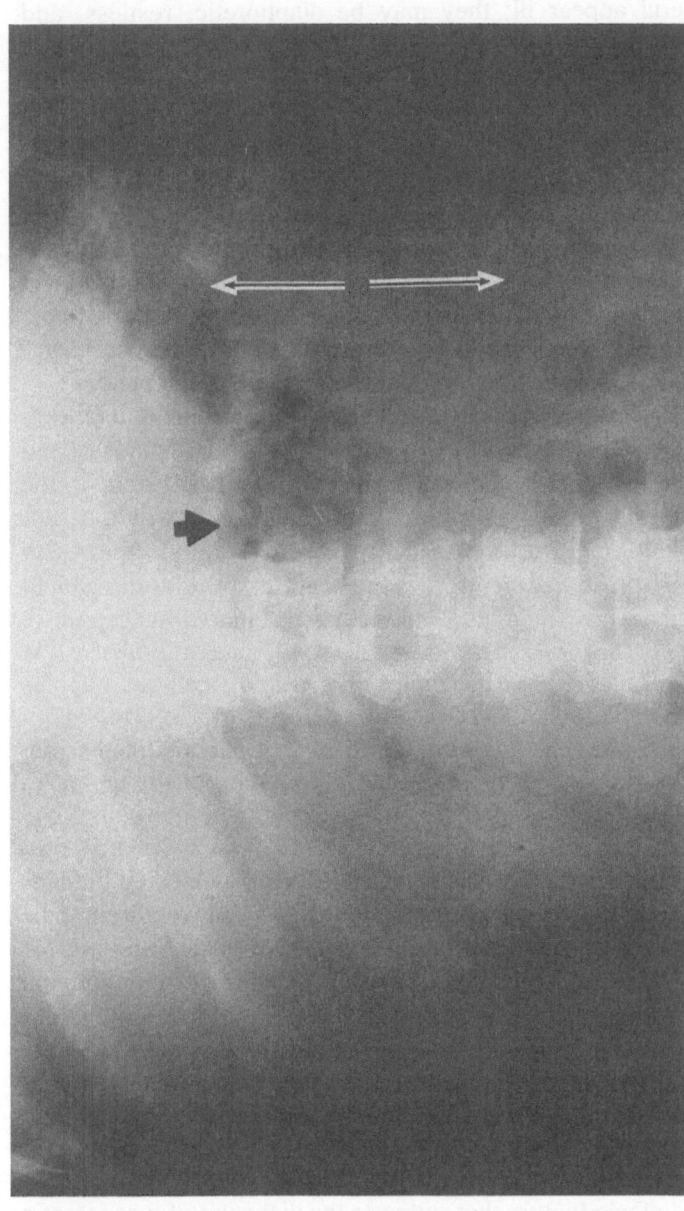

FIGURE 26 Plain Roengtenogram of the Abdomen: Pancreatic Abscess. Amorphous air bubbles are visible in the pancreatic bed especially to the left of the spine (short black arrow). Note also that the contour of the transverse colon in the lower left is widely separated from the gastric contour in the upper left (vertical arrows) indicating marked pancreatic exudation. At surgery, a very large pancreatic abscess was encountered that extended behind both the ascending and descending colon. Years later, a fecal fistula that had undoubtedly originated as a result of suppuration behind the mid-descending colon eroded to the skin. This pancreatic abscess was a result of pancreatitis in association with biliary tract disease.

or Tylenol has been given on a regular basis and has suppressed fever. The pulse is usually in excess of 100, and frequently 120–130. Blood pressure is variable. Many patients have an increased respiratory rate. All patients in general appear ill; they may be diaphoretic, restless, and uncomfortable.

The level of abdominal pain ranges from severe to relatively mild. Anorexia, nausea, and vomiting are common. A tender abdominal mass is palpable in less than one half of patients. Abdominal tenderness is frequent even in the absence of a mass.

White blood count is almost always increased to levels of 13,000 to 25,000, occasionally higher and rarely lower. Serum amylase and lipase values are increased in only 30% to 50% of patients. Serum albumin level may be surprisingly low (at times below 2.5 gm%); serum alkaline phosphatase and bilirubin are likely to be increased. Serum glucose is frequently increased perhaps as a result of severe necrosis of the pancreas.

Pancreatic abscess should be suspected if there is clinical deterioration associated with fever, leukocytosis, and tender abdominal mass, and especially if there had been a short interval of improvement prior to the deterioration. The diagnosis is strongly supported by the growth of organisms on blood cultures. The importance of positive blood cultures in confirming pancreatic abscess reinforces the belief that antibiotics should not be used routinely for pancreatitis unless there is biliary tract sepsis.

(d) Radiologic Diagnosis. The presence of a pancreatic abscess is confirmed by the radiologic visualization of multiple small gas bubbles behind the stomach on plain film of the abdomen (Figure 26). This radiologic feature can be demonstrated in 20% to 25% of pancreatic abscesses.[23,24] If a pancreatic abscess is suspected, a daily film of the abdomen should be obtained and scrutinized for the characteristic mottled "soap bubble" appearance of gas in a pancreatic abscess. If an abdominal radiograph is underexposed, air bubbles may not be visible. Once air bubbles are identified, additional views of the abdomen may be required to be certain that the air is extraluminal and behind the stomach, and not for example in transverse colon or splenic flexure. One view is an upright film of the abdomen, which may cause coalescence of multiple air bubbles into a convincing air–fluid level. A lateral film in the upright position is particularly helpful especially if the posterior wall of the stomach is outlined by a nasogastric tube (Figure 27). Another method is to instill a small amount of Gastrografin and rotate the patient laterally in order to confirm localization of gas bubbles in a retrogastric position (Figure 28).

Another radiologic feature that supports the diagnosis of a pancreatic abscess is extravasation of barium into the abscess cavity (Figure 23). This results from prior fistulization of the abscess into the gastrointestinal

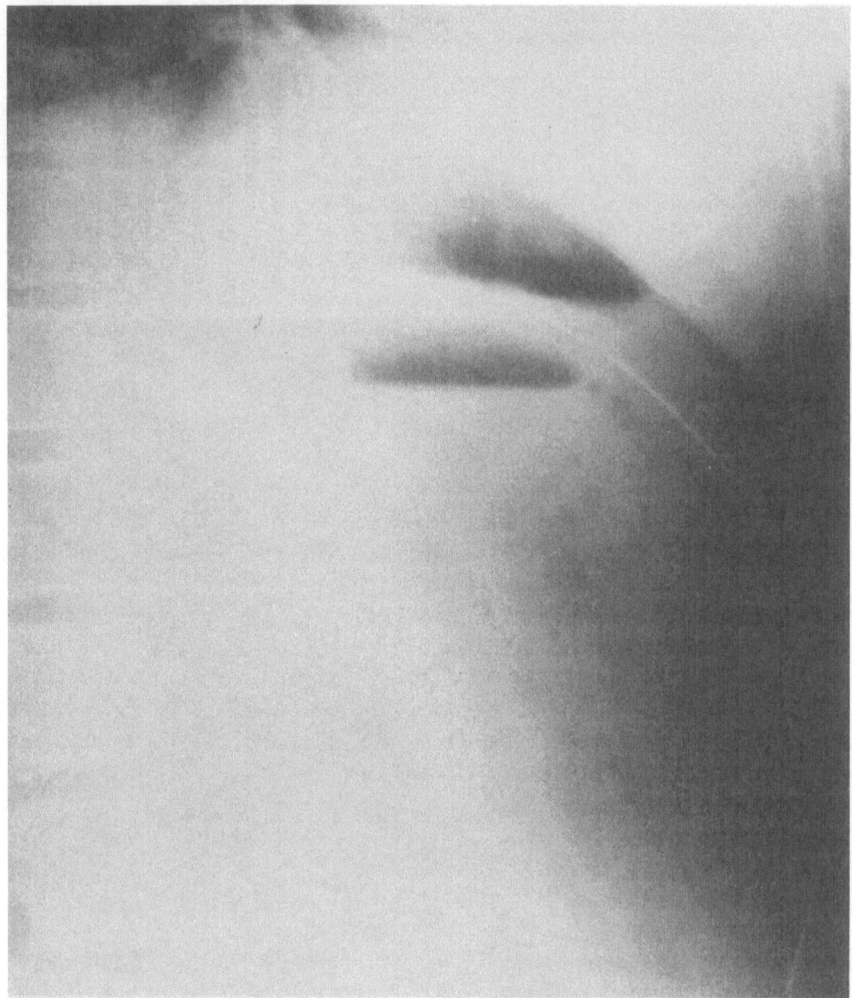

FIGURE 27 *Upright View of Abdomen with Lateral Projection: Pancreatic Abscess.* Two air–fluid levels are visible. Small scattered bubbles of gas are also visible just behind the radiopaque nasogastric tube which is displaced far anteriorly by a retrogastric mass. The air–fluid level above the nasogastric tube is within stomach. The air–fluid level beneath the nasogastric tube represents a large pancreatic abscess that was drained surgically. There is inflammation and fluid at the lung bases.

tract. Other radiologic features that may occur include anterior displacement of the stomach, depression of the ligament of Treitz, depression of the transverse colon and splenic flexure, and stretching and widening of the duodenal loop with intense mucosal inflammatory changes of the duodenum. These various changes may also occur on the basis of a large

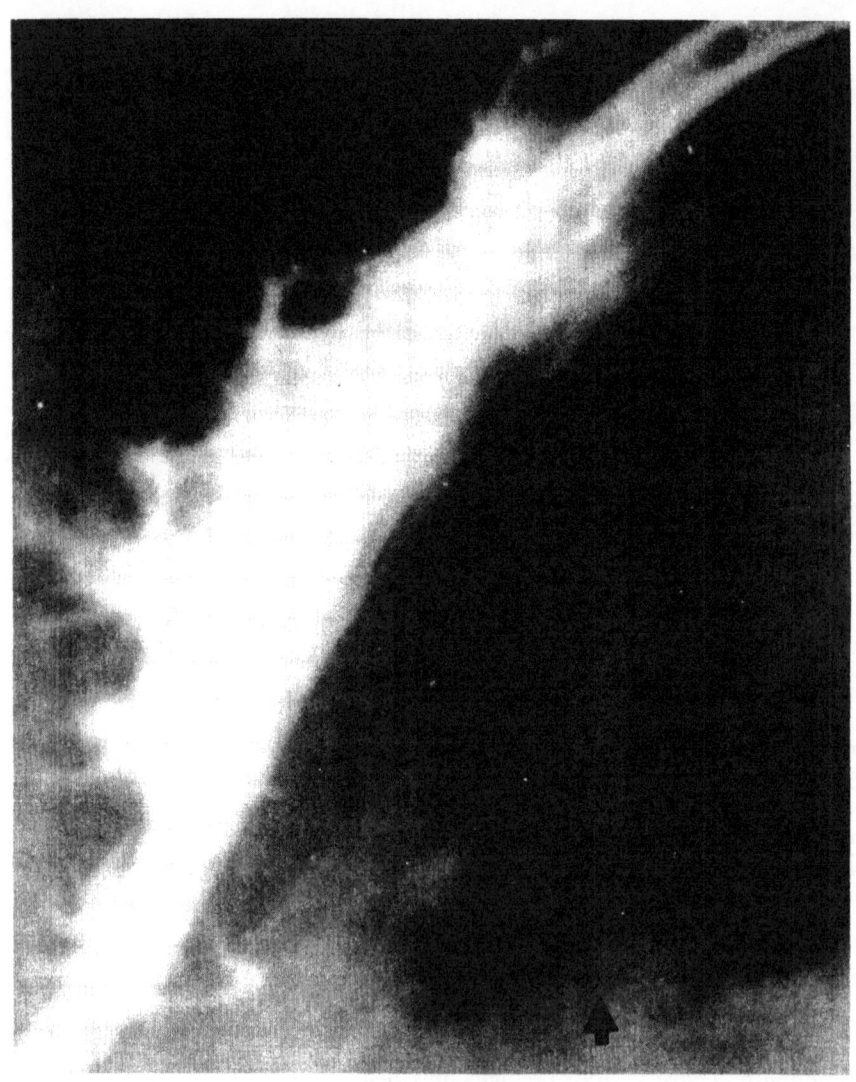

FIGURE 28 Pancreatic Abscess. There is a large collection of mottled air (arrow). Radiologic confirmation that this abscess is behind the stomach and therefore originates in the pancreas was accomplished by rotating the patient laterally and delineating the posterior wall of the stomach with Gastrografin and a nasogastric tube. This pancreatic abscess was a result of alcoholic pancreatitis.

phlegmon of the pancreas. A pancreatic abscess may cause changes on chest x-ray.

These include elevation of the left hemidiaphragm, pleural effusion, and poor motion of either diaphragm on fluoroscopy if there is associated subphrenic abscess.

Abdominal ultrasound may reveal an echo-free area that is compatible with either a pancreatic pseudocyst or abscess. This appearance coupled with a septic clinical course is strong evidence in favor of an abscess even if blood cultures are not positive and air bubbles are not visualized.

(e) Differential Diagnosis. It is important to distinguish between a pancreatic abscess and a pancreatic pseudocyst. A pseudocyst is not usually associated with a septic course and severe leukocytosis. An ultrasonic study showing a fluid-filled mass should be considered as confirmatory of an infected pseudocyst (i.e., abscess) in the presence of high fever, leukocytosis, and clinical deterioration.

A second problem is to distinguish a pancreatic abscess from severe necrotizing pancreatitis without secondary infection. Fever, leukocytosis, and tender abdominal mass may occur in either clinical setting. If a pancreatic abscess is strongly suspected but blood cultures are negative, air bubbles are not visualized, and diagnostic ultrasound does not reveal a fluid-filled structure, a laparotomy is required if there is clinical deterioration. Whether a pancreatic abscess or severe necrotizing pancreatitis is discovered, devitalized pancreatic tissue should be removed and surgical drainage provided.

(f) Complications of Pancreatic Abscess. Fistulization into an adjacent structure is a very serious complication. An abscess may perforate into the stomach, duodenum, jejunum, transverse colon, pleural space via the diaphragm, bronchus, bile duct, or skin.[24,71-74,126] Following fistulization, the septic course usually persists and massive bleeding may occur. This relentless virulent course should be contrasted with the occasional amelioration of toxicity when a pancreatic pseudocyst fistulizes into a nearby structure. Fistulization to the skin may occur directly from the pancreas or a visceral perforation. An abscess that tracks behind the ascending or descending colon may give rise to a perforation in either location. Not infrequently there are multiple abscesses and multiple perforations.

Massive bleeding may occur after fistulization or by dissolution of a retroperitoneal artery in an abscess.

An empyema may occur if a subphrenic abscess perforates into the pleural space through the diaphragm.

(g) Treatment of Pancreatic Abscess. The use of antibiotics in the hope of curing or suppressing a pancreatic abscess medically is futile.

Without appropriate surgical drainage, the mortality owing to a pancreatic abscess is 100%.[120] Early aggressive surgical drainage enhances chances of survival.[120,121,123] Important surgical principles include removal of necrotic and suppurative tissue, drainage of frank pus where visible, and thorough intraabdominal search for nearby and distant abscesses including reflection of both the hepatic and splenic flexures to be sure there are no foci of infection tracking down both gutters.[24,95,126] Ample drainage to the outside must be achieved with soft tubes to facilitate removal of additional amounts of necrotic infected material.

In many instances, two and even three operative approaches are required to remove infected tissue completely. Serious postoperative complications include liver failure, renal insufficiency, respiratory insufficiency, and postoperative bleeding caused by enzymatic destruction of nearby blood vessels.

Use of antibiotics in conjunction with surgery is desirable in an effort to sterilize the bloodstream and contain infection. Since most of the organisms are coliforms with E. coli predominating,[22,23,120–122] antibiotic coverage should be directed primarily to this flora until results of cultures are available. An effective antibiotic is Gentamicin in a dosage of 1.5 mg/kg intramuscularly every 8 hr.[127] For broader coverage for severe sepsis and especially if an anaerobic organism is also suspected, one alternative would be the combination of Gentamicin and Clindamycin (600 mg intravenously every 6 hr); another would be Chloramphenicol in a dosage of 500 mg intravenously every 6 hr.

(h) Prognosis. A pancreatic abscess is one of the most formidable complications of acute pancreatitis. Mortality without surgery is usually 100%. Survival after surgery is of the order of 40% to 60%.[24,120–122] The earlier the surgical approach, the more favorable the prognosis.[120,121,123] The prognosis of a pancreatic abscess following pancreatitis caused by biliary tract disease or surgery (i.e., postoperative pancreatitis) is more serious than following alcoholic pancreatitis.[120,121] The reason for this is not clear but may be related to more extensive enzymatic destruction of the pancreas in both gallstone and postoperative pancreatitis than in chronic alcoholic pancreatitis.

There is no known way to prevent a pancreatic abscess since there is no known method of preventing pancreatic necrosis. The intensity of pancreatic inflammation can perhaps be minimized by protecting the microcirculation of the pancreas with sufficient quantities of intravenous fluids (including colloid and blood if needed) and other medical strategies outlined in Chapter 8. Antibiotic agents have no proven value in preventing an abscess and may prevent the early recognition of a pancreatic abscess. Since a delay in surgery increases mortality, use of antibiotic agents in pancreatitis should be restricted to specific indications such as biliary tract sepsis, pulmonary infection, and as an adjunct to the prompt surgical treatment of a pancreatic abscess.

9.2.5 Pancreatic Ascites

(a) Chronic Pancreatic Ascites Following Severe Acute Pancreatitis. Pancreatic exudate causes severe irritation of retroperitoneal and peritoneal surfaces, an effect that has been likened to a chemical burn. The result is an accumulation of ascitic fluid which usually is minimal to moderate in amount, and on rare occasions is massive. Once the acute inflammation subsides, ascites usually is completely reabsorbed. Occasionally, ascites persists indefinitely after an episode of severe acute pancreatitis. There are several possible explanations for chronic pancreatic ascites. First, there may be pancreatic ductal disruption as a result of severe parenchymal necrosis permitting extravasation of pancreatic fluid into the peritoneal cavity.[128] This mechanism rarely causes chronic ascites, presumably because agglutination of retroperitoneal tissues in the form of a phlegmon or a pseudocyst contains pancreatic fluid relatively well even if there is significant ductal disruption.[52] Since a pancreatic pseudocyst occurs in perhaps 50% of patients with severe necrotizing pancreatitis, it is likely that ductal disruption is quite common but usually well contained.

A second explanation for chronic ascites following clinical subsidence of acute pancreatitis is continuing release of small amounts of pancreatic enzymes by mild residual pancreatitis. This formulation is supported by the discovery of an occasional patient with amylase-rich tense ascites without demonstrable ductal rupture or leaking pseudocyst.[128] Alternatively, one might reason that a pseudocyst or rupture of a pancreatic duct was present but not identified at surgery or that it had resolved spontaneously before surgery. On occasion, the amylase in ascitic fluid is uncharacteristically dilute, suggesting marked peritoneal exudation in response to very mild smoldering pancreatitis. In this situation, several abdominal paracenteses may be successful in removing the bulk of fluid without substantial reaccumulation.

(b) Chronic Pancreatic Ascites without Acute Pancreatitis. When chronic pancreatic ascites develops after acute pancreatitis, there is sufficient peritoneal irritation by pancreatic enzymes to cause diffuse abdominal pain. When chronic pancreatic ascites occurs in the absence of recognizable acute pancreatitis, there is little or no abdominal pain because the extravasated pancreatic juice contains enzymes that have not been activated. The syndrome of chronic pancreatic ascites without acute pancreatitis has been reported on many occasions, and clinical features can be readily summarized.[51,128-136] The patient is a relatively young chronic alcoholic, usually a male aged 20 to 50, frequently without a background of pancreatic disease, who presents with painless tense ascites, cachexia, and profound weight loss. The abdomen is usually not tender. In about 10% to 30% of patients there is an associated pleural effusion.[52,129,134,136] Passage of fluid to the pleural space presumably occurs either via lympathic channels or through the aortic or esophageal hiatus to the mediastinum and from there to the pleural spaces. Subcutaneous fat necrosis suggestive of ongoing pancreatic inflammation has been noted in several instances,[129] but at the time of surgery there is usually little intraabdominal fat necrosis or evidence of significant intraabdominal inflammation caused by extravasation of pancreatic enzymes.

The development of painless ascites in a chronic alcoholic may lead to the erroneous diagnosis of cirrhosis with portal hypertension. A diagnosis of chronic pancreatic ascites is strongly suggested if serum amylase is increased, although on rare occasions serum amylase is also elevated in acute or chronic liver disease. The diagnosis of pancreatic ascites is reinforced by a detailed history that elicits a prior episode of abdominal discomfort suggestive of acute pancreatitis.

The most accurate way to distinguish chronic pancreatic ascites from other causes of ascites is a diagnostic paracentesis. In chronic pancreatic ascites, the fluid is either clear, straw colored, serosanguineous, or occasionally chylous[129]; ascitic fluid protein levels are almost always above 2.5 gm/100 ml and usually greater than 3 gm/100 ml indicating that the fluid is an exudate rather than a transudate; there are variable numbers of red blood cells and white blood cells. The most important measurement is the ascitic fluid amylase, which is increased in all cases of chronic pancreatic ascites and is invariably normal in ascitic fluid transudates such as cirrhosis. On very rare occasions, ascitic fluid amylase is increased in conditions other than chronic pancreatic ascites. These include intraabdominal malignancies that secrete amylase, and either primary carcinoma of the pancreas or metastatic carcinoma to the pancreas associated with pancreatic ductal disruption or a leaking pseudocyst (see Chapter 6). Abdominal fluid lipase as well as amylase is elevated in chronic pancreatic ascites,[133] and is not increased in intraabdominal malignancies that secrete amylase, but may be increased in carcinomas involving the pancreas.

The cause of chronic pancreatic ascites is usually either ductal disruption or leakage from a pancreatic pseudocyst. Presumably a prior episode of pancreatitis or pancreatic trauma occurred but was not recognized by the patient as an important event. A gastrointestinal series usually fails to reveal a retrogastric mass suggestive of a pseudocyst

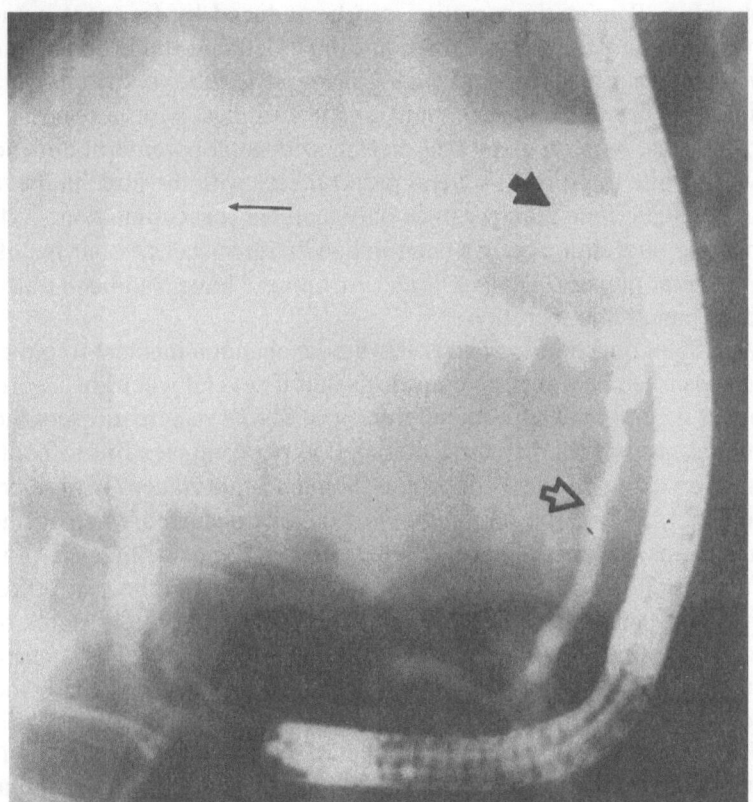

FIGURE 29 ERCP: Pancreatic Pseudocyst and Ductal Disruption. ERCP with visualization of the main pancreatic duct (short clear arrow), a large pseudocyst of the tail of the pancreas (short black arrow), and extravasation of contrast material from the region of the pseudo-cyst posteriorly in an irregular horizontal column until it forms a vertical column over the spine (long horizontal arrow). A second pseudocyst on the bottom right of the figure is obscured in this projection by the endoscope. At surgery, several pseudocysts were visual-ized, one with recent perforation. A distal two-thirds pancreatectomy and splenectomy were performed with an excellent postoperative course. A perforation that extends posteriorly as in this case may reach the mediastinum and erode into a pleural space causing intractable pleural effusion. A perforation that extends anteriorly causes pancreatic ascites. (Courtesy of Dr. R. Norton.)

probably because leakage from the cyst keeps it small. Diagnostic ultra-sound may reveal a pseudocyst, but frequently is unsuccessful owing to its small size. ERCP has been a very successful and safe preoperative method of visualizing either ductal disruption or pseudocyst[52,134,136-141] (Figure 29).

A medical trial to eliminate ascites is usually warranted. There are two goals: prevention of pancreatic secretion and improvement in nutritional status. Pancreatic secretion can be reduced by frequent antacid administration, by the use of Cimetidine or Cimetidine and Propantheline, or by aspiration of gastric acid with a nasogastric tube. Nutrition can be provided in the form of frequent small feedings with emphasis on carbohydrates, with an elemental diet, or with total parenteral nutrition. It is worthwhile to perform several paracenteses with the hope that evacuation of ascitic fluid may result in only minimal reaccumulation. External thoracic duct drainage has been utilized with success,[142] but is not in general use at present. Diamox[134] and Atropine[134] have also been utilized to reduce pancreatic secretion.

A difficult question to answer is when to abandon medical treatment. There appears to be a general consensus that if several weeks of vigorous treatment including efforts to suppress gastric and pancreatic secretion, nutritional support, and several therapeutic paracenteses fail to control pancreatic ascites, surgical correction should be undertaken. In one series of patients, most of the nonoperative fatalities occurred when medical treatment was prolonged more than 2 weeks.[134] The guidelines are not as yet fully established. A strong case can be made for the use of total parenteral nutrition for at least several weeks to improve the status of a cachectic debilitated patient. Once nutritional improvement has occurred, surgical intervention can be approached with less risk and more confidence.

ERCP should be performed preoperatively to define the location of ductal disruption or pseudocyst even if abdominal ultrasound has already revealed the presence of one or more pseudocysts. The reason for this is that pancreatic fluid may be leaking from a pseudocyst not visualized by ultrasound. Because of the occasional pancreatic abscess or severe pancreatitis caused by ERCP, this technique should be utilized only when it is clear that a surgical approach is necessary. If a ductal disruption is visualized, it is desirable to provide antibiotic coverage since bacteria that may have been instilled into the pancreatic duct now have ready access to the retroperitoneal area. A reasonable choice would be Ampicillin in a dosage of 1 gm intravenously every 4 hr. On occasion, antibiotics have been infused prophylactically into the pancreatic duct at the time of the injection of the contrast material,[137] or administered parenterally prior to instrumentation.[138] Visualization of a small pseudocyst without demonstration of leakage of contrast material probably does not require antibiotic coverage in an otherwise uncomplicated endoscopic study. In general, complications have been rarely reported following ERCP for pancreatic ascites. Surgery has usually been performed electively within several days of the endoscopic procedure. The usual surgical treatment of a cyst has been internal drainage to an adjacent hollow viscus or pancreatic resection if the pseudocyst was in the tail of the pancreas. Surgical management of a ductal disruption has included a Roux-en-Y anastomosis with a loop of jejunum or resection of distal body and tail when the disruption occurred in this location.

Mortality in chronic pancreatic ascites has been approximately 20%[129,134,136] Some patients have been extremely debilitated when first seen and could not be helped; others have expired following surgery. In one series, there was neither postoperative mortality nor postoperative recurrence of ascites if the ductal pathology could be accurately visualized either by preoperative ERCP or operative ductography and if proper surgical aproach could be carried out.[136] This information reinforces the belief that nutritional support and identification of ductal pathology by ERCP are essential for successful surgery.

REFERENCES

1. Guerrier K, Persky L: Pancreatic disease stimulating renal abnormality. *Am J Surg* 120:46–49, 1970.
2. Goldstein DA, Llach F, Massry SG: Acute renal failure in patients with acute pancreatitis. *Arch Intern Med* 136:1363–1365, 1976.
3. Gordon D, Calne RY: Renal failure in acute pancreatitis. *Br Med J* 3:801–802, 1972.
4. Simon GT, Giacobino JP: Pathogenesis of the glomerular lesions in acute pancreatitis. *Lancet* 2:669–670, 1970.
5. Werner MH, Hayes DF, Lucas CE, et al: Renal vasoconstriction in association with acute pancreatitis. *Am J Surg* 127:185–190, 1974.
6. Sankaran S, Lucas CE, Walt AJ: Transient hypertension with acute pancreatitis. *Surg Gynecol Obstet* 138:235–238, 1974.
7. Gregory PB, Klatskin G: Splenomegaly in uncomplicated biliary tract and pancreatic disease. *Gastroenterology* 62:436–440, 1972.
8. Longstreth GF, Newcomer AD, Green PA: Extrahepatic portal hypertension caused by chronic pancreatitis. *Ann Intern Med* 75:903–908, 1971.
9. Warshaw AL, Chesney TMcH, Evans GW, et al: Intrasplenic dissection by pancreatic pseudocysts. *N Engl J Med* 287:72–75, 1972.
10. Yale CE, Crummy AB: Splenic vein thrombosis and bleeding esophageal varices. *JAMA* 217:317–320, 1971.
11. Sutton JP, Yarborough DY, Richards JT: Isolated splenic vein occlusion. *Arch Surg* 100:623–626, 1970.
12. Moreaux J, Bismuth H: Les complications spleniques des pancreatitis chroniques. *Presse Med* 77:1467–1470, 1969.
13. Catanzaro FP, Abiri M, Allegra S: Spontaneous rupture of spleen and pleural effusion complicating pancreatitis. *R I Med J* 51:328–329, 1968.
14. Shafiroff BB, Berkowitz D, Li JK: Splenic erosion and hemorrhage secondary to pancreatic pseudocyst. *Am J Gastroenterol* 68:145–153, 1977.
15. Sahebjami H, Gillespie L, Ferris PJ, et al: Rectal bleeding as the presenting symptom of acute pancreatitis. *Am J Gastroenterol* 54:388–394, 1970.
16. Sandblom P: Gastrointestinal hemorrhage through the pancreatic duct. *Ann Surg* 171:61–66, 1970.

17. Seeff LB, Zimmerman HJ: Relationship between hepatic and pancreatic disease. In *Progress in Liver Diseases,* Volume 5, H. Popper and F. Schaffner (eds) Grune and Stratton, New York. Chapter 35, pp. 590–608, 1976.

18. Sarles H: Alcholism in pancreatitis. *Scand J Gastroenterol* 6:193–198, 1971.

19. Marks IN, Bank S: The etiology, clinical features and diagnosis of pancreatitis in the southhwestern Cape. *S Afr Med J* 37:1039–1053, 1963.

20. Strum WB, Spiro HM: Chronic pancreatitis. *Ann Intern Med* 74:264–277, 1971.

21. Dutta SK, Mobrahan S, Iber FL: Associated liver disease in alcoholic pancreatitis. Presented at the annual meeting of the American Pancreatic Association, Chicago, November, 1977.

22. Candido FM, Pitchumoni CS, Panchacharam P, et al: Coexistent pancreatitis and cirrhosis in alcoholics: a clinical and histopathological survey. *Gastroenterology* 72:1035, 1977.

23. Camer SJ, Tan EGC, Warren KW, et al: Pancreatic abscess. *Am J Surg* 129:426–431, 1975.

24. Holden JL, Berne TV, Rosoff L: Pancreatic abscess following acute pancreatitis. *Arch Surg* 111:858–861, 1976.

25. Frieden JH: The significance of jaundice in acute pancreatitis. *Arch Surg* 90:422–426, 1965.

26. McCollum WB, Jordan PH Jr: Obstructive jaundice in patients with pancreatitis without associated biliary tract disease. *Ann Surg* 182:116–120, 1975.

27. Wapnick S, Purow E, Grosberg S, et al: Obstructive jaundice due to pancreatitis. *Gastroenterology* 27: A–122/1145, 1977.

28. Falko JM, Mekhjian HS, Thomas FB: Silent pancreatic pseudocyst. *Am J Dig Dis* 20:583–587, 1975.

29. Christensen NM, Demling R, Mathewson C Jr: Unusual manifestations of pancreatic pseudocysts and their surgical management. *Am J Surg* 130:199–205, 1975.

30. Weinstein BR, Korn RJ and Zimmerman HJ: Obstructive jaundice as a complication of pancreatitis. *Ann Intern Med* 58:245–258, 1963.

31. Lukash WM, Bishop RP, Nielsen OF: Transaminase levels in acute pancreatitis and after secretin stimulation. *JAMA* 197:927–929, 1966.

32. Chawla SK, Chawla K, Sossi AJ, et al: Uncommon presentation of pancreatic pseudocyst. *Am J Gastroenterol* 68:154–160, 1977.

33. Foulk WT, Fleisher GA: Serum glutamic-oxalacetic transaminase in acute pancreatitis. *Gastroenterology* 35:375–380, 1958.

34. Warshaw AL, Schapiro RH, Ferrucci JT, et al: Persistent obstructive jaundice, cholangitis, and biliary cirrhosis due to common bile duct stenosis in chronic pancreatitis. *Gastroenterology* 70:562–567, 1976.

35. Snape WJ, Jr., Long WB, Trotman BW, et al: Marked alkaline phosphatase elevation with partial common bile duct obstruction due to calcific pancreatitis. *Gastroenterology* 70:70–73, 1976.

36. Harris AJ, Korsten MA: Acute suppurative cholangitis secondary to calcific pancreatitis. *Gastroenterology* 71:847–850, 1976.

37. Scott J, Summerfield JA, Elias E, et al: Chronic pancreatitis: a cause of cholestasis. *Gut* 18:196–201, 1977.

38. Read G, Braganza JM, Howat HT: Pancreatitis—a retrospective study. *Gut* 17:945–952, 1976.

39. Pereiras R, Jr., Chiprut RO, Greenwald RA, et al: Percutaneous transhepatic cholangiography with the "skinny" needle. *Ann Intern Med* 86:562–568, 1977.

40. Schulte WJ, LaPorta AJ, Condon RE, et al: Chronic pancreatitis: a cause of biliary stricture. *Surg* 82:303–309, 1977.

41. Falkenstein DB, Hsu KD, Abrams RM, et al: Influence of endoscopic manipulation

and patient position on cholangiographic interpretation in endoscopic retrograde cholangiopancreatography. *Radiology* 122:836–838, 1977.

42. Potts DE, Mass MF, Iseman MD: Syndrome of pancreatic disease, subcutaneous fat
    necrosis and polyserositis. *Am J Med* 58:417–423, 1975.

43. Hodson-Walker NJ, Woods JM: Acute pancreatitis with peripheral fat necrosis. *CMA
    Journal* 103:382–384, 1970.

44. Mullin, GT, Caperton EM, Crespin SR, et al: Arthritis and skin lesions resembling
    erythema nodosum in pancreatic disease. *Ann Intern Med* 68:75–86, 1968.

45. Zeller M, Hetz HH: Rupture of a pancreatic cyst into the portal vein. Report of a case
    of subcutaneous nodular and generalized fat necrosis. *JAMA* 195:181–183, 1966.

46. Morgan JE, Robbins AH, Matsumoto G, et al: Total pancreatectomy for recurrent
    medullary fat necrosis. *Arch Surg* 111:1394–1398, 1976.

47. Achord JL, Gerle RD: Bone lesions in pancreatitis. *Am J Dig Dis* 11:453–460, 1966

48. Sperling MA: Bone lesions in pancreatitis. *Aust Ann Med* 17:334–340, 1968.

49. Bank S, Marks IN, Farman J, et al: Further observations on calcified medullary bone
    lesions in chronic pancreatitis. *Gastroenterology* 51:224–230, 1966.

50. Tombroff M, Loicq A, De Koster JP, et al: Pleural effusion with pancreaticopleural
    fistula. *Br Med J* 1:330–331, 1973.

51. Razzaque MA, Hussain SA, Hossain Z, et al: Pleural effusion with pancreaticopleural
    fistula. *Am J Gastroenterol* 68:84–87, 1977.

52. Cameron JL: Chronic pancreatic ascites and pancreatic pleural effusions. *Gastroenter-
    ology* 74:134–140, 1978.

53. Mitchell CE: Relapsing pancreatitis with recurrent pericardial and pleural effusions. A
    case report and review of the literature. *Ann Intern Med* 60:1047–1052, 1964.

54. Rovner AJ, Westcott JL: Pulmonary edema and respiratory insufficiency in acute
    pancreatitis. *Radiology* 118:513–520, 1976.

55. Warshaw AL, Lesser PB, Rie M, et al: The pathogenesis of pulmonary edema in acute
    pancreatitis. *Ann Surg* 182:505–510, 1975.

56. Interiano B, Stuard ID, Hyde RW: Acute respiratory distress syndrome in pancreatitis.
    Ann Intern Med 77:923–926, 1972.

57. Petty TL, and Ashbaugh DG: The adult respiratory distress syndrome. Clinical fea-
    tures, factors influencing prognosis and principle of management. *Chest* 60:233–239,
    1971.

58. Morgan AP, Jenning ME, Haessler H: Phospholipids, acute pancreatitis and the lungs.
    Ann Surg 167:329–335, 1968.

59. Ranson JHC, Roses DF, Fink SD: Early respiratory insufficiency in acute pancreatitis.
    Ann Surg 178:75–79, 1973.

60. Ranson JHC, Turner JW, Roses DF, et al: Respiratory complications in acute pancrea-
    titis. *Ann Surg* 179:557–566, 1974.

61. Fulton MC, Marriott HJL: Acute pancreatitis simulating myocardial infarction in the
    electrocardiogram. *Ann Intern Med* 59:730–732, 1963.

62. Shamma'a MH, Rubeiz GA: Acute pancreatitis with electrocardiographic findings of
    myocardial infarction. *Am J Med* 32:827–830, 1962.

63. Ranson JHC, Lackner H, Berman IR, et al: The relationship of coagulation factors to
    clinical complications of acute pancreatitis. *Surg* 81:502–511, 1977.

64. Greipp PR, Brown JA, Gralnick HR: Defibrination in acute pancreatitis. *Ann Intern
    Med* 76:73–76, 1972.

65. Kwaan HC, Anderson MC, Gramatica L: A study of pancreatic enzymes as a factor in
    the pathogenesis of disseminated intravascular coagulation during acute pancreatitis.
    Surg 69:663–672, 1971.

66. Thompson WM, Kelvin FM, Rice RP: Inflammation and necrosis of the transverse
    colon secondary to pancreatitis. *Am J Roentgenol* 128:943–948, 1977.

67. Mair WSJ, McMahon MJ, Goligher JC: Stenosis of the colon in acute pancreatitis. *Gut* 17:692–695, 1976.
68. Lukash WM, Bishop RP: Acute pancreatitis affecting the transverse colon. Report of a case. *Am J Dig Dis* 12:734–736, 1967.
69. DeFord JW, Major, Kolts BE: Stenosis of the colon secondary to pancreatitis. *Am J Dig Dis* 18:630–632, 1973.
70. Mohiuddin S, Sakiyalak P, Gullick HD, et al: Stenosing lesions of the colon secondary to pancreatitis. *Arch Surg* 102:229–231, 1971.
71. Hunt Dr, Mildenhall P: Etiology of stricture of the colon associated with pancreatitis. *Am J Dig Dis* 20:941–946, 1975.
72. Katz P, Dorman MJ, Aufses AH, Jr.: Colonic necrosis complicating postoperative pancreatitis. *Ann Surg* 179:403–405, 1974.
73. Corlette MB, Jr., and Lynch JA: Pancreatitis presenting as a colonic fistula. *Arch Surg* 104:708–709, 1972.
74. Berne TV, Edmondson HA: Colonic fistulization due to pancreatitis. *Am J Surg* 111:359–363, 1966.
75. Hodson–Walker NJ, Woods JM: Acute pancreatitis with peripheral fat necrosis. *Can Med Assoc J* 103:382–384, 1970.
76. Griffiths RW, Brown PW, Jr.: Jejunal infarction as a complication of pancreatitis. *Gastroenterology* 58:709–712, 1970.
77. Collins JJ, Peterson LM, Wilson RE: Small intestinal infarction as a complication of pancreatitis. *Ann Surg* 167:433–436, 1968.
78. Simon M, Lerner MA: Duodenal compression by the mesenteric root in acute pancreatitis and inflammatory conditions of the bowel. *Radiology* 79: #1:75–81, 1962.
79. Bradley EL, III: Pathophysiology of ruptured pseudocysts. *Gastroenterology* 72:A-9/1032, 1977.
80. Anderson MC: Management of pancreatic pseudocysts. *Am J Surg* 123:209–221, 1972.
81. Winship D, Trenbeath M, Smith N, et al: Pancreatitis: pancreatic pseudocysts and their complications. *Gastroenterology* 73:593–603, 1977.
82. Gee W, Lt. Cmdr., Foster ED, Lt., Doohen DJ, Capt.: Mediastinal pancreatic pseudocyst. *Ann Surg* 169:420–424, 1969.
83. Silvis SE, Vennes JA, Rohrmann CA: Endoscopic pancreatography in the evaluation of patients with suspected pancreatic pseudocyst. *Am J Gastroenterology* 61:452–459, 1974.
84. Hancke S, Pedersen JF: Percutaneous puncture of pancreatic cysts guided by ultrasound. *Surg Gynecol Obstet* 142:551–552, 1976.
85. Andersen BN, Hancke S, Nielsen SAD, et al: The diagnosis of pancreatic cyst by endoscopic retrograde pancreatography and ultrasonic scanning. *Ann Surg* 185:286–289, 1977.
86. Sybers HD, Shelp WD, Morrissey JF: Pseudocyst of the pancreas with fistulous extension into the neck. *N Engl J Med* 278:1058–1059, 1968.
87. Elliott DW: Pancreatic pseudocyst. Symposium on Surgery of the Liver, Spleen and Pancreas. *Surg Clin North Am* 55:339–362, 1975.
88. Grace RR, Jordan PH, Jr.: Unresolved problems of pancreatic pseudocysts. *Ann Surg* 184:16–21, 1976.
89. Bradley EL, Gonzalez AC, Clements JL, Jr.: Acute pancreatic pseudocysts: incidence and implications. *Ann Surg* 184:734–737, 1976.
90. Hastings PR, Nance FC, Becker WF: Changing patterns in the management of pancreatic pseudocysts. *Ann Surg* 181:546–551, 1975.
91. Gonzalez AC, Bradley EL, Clements JL, Jr.: Pseudocyst formation in acute pancreati-

tis: ultrasonographic evaluation of 99 cases. *Am J Roentgenol* 127:315–317, 1976.
92. Haaga JR, Alfidi RJ, Zelch MG, et al: Computed tomography of the pancreas. *Radiology* 120:589–595, 1976.
93. Niccolini DG, Graham JH, Banks PA: Tumor-induced acute pancreatitis. *Gastroenterology* 71:142–145, 1976.
94. Sarles H: Pancreatic pseudocysts—high percentage of 47 patients. *Gut* 6:545–559, 1965.
95. Warshaw AL: Inflammatory masses following acute pancreatitis. Phlegmon, pseudocyst, and abscess. *Surg Clin North Am* 54:621–636, 1974.
96. Bradley EL, III, Clements JL, Jr.: Implications of diagnostic ultrasound in the surgical management of pancreatic pseudocysts. *Am J Surg* 127:163–173, 1974.
97. Doust BD: The use of ultrasound in the diagnosis of gastroenterological disease. *Gastroenterology* 70:602–610, 1976.
98. Barnardo DE, Grogono JL, Parks AG: Spontaneous rupture of a pancreatic pseudocyst into the colon. *Am J Dig Dis* 19:1165–1167, 1974.
99. Bohlman TW, Katon RM, Lee TG, et al: Use of endoscopic retrograde cholangiopancreatography in the diagnosis of pancreatic fistula. A case report and review of the literature. *Gastroenterology* 70:582–584, 1976.
100. Clements JL, Jr., Bradley EL, III, Eaton SB: Spontaneous internal drainage of pancreatic pseudocyst. *Am J Roentgenol* 126:985–991, 1976.
101. Hartong WA, Skibba RM, Greenberger NJ: Spontaneous pseudocystogastrostomy associated with pancreatitis. Detection by endoscopy. *Arch Intern Med* 136:1287–1289, 1976.
102. Dalton WE, Lee HM, Williams GM et al: Pancreatic pseudocyst causing hemobilia and massive gastrointestinal hemorrhage. *Am J Surg* 120:106–107, 1970.
103. Jacobs E: Spontaneous perforation of the left diaphragm by a pancreatic pseudocyst. *Gastroenterology* 55:311, 1968.
104. Merikas G, Stathopoulos G, Katsas A: Painless pancreatic pseudocyst ruptured into the thoracic cavity. *Gastroenterology* 54:101–104, 1968.
105. Gee W, Foster ED, Doohen DJ: Mediastinal pancreatic pseudocyst. *Ann Surg* 169:420–424, 1969.
106. Weidmann P, Rutishauser W, Siegenthaler W, et al: Mediastinal pseudocyst of the pancreas. *Am J Med* 46:454–459, 1969.
107. Kirschner SG, Heller RM, Smith CW: Pancreatic pseudocyst of the mediastinum. *Radiology* 123:37–42, 1977.
108. Bardenheier JA, Quintero O, Barner HG: False aneurysm in a pancreatic pseudocyst. *Ann Surg* 172:53–55, 1970.
109. Greenstein A, DeMaio EF, Nabseth DC: Acute hemorrhage associated with pancreatic pseudocysts. *Surg* 69:56–62, 1971.
110. Stanley JC, Frey CF, Miller TA, et al: Major arterial hemorrhage. A complication of pancreatic pseudocysts and chronic pancreatitis. *Arch Surg* 111:435–440, 1976.
111. Wu TK, Zaman SN, Gullick HD, et al: Spontaneous hemorrhage due to pseudocysts of the pancreas. *Am J Surg* 134:408–410, 1977.
112. Brintnall BB, Laidlaw WW, Papp JP: Hemobilia: Pancreatic pseudocyst hemorrhage demonstrated by endoscopy and arteriography. *Am J Dig Dis* 19:186–188, 1974.
113. Bradley EL, Clements LJ: Spontaneous resolution of pancreatic pseudocysts. Implications for timing of operative intervention. *Am J Surg* 129:23–28, 1975.
114. Goldstein HM, Zornoza J, Wallace S, et al: Percutaneous fine needle aspiration biopsy of pancreatic and other abdominal masses. *Radiology* 123:319–322, 1977.
115. Haff RC, Page CP, Andrassy RJ, et al: Splenectomy: its place in operations for inflammatory disease of the pancreas. *Am J Surg* 134:555–557, 1977.

116. Voitk A, Brown RA, Echave V, et al: Use of an elemental diet in the treatment of complicated pancreatitis. *Am J Surg* 125:223–227, 1973.

117. Lenggenhager K: Therapy and origin of large pancreatic pseudocysts. *Am J Surg* 125:542–545, 1973.

118. Hopkins RW, Fratianne RB, Abrams JS, et al: Controlled hypotension for uncontrolled hemorrhage. *Arch Surg* 95:517–530, 1967.

119. Lutwick LI: Pancreatic abscess with haemophilus influenzae and eikenella corrodens. *JAMA* 236:2091–2092, 1976.

120. Miller TA, Lindenauer SM, Frey CF, et al: Pancreatic abscess. *Arch Surg* 108:545–551, 1974.

121. Bolooki H, Jaffe B, Gliedman ML: Pancreatic abscesses and lesser omental sac collections. *Surg Gynecol Obstet* 125:1301–1308, 1968.

122. Evans FC: Pancreatic Abscess. *Am J Surg* 117:537–540, 1969.

123. Jones CE, Polk HC, Fulton RL: Pancreatic Abscess. *Am J Surg* 129:44–47, 1975.

124. Miller TA, Lindenauer M, Frey CF, et al: Pancreatic Abscess. *Arch Surg* 108:545–551, 1974.

125. Owens BJ, Hamit HF: Pancreatic abscess and pseudocyst. *Arch Surg* 112:42–45, 1977.

126. Mason HDW, Forgash A, Balch HH: Intestinal fistula complicating pancreatic abscess. *Surg Gynecol Obstet* 140:39–43, 1975.

127. The Choice of Antimicrobial Drugs in *The Medical Letter* 20:1–8, January 13, 1978.

128. Paloyan D, Skinner DB: Clinical significance of pancreatic ascites. *Am J Surg* 132:114–117, 1976.

129. Donowitz M, Kerstein MD, Spiro HM: Pancreatic ascites. *Medicine* 53:183–195, 1974.

130. Wagner RB, Tolins SH: Pancreatic ascites. Case report: ascitic fluid lipase utilized for diagnosis. *J M Sinai Hosp* 36:216–220, 1969.

131. Cameron JL, Brawley RK, Bender HW, et al: The treatment of pancreatic ascites. *Ann Surg* 170:668–676, 1969.

132. Schindler SC, Schaefer JW, Hull D, et al: Chronic pancreatic ascites. *Gastroenterology* 59:453–459, 1970.

133. Sileo AV, Chawla SK, LoPresti PH: Pancreatic ascites: diagnostic importance of ascitic lipase. *Am J Dig Dis* 20:1110–1114, 1975.

134. Cameron JL, Kieffer RS, Anderson WJ, et al: Internal pancreatic fistulas: pancreatic ascites and pleural effusions. *Ann Surg* 184:587–593, 1976.

135. Munoz JN, Bose S: Pancreatic ascites. A case report and review of the literature. *Am J Dig Dis* 20:1178–1183, 1975.

136. Sankaran S, Walt AJ: Pancreatic ascites. Recognition and management. *Arch Surg* 111:430–434, 1976.

137. Davis RE, Graham DY: Pancreatic ascites. The role of endoscopic pancreatography. *Am J Dig Dis* 20:977–980, 1975.

138. Rawlings W, Bynum TE, Pasternak G: Pancreatic ascites: Diagnosis of leakage site by endoscopic pancreatography. *Surg* 81:363–365, 1977.

139. Paloyan D, Simonowitz D, Blackstone M: Pancreatic fistula. Management guided by endoscopic retrograde cholangiopancreatography. *Arch Surg* 112:1139–1140, 1977.

140. Ward PA, Raju S, Suzuki H: Preoperative demonstration of pancreatic fistula by endoscopic pancreatography in a patient with pancreatic ascites. *Ann Surg* 185:232–234, 1977.

141. Levine JB, Warshaw AL, Falchuk KR, et al: The value of endoscopic retrograde pancreatography in the management of pancreatic ascites. *Surg* 81:360–362, 1977.

142. Dreiling DA: The lymphatics, pancreatic ascites and pancreatic inflammatory disease. *Am J Gastroenterol* 53:119–131, 1970.

10

Prognosis of Acute Pancreatitis

The overall mortality in acute pancreatitis is approximately 13% to 15%.[1,2] The mortality of hemorrhagic pancreatitis is far greater than edematous pancreatitis, at least 20%[3] and in some series greater than 50%.[4] Fatalities do occur on the basis of edematous pancreatitis,[4-6] usually from hypovolemia leading to shock and renal shutdown.[2]

Mortality is influenced by what has caused the pancreatitis. Overall mortality in pancreatitis associated with biliary tract disease is approximately 10%,[2] with alcohol 7% to 8%, and with idiopathic pancreatitis 17%.[2] Pancreatitis caused by trauma has a mortality of approximately 20%.[7] Pancreatitis associated with use of adrenocorticosteroid hormones is reported to have a very high mortality, but this may be related to the severity of the underlying illness.[8] Postoperative pancreatitis was associated with a mortality of 42% in one study.[9]

Various factors other than etiology influence prognosis. A patient is more vulnerable to death during the first clinical episode of pancreatitis than in subsequent episodes.[1] Prognosis is also worse in the presence of shock,[2,5,6,10] renal shutdown,[2] and severe hypocalcemia.[4,11-14] The level of serum amylase has no prognostic significance.[1,2,5,12,13,15] The development of subcutaneous fat necrosis is associated with a 50% mortality in published reports,[16] but it is possible that there are many patients who have survived and have not been reported. As noted in earlier chapters, serious complications such as rupture of a pancreatic pseudocyst, massive bleeding associated with a pseudocyst, development of a pancreatic abscess, or severe respiratory insufficiency carry a mortality of at least 50%.[1,2]

Two recent reports have attempted to cull information that could be of prognostic significance.[1,2] In one report, physical examination did not yield prognostic information, but analysis of eleven variables did such that a 62% mortality was recorded if three or more of these signs were positive and only a 3% mortality if fewer than three variables were positive.[1] The eleven signs that exhibited prognostic significance were: age of patient in excess of 55 years, blood glucose greater than 200 mg%, white blood count greater than 16,000, serum lactic dehydrogenase level greater than 700 IU%, glutamic oxaloacetic transaminase (SGOT) greater than 250 units, serum calcium less than 8 mg%, BUN rise greater than 5 mg%, a decrease in hematocrit more than 10%, a base deficit greater than 4 mEq/liter, arterial pO_2 below 60 mm Hg, and an estimated fluid sequestration of greater than 6 liters. In the second report, abnormalities on physical examination as well as laboratory results correlated with a poor prognosis.[2] These included severe systemic hypotension, severe hypertension, temperature elevation greater than 101°F, abnormalities on auscultation of the lungs, presence of abdominal mass, serum albumin less than 3 gm/100 ml, maximum prothrombin time greater than 14 sec, maximum white blood cell count greater than 20,000/ml, maximum hematocrit less than 30%, maximum serum bilirubin greater than 4 mg%, serum calcium less than or equal to 8 mg%, and evidence of renal insufficiency with maximum BUN greater than 30 mg% and maximum creatinine greater than 2 mg%. Many of these abnormalities are common in severe pancreatitis associated with hemorrhage and necrosis, including unstable vital signs, evidence of organ failure including respiratory and renal, decreases in serum hematocrit and calcium, and increases in white blood count and glucose.

The role of early surgery in altering prognosis remains uncertain. In one report, there was no mortality among patients treated medically or surgically in a controlled fashion, but respiratory difficulties appeared to be more severe among those treated surgically.[1] In two other reports, an early surgical approach was utilized because of very severe pancreatitis culminating at times in a moribund state. The operative procedure, consisting of cholecystostomy, gastrostomy, feeding jejunostomy, and drainage of the lesser sac, was believed to be extremely beneficial.[14] The role of early surgery for a seriously ill patient can be defined more precisely only after carefully controlled randomized clinical trials involving large numbers of patients.

REFERENCES

1. Ranson JHC, Rifkind KM, Roses DF, et al: Prognostic signs and the role of operative management in acute pancreatitis. *Surg Gynecol Obstet* 139:69–81, 1974.
2. Jacobs ML, Dagget WM, Civetta JM, et al: Acute pancreatitis: analysis of factors influencing survival. *Ann Surg* 185:43–51, 1977.
3. White TT, Heimbach DM: Sequestrectomy and hyperalimentation in the treatment of hemorrhagic pancreatitis. *Am J Surg* 132:270–275, 1976.
4. Geokas MC, Rinderknecht H, Walberg CB, et al: Methemalbumin in the diagnosis of acute hemorrhagic pancreatitis. *Ann Intern Med* 81:483–486, 1974.

5. Whalen J, Rush B, Albano E, et al: Fatal acute pancreatitis a clinicopathologic analysis. *Am J Surg* 121:16–19, 1971.
6. Shader AE, Paxton JR: Fatal pancreatitis. *Am J Surg* 111:369–373, 1966.
7. Karl HW, Chandler JG: Mortality and morbidity of pancreatic injury. *Am J Surg* 134:549–554, 1977.
8. Nakashima Y, Howard JM: Drug-induced acute pancreatitis. *Surg Gynecol Obstet* 145:105–109, 1977.
9. White TT, Morgan A, Hopton D: Postoperative pancreatitis. *Am J Surg* 120:132–137, 1970.
10. Toffler AH, Spiro HM: Shock or coma as the predominant manifestation of painless acute pancreatitis. *Ann Intern Med* 57:655–659, 1962.
11. Edmondson HA, Berne CJ: Calcium changes in acute pancreatic necrosis. *Surg Gynecol Obstet* 79:240–243, 1944.
12. Read G, Braganza JM, Howatt HT: Pancreatitis—a retrospective study. *Gut* 17:945–952, 1976.
13. Feller JH, Brown RA, MacLaren Toussaint GP, et al: Changing methods in the treatment of severe pancreatitis. *Am J Surg* 127:196–201, 1974.
14. Warshaw AL, Imbembo AL, Civetta JM, et al: Surgical intervention in acute necrotizing pancreatitis. *Am J Surg* 127:484–491, 1974.
15. Edmondson HA, Berne CJ, Homann RE, et al: Calcium, potassium, magnesium and amylase disturbance in acute pancreatitis. *Am J Med* 12:34–42, 1952.
16. Potts DE, Mass MF, Iseman MD: Syndrome of pancreatic disease, subcutaneous fat necrosis and polyserositis. *Am J Med* 58:417–423, 1975.

CHRONIC PANCREATITIS

Etiology of Chronic Pancreatitis

11.1 ACUTE VS. CHRONIC PANCREATITIS

At a symposium held in Marseilles, France, in 1962, a classification of pancreatitis was developed that correlated histologic and clinical features.[1] By this classification, the term acute pancreatitis is reserved for an acute inflammation of the pancreas that resolves completely both clinically and histologically. The term relapsing acute pancreatitis is reserved for recurring episodes of pancreatitis that also resolve completely both clinically and histologically. The best example of acute and relapsing acute pancreatitis is the illness associated with biliary tract disease. Each episode of pancreatitis usually resolves completely, and after corrective surgery no further episodes of pancreatitis occur. Only rarely is there evidence of residual histologic damage, and on these occasions there has usually been a serious complication such as a pseudocyst or abscess. Other examples of acute and relapsing acute pancreatitis include pancreatitis associated with hyperlipidemia, medication, infectious agents, pregnancy, endoscopic procedures, operations, and structural abnormalities of the common bile duct, ampullary region, and duodenum.

The term chronic pancreatitis means the persistence of histologic changes even after the etiologic agent has been removed. In the United States, the most common cause of chronic pancreatitis is alcohol. At the time of the first clinical episode of alcoholic pancreatitis, histologic damage has already taken place,[2] and, according to the classification adopted at the Marseilles conference, the illness should be characterized as chronic pancreatitis. Each additional episode of painful alcoholic pancreatitis should then be classified as chronic relapsing pancreatitis rather than relapsing acute pancreatitis. Other examples of chronic and chronic relapsing pancreatitis include hyperparathyroidism and hereditary pancreatitis.

From a clinical viewpoint, the transition from acute to chronic pancreatitis is rarely identified. Episodes of acute pancreatitis, as typified by biliary tract disease, tend to occur in patients in the 40 to 50 age group and rarely progress to chronic pancreatitis. The first clinical episode of alcoholic pancreatitis usually takes place in the 30 to 40 age group and is already chronic by histologic criteria (see Chapter 2).

11.2 CHRONIC AND CHRONIC RELAPSING PANCREATITIS

The distinction between chronic and chronic relapsing pancreatitis is clinical. It depends on whether there are recurring episodes of pain. Some patients with chronic pancreatitis experience no pain at all. This is typical of protein-calorie malnutrition, which is characterized by atrophy of acinar cells and fibrosis of the gland without ductal obstruction.[3] On occasion, chronic pancreatitis occurs on the basis of alcohol, hyperparathyroidism, or hyperlipidemia without episodes of pain.

Almost all diseases that cause chronic pancreatitis give rise to recurrent episodes of pain and are thus characterized as chronic relapsing pancreatitis. This includes alcohol, hyperparathyroidism, and hereditary pancreatitis. It is of interest that the first clinical episode of pancreatitis may occur long after very severe histologic abnormalities of chronic pancreatitis have evolved. The reason for this unexpectedly long latent period is not clear, nor is it clear what local factors precipitate the first painful attack.

The presence of intraductal calcification is evidence of a particularly severe form of chronic pancreatitis of many years duration, whether associated with symptoms or not. In the United State, France, and South Africa, the most common cause of calcific pancreatitis is alcohol.[4-6] Other causes of calcific pancreatitis are hyperparathyroidism and hereditary pancreatitis. Calcific pancreatitis has also been documented in other locations throughout the world, occasionally on the basis of alcohol but frequently not.[7-25] Since at least some cases of calcific pancreatitis occur in areas in which protein-calorie malnutrition is prevalent, it has been suggested that protein-calorie malnutrition may be a precursor of this form of pancreatitis. Detailed studies of patients with calcific pancreatitis in southwestern India[7-9] indicate that protein-calorie malnutrition is probably not a cause of calcific pancreatitis in India. First, protein-calorie malnutrition is endemic throughout India whereas calcific pancreatitis is localized to the southwestern portion in the state of Kerala. Second, calcification is not a feature of pancreatic insufficiency associated with protein-calorie malnutrition. Finally, in protein-calorie malnutrition, there is a reduction in bicarbonate concentration,[3] whereas in calcific pancreatitis bicarbonate concentration has been found to be normal.[9] It seems unlikely that the development of calcific pancreatitis on the basis of protein-calorie malnutrition would be heralded by an improvement in pancreatic bicarbonate secretion.

REFERENCES

1. Symposium on the etiology and pathological anatomy of chronic pancreatitis: Marseilles, 1963. *Am J Dig Dis* 9:371–376, 1964.
2. Strumm WB, Spiro HM: Chronic pancreatitis. *Ann Intern Med* 74:264–277, 1971.
3. Tandon BN, Banks PA, George PK, et al: Recovery of exocrine pancreatic function in adult protein-calorie malnutrition. *Gastroenterology* 58:358–362, 1970.
4. Sarles H, Sahel J: Pathology of chronic calcifying pancreatitis. *Am J Gastroenterol* 66:117–139, 1976.
5. Howard JM, Ehrlich EW: The etiology of pancreatitis. *Ann Surg* 152:135–146, 1960.
6. Marks IN, Bank S: The etiology, clinical features and diagnosis of pancreatitis in the South Western Cape. *S Afr Med J* 19 October, 1963:1039–1053.
7. Geevarghese PJ: *Pancreatic Diabetes: A Clinico-pathologic Study of Growth Onset Diabetes with Pancreatic Calculi.* G. R. Bhatkal for *Popular Prakashan*, Bombay, 1968.
8. Narayana Pai K, Soman CR, Varghese R: *Pancreatic Diabetes.* Printed at Geo Printers Medical College P. O. Trivandrum, 1970.
9. George PK, Banks PA, Pai KN, et al: Exocrine pancreatic function in calcifice pancreatitis in India. *Gastroenterology* 60:858–863, 1971.
10. Wye Poh Fung AM, Aw SE, Khoo OT: Chronic pancreatitis in Asian patients in Singapore. *Med J Aust* March 28, 1970:653–656.
11. Rajasuriya K, Thenabadu PN, Munasinghe DR: Pancreatic calcification in Ceylon with special reference to its etiology. *Ceylon Med J* March, 1970:11–24.
12. Banwell JG, Campbell J: Pancreatic exocrine function in African patients. *Trans R Soc Trop Med Hyg* 61:390–398, 1967.
13. Shaper AG: Chronic pancreatic disease and protein malnutrition. *Lancet* June 4, 1960:1223–1224.
14. Nagaratnam N, Gunawardene KRW: Aetiological factors in pancreatic calcification in Ceylon. *Digestion* 5:9–16, 1972.
15. Banwell JG, Hutt MRS. Leonard PJ, et al: Exocrine pancreatic disease and the malabsorption syndrome in tropical Africa. *Gut* 8:388–399, 1967.
16. Olurin EO, Olurin O: Pancreatic calcification: a report of 45 cases. *Br Med J* 4:534–539, 1969.
17. Shaper AG: Aetiology of chronic pancreatic fibrosis with calcification seen in Uganda. *Br Med J* 1:1607–1609, 1964.
18. Zuidema PJ: Cirrhosis and disseminated calcification of the pancreas in patients with malnutrition. *Trop Geog Med* 11:70–74, 1959.
19. Kinnear TWG: The pattern of diabetes mellitus in a Nigerian teaching hospital. *East Afr Med J* 40:288–294, 1963.
20. Wicks ACB, Clain DJ: Chronic pancreatitis in African diabetics. *Am J Dig Dis* 20:1–8, 1975.
21. Moshal MG: A study of chronic pancreatitis in Natal. *Digestion* 9:438–446, 1973.

22. Gastard J, Joubaud F, Farbos T, et al: Etiology and course of primary chronic pancrea-titis in Western France. *Digestion* 9:416–428, 1973.
23. Ammann RW, Hammer B, Fumagalli I: Chronic pancreatitis in Zurich, 1963–1972. *Digestion* 9:404–415, 1973.
24. Marks IN, Bank S, Louw JH: Chronic pancreatitis in the Western Cape. *Digestion* 9: 447–453, 1973.
25. Ishii K, Nakamura K, Takeuchi T, et al: Chronic calcifying pancreatitis and pancreatic carcinoma in Japan. *Digestion* 9:429–437, 1973.

12

Pathology of Chronic Pancreatitis

The pathology of alcoholic pancreatitis has been studied in great detail. The earliest changes are the deposition of protein plugs within pancreatic ductules.[1] At first, protein plugs are deposited in random fashion within some lobules but not in others, but eventually this process becomes relatively diffuse. Various histologic abnormalities follow the deposition of enzymic protein in the form of plugs and probably occur on the basis of other toxic effects of alcohol as yet not clarified.[1-5] At points of contact with proteinaceous material, ductal epithelium may undergo squamous metaplasia and ulceration. Inspissation of protein plugs causes ductular dilatation followed by acinar atrophy. An inflammatory process may occur in the interstitium. Eventually, a considerable amount of fibrous tissue is deposited in the vicinity of pancreatic ducts, between pancreatic lobules, and within lobules cleaving acinar tissue. As this process becomes more extensive, acinar tissue may disappear leaving dense scar tissue associated with a scant number of inflammatory cells. Pancreatic ducts may be widely dilated as a result of obstruction by protein plugs or intraductal stones (Figure 30). At times, however, pancreatic ducts are widely dilated with no apparent major obstruction. It is possible that periductular fibrosis distorts the architecture by actually pulling the ductal wall into a pseudosacculation. At other times, zones of marked stenosis of pancreatic ducts alternate with zones of marked dilatation producing the so-called "chain-of-lakes" appearance. Very high intraductal pressure secondary to one or more stenoses may even cause ductal cul-de-sacs. Eventually, there may be such marked parenchymal destruction that only some hardy islets cells and a few nests of acinar tissue remain imbedded in dense fibrous tissue (Figure 31). Fibrous tissue may encase

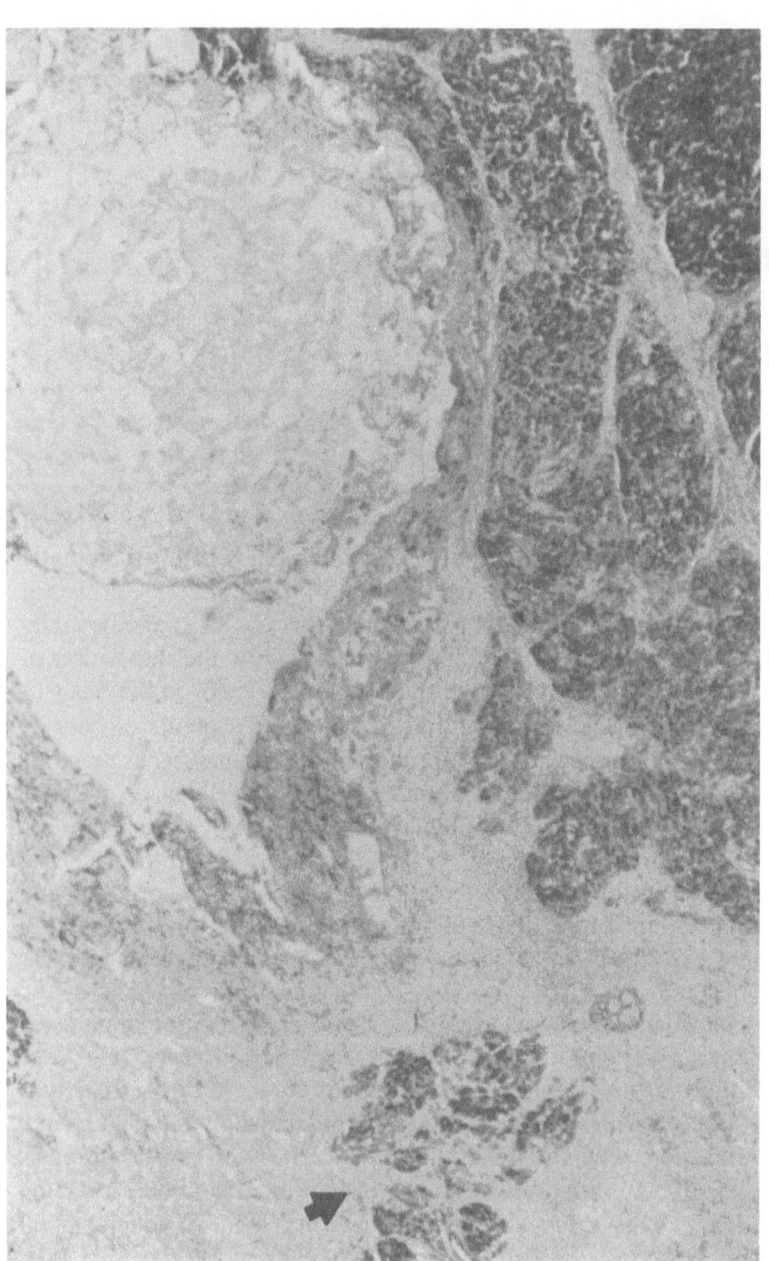

FIGURE 30 *Chronic Pancreatitis.* A large pancreatic duct with inspissated material is visible on the right. There is considerable periductular fibrosis. Residual acinar tissue is undergoing dissolution at the far left (arrow). In the lower right, acinar tissue is being cleaved by bands of fibrosis.

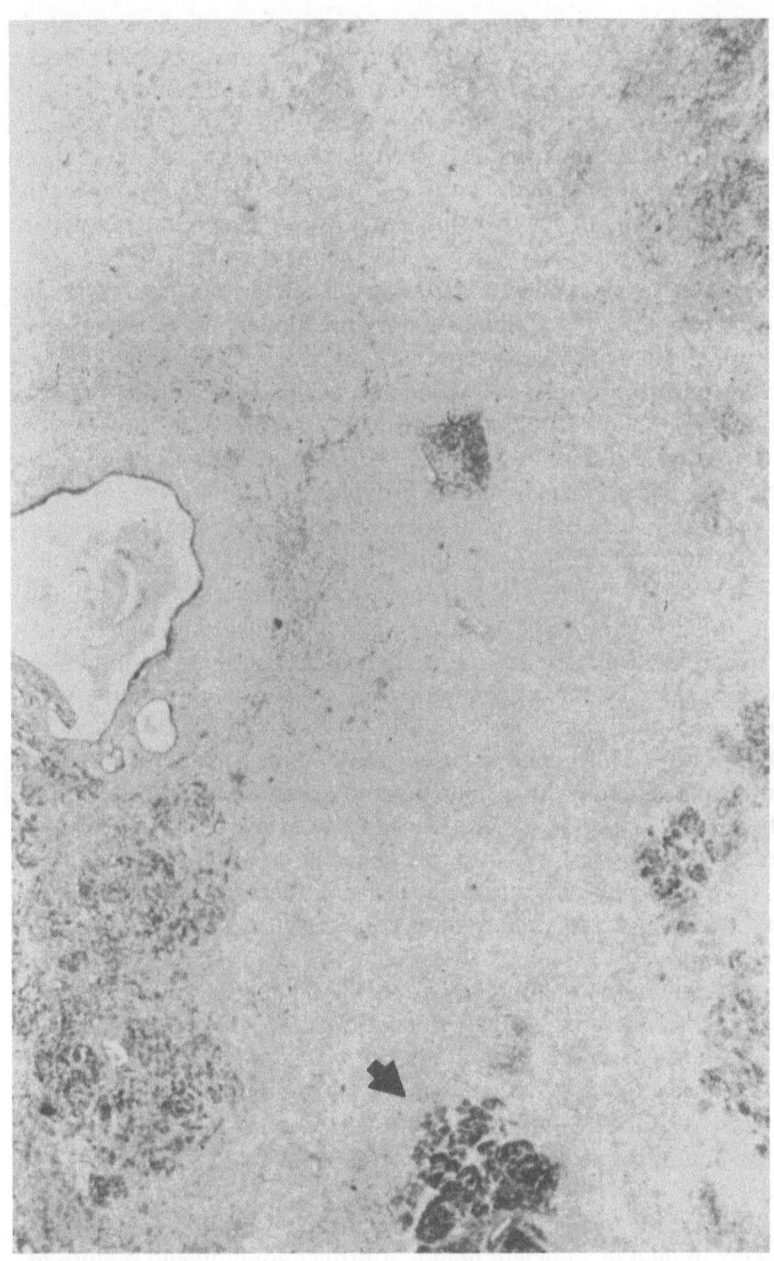

FIGURE 31 *Severe Chronic Pancreatitis*. There is substantial fibrosis throughout. A small irregular ductule contains inspissated material in the upper center. Zones of chronic inflammation containing lymphocytes are visible to the left of the duct, in the lower right, and lower left. Remnants of acinar tissue remain at the far left (arrow).

nerves and be responsible for severe chronic pain. Characteristically, there is only a scant round cell infiltrate.

One early abnormality of some interest is the formation of rounded cavities surrounded by cuboidal epithelium.[1,4] The suggestion has been made that this represents ductular proliferation and as such constitutes one of the earlier responses of the pancreas to injury. Ductal reduplication in response to alcohol has also been documented in the dog.[6] The increased bicarbonate and fluid secretion of early alcoholic pancreatitis in the dog[6] and in man[7] may result from such pancreatic ductular reduplication.

There is general agreement that intraductal calcification occurs late in alcoholic pancreatitis.[4,5,8,9] Calcification is predominantly if not exclusively intraductal and is composed primarily of calcium carbonate.[1,3,8,10–12] Intraductal stones are formed by secondary calcification of protein plugs, desquamated epithelium, and other intraductal debris. The process of calcification may be facilitated by the secretion of ionized calcium in pancreatic juice in chronic pancreatitis (Chapter 2, p. 23).

The natural history of alcoholic pancreatitis appears to be progressive histologically and functionally. First, even with total abstention from alcohol, once the patient has far advanced pancreatic lesions associated with pain, there is relentless progression of histologic abnormalities.[13] Second, pancreatic function appears to deteriorate so that abnormalities of pancreatic secretion are in general more severe among patients with long-standing chronic pancreatitis than those in whom the disease is of briefer duration.[14,15] Third, there is often greater impairment of pancreatic secretion among patients with calcific than noncalcific pancreatitis.[15,16] (In one study in which pancreatic secretion was very severely impaired, however, there was no apparent difference.[9]) Finally, as will be discussed in Chapter 13, steatorrhea and diabetes mellitus, markers of very severe pancreatic destruction, are much more common in calcific than noncalcific pancreatitis.

There probably are many factors that limit recovery in alcoholic pancreatitis. One is that most patients continue to consume alcohol in excess. Another is that once there has been substantial intraductal obstruction, pancreatic inflammation and atrophy become self-perpetuating and progressive. A third is that the fibrotic process obstructs subcapsular lymphatics, and prevents drainage of pancreatic inflammation and exudation by this route.[17]

The ability of the pancreas to regenerate after alcohol-induced injury has not been studied in sufficient detail. A proper study would require at the very least a long-term surveillance of pancreatic secretion in patients with alcoholic pancreatitis, some of whom abstain from alcohol and others of whom do not. In one very small study, abstinence appeared to improve pancreatic secretion at least a little, whereas continued alcohol-ism appeared to be associated with deterioration in pancreatic function.[18] Additional studies of this type with statistical analysis would be of great interest. Pancreatic function studies would also be of interest among patients who have undergone surgical procedures for relief of pain (such as lateral pancreaticojejunostomy.) For example, 72-hr stools for fat should be collected to determine whether there was improvement in fat absorption. If that were the case, one might suspect that regeneration of pancreatic tissue had occurred once obstruction of the main pancreatic duct was relieved. An alternative explanation is that pancreatic secretion was no longer sequestered within an obstructed duct and could now reach the small intestine in reasonable quantity.

It should be emphasized that the histologic features of alcoholic pan-creatitis bear no resemblance to the diffuse fibrosis and atrophy that occur when the pancreatic duct of the dog is subjected to ligation,[19-22] or when the pancreatic duct of man is obstructed either by a carcinoma or by ductal stenosis at the head of the pancreas.[11]

Histologic features of chronic pancreatitis associated with cystic fi-brosis include dilatation of ducts with inspissated secretions, loss of acini, increase in islet cells, and fibrosis.[23,24] In protein-calorie malnutrition, there is marked atrophy of acinar cells associated with fibrosis with spar-ing of islet cells. Secretory abnormalities including reduction in bicarbon-ate and enzyme secretion are markedly improved within weeks of institu-tion of a high-protein diet.[25,26]

Although regeneration of pancreatic tissue has been demonstrated in the experimental animal following partial resection of the pancreas or removal of ductal obstruction,[27-30] and although functional recovery has been suggested in man following pancreatic resection,[31] it bears repeating that these situations bear no resemblance to the unique histology of alco-holic pancreatitis, and there is as yet no evidence of regeneration of the pancreas after the first clinical episode of alcoholic pancreatitis. Evidence will be cited in Chapter 14 of at least temporary improvement in secretory function once alcohol is discontinued or a nutritious diet is provided. This improvement may relate to a correction of protein-calorie malnutrition rather than an improvement in histologic features of alcoholic pancreatitis.

REFERENCES

1. Sarles H, Sahel J: Pathology of chronic calcifying pancreatitis. *Am J Gastroenterol* 66:117–139, 1976.

2. Howard JM, Nedwich A: Correlation of the histologic observations and operative findings in patients with chronic pancreatitis. *Surg Gynecol Obstet* 132:387–395, 1971.

3. Edmondson HA, Bullock WK, Mehl JW: Chronic pancreatitis and lithiasis II. Pathology and pathogenesis of pancreatic lithiasis. *Am J Pathol* 26:37–49, 1950.

4. Sarles H: Chronic calcifying pancreatitis—chronic alcoholic pancreatitis. *Gastroenterology* 66:604–616, 1974.

5. Uys CJ, Bank S, Marks IN: The pathology of chronic pancreatitis in Cape Town. *Digestion* 9:454–468,1973.

6. Sarles H, Tiscornia O, Palasciano G: Chronic alcoholism and canine exocrine pancreas secretion. A long term follow-up study. *Gastroenterology:* 72:238–243, 1977.

7. Dreiling DA, Bordalo O: Secretory pattern in minimal pancreatic inflammatory pathology. *Am J Gastroenterol* 60:60–69, 1973.

8. Owens JL Jr., Howard JM: Pancreatic calcification: a late sequel in the natural history of chronic alcoholism and alcoholic pancreatitis. *Ann Surg* 147:326–338, 1958.

9. Bank S, Marks IN, Lurie B, et al: Precalcific pancreatitis. *S Afr Med J* 46:2093–2097, 1972.

10. Lagergren C: Calcium carbonate precipitation in the pancreas, gallstones and urinary calculi. *Acta Chir Scand* 124:320–325, 1962.

11. Stobbe KC, ReMine WH, Baggenstoss AH: Pancreatic lithiasis. *Surg Gynecol Obstet* 131:1090–1099, 1970.

12. McGeorge CK, Widmann BP, Ostrum H, et al: Diffuse calcification of the pancreas. *Am J Roentgenol* 78:599–606, 1957.

13. Strumm WB, Spiro HM: Chronic pancreatitis. *Ann Intern Med* 74:264–277, 1971.

14. DiMagno EP, Malagelada J–R, Go VLW: Relationship between alcoholism and pancreatic insufficiency. *Ann NY Acad Sci* 252:200–207, 1975.

15. Vagne M, Descos L: Pancreatic secretion of bicarbonate in patients with chronic pancreatitis. *Digestion* 3:350–356, 1970.

16. Janowitz HD, Dreiling DA: Is there pancreatic ductal obstruction in chronic pancreatitis? *Gastroenterology* 13:12–16, 1959.

17. Reynolds BM: Observations of subcapsular lymphatics in normal and diseased human pancreas. *Ann Surg* 171:559–566, 1970.

18. Dreiling DA, Greenstein AJ, Bordalo O: The hypersecretory states of the pancreas. Implications in the pathophysiology of pancreatic inflammation and that pathogenesis of peptic ulcer diathesis. *Am J Gastroenterol* 59:505–511, 1973.

19. Pairent FW, Trapnell JE, Howard JM: The treatment of pancreatic exocrine insufficiency: III. The effects of pancreatic ductal ligation and oral pancreatic enzyme supplements on fecal lipid excretion in the dog. *Ann Surg* 170:737–746, 1969.

20. Ambromovage AM, Pairent FW, Howard JM: Pancreatic exocrine insufficiency: The effects of long-term pancreatic duct ligation on serum insulin levels and glucose metabolism in the dog. *Ann Surg* 177:338–343, 1973.

21. Tiscornia OM, Dreiling DA: Recovery of pancreatic exocrine secretory capacity following prolonged ductal obstruction. *Ann Surg* 164:267–270, 1966.

22. Hiebert JM, Mack E, Goodman ML, et al: Immunofluorescent studies after ligation of the pancreatic duct. *Surg Gynecol Obstet* 130:72–76, 1970.

23. Scully RE, Galdabini JJ, McNeely BU: Case records of the Massachusetts General Hospital: Case 26–1977. *N Engl J Med* 296:1519–1526, 1977.

24. Kopito LE, Shwachman H: The pancreas in cystic fibrosis: chemical composition and comparative morphology. *Pediatr Res* 10:742–749, 1976.

25. Tandon BN, Banks PA, George PK, et al: Recovery of exocrine pancreatic function in adult protein-calorie malnutrition. *Gastroenterology* 58:358–362, 1970.

26. Kumar R, Banks PA, George PK, et al: Early recovery of exocrine pancreatic function in adult protein-calorie malnutrition. *Gastroenterology* 68:1593–1595, 1975.
27. Pearson KW, Scott D, Torrance B: Effects of partial surgical pancreatectomy in rats. I. Pancreatic regeneration. *Gastroenterology* 72:469–473, 1977.
28. Fitzgerald PJ, Herman L, Carol B, et al: Pancreatic acinar cell regeneration. I. Cytologic, cytochemical and pancreatic weight changes. *Am J Pathol* 52:983–1011, 1968.
29. Lehv M, Fitzgerald PJ: Pancreatic acinar cell regeneration. IV. Regeneration after surgical resection. *Am J Pathol* 53:513–535, 1968.
30. Tiscornia OM, Dreiling DA: Editorial: Does the pancreatic gland regenerate? *Gastroenterology* 51:267–270, 1966.
31. Dreiling DA: Pancreatic secretory testing in 1974. Symposium on Diagnosis of Pancreatic Disease. *Gut* 16:653–657, 1975.

13

Clinical Features of Chronic Pancreatitis

13.1 ABDOMINAL PAIN

The clinical features of chronic relapsing pancreatitis as typified by alcoholic pancreatitis may be identical to acute pancreatitis as typified by biliary tract disease. The reader is referred to Chapter 5 for a full discussion. The relationship of pain to alcohol consumption is variable. Some patients claim no recent alcohol ingestion whatsoever, some have clearly ingested alcohol in an effort to relieve the pain of pancreatitis, and others have clearly consumed alcohol and then experienced an episode of pancreatitis. The time lag may be variable. One interesting pattern that has been observed is the development of pain during the afternoon following an evening of heavy alcohol consumption.[1] This prolonged latent period cannot be explained on the basis of the known metabolic and physiologic effects of alcohol. Another interesting observation is that in severe chronic pancreatitis pain may recur after consumption of only modest amounts of alcohol whereas in earlier years considerably more alcohol was required. The explanation for this phenomenon may involve the progressive blockade of pancreatic ductules in severe chronic pancreatitis such that eventually any stimulus of pancreatic secretion, even a relatively weak one such as alcohol, causes pain on the basis of ductal distention.

In general, episodes of pain tend to occur with increasing frequency, but are milder and briefer in duration, presumably as a result of progressive destruction of acinar tissue. It is for this reason that an episode of hemorrhagic pancreatitis is more likely to occur during an earlier clinical episode of alcoholic pancreatitis than a later one.

An important question is whether abstinence from alcohol amelio-rates the discouraging pattern of recurrent episodes of pain and disability. While a carefully controlled clinical study involving large numbers of patients has not been performed and perhaps would be impossible owing to patient noncompliance, there have been suggestions that episodes of pain may be curtailed by total abstinence from alcohol.[2]

One of the most serious problems in chronic pancreatitis is persistent abdominal pain which leads to narcotic addiction. Several potential mech-anisms should be kept in mind. One is that there is residual pancreatic inflammation following a bout of chronic relapsing pancreatitis that re-quires more intensive treatment, including at times total parenteral nutri-tion. Another is that a complication of pancreatitis has occurred. The most important complications of chronic pancreatitis which are asso-ciated with abdominal pain are pancreatic pseudocyst, stricture and ob-struction of the common bile duct or pancreatic duct, and, rarely, a carci-noma of the pancreas (Chapter 16). Another mechanism is marked perineural inflammation and fibrosis which causes unrelenting abdominal pain refractory to even large amounts of narcotic agents. This type of pain tends to be steady, severe, boring, and not influenced by meals. At times, the patient has abdominal pain lasting for several hours specifically after meals. He then remains relatively asymptomatic until the next meal. In these circumstances, there is likely to be substantial pancreatic ductal obstruction so that postprandial pancreatic secretion aggravates existing ductal dilatation and perhaps causes extravasation of some pancreatic fluid into interstitial spaces. Finally, if the patient is already addicted to the regular use of narcotic agents, complaints of pain may reflect this dependence.

Abdominal pain constitutes the most important clinical problem in chronic pancreatitis. It may be responsible for severe weight loss, malnu-trition, and general debility of the patient, and represents the most com-mon indication for surgery in chronic pancreatitis.

13.2 STEATORRHEA

Steatorrhea does not occur unless the secretion of pancreatic lipase is reduced to less than 10% of normal.[3] Therefore, fat digestion remains normal until there is either very far-advanced pancreatic destruction or, in rare circumstances, complete blockage of the main pancreatic duct. In the absence of abdominal pain, the patient is frequently able to increase caloric intake substantially and avoid significant weight loss.

If steatorrhea is massive, the patient may pass loose oily stools and even droplets of oil. The presence of oil in the stool imparts a characteristic soft greasy consistency that is easily appreciated when the physician performs a rectal examination. It is of interest that diarrhea tends not to be excessive even if steatorrhea is significant. In one recent study, stool frequency was less than 3 times per 24 hr among patients losing between 50 to 80 gm of fat in their stool each 24 hr.[4] Patients with relatively severe steatorrhea may pass only one stool per day and at times are constipated (a pattern which can occur in the absence of narcotic agents for pain).

The absence of severe diarrhea in steatorrhea of pancreatic insufficiency is in contrast to severe diarrhea in steatorrhea caused by mucosal injury of the small intestine, as in sprue. The explanation appears to be as follows. In steatorrhea of pancreatic insufficiency, unabsorbed triglyceride passes into the colon in quantity. Some is excreted in stool as triglyceride,[5] the rest undergoes hydrolysis by bacterial lipases,[6] and are excreted as fatty acids but not as hydroxylated fatty acids.[7] The stool in pancreatic insufficiency therefore contains a mixture of triglyceride and nonhydroxylated fatty acid. In contrast, in sprue and other diseases of the small intestine, pancreatic lipase hydrolyzes dietary fat to free fatty acids almost completely.[5] Some of the free fatty acids that are delivered to the colon are hydrated by bacteria to hydroxy fatty acids and are excreted as such.[7] Hydroxy fatty acids stimulate cyclic AMP in the colon,[8] and thereby cause colonic secretion of water and electrolytes.[9]

Deficiency of fat-soluble vitamins is rarely of clinical importance in chronic pancreatitis.[10] Many patients are able to overeat and thereby prevent vitamin deficiency. Furthermore, in chronic pancreatitis, the small intestinal absorptive surface is normal as is secretion of bile. Also, the bulk of the fat that traverses the small intestine is in the form of triglyceride, which does not bind fat-soluble vitamins, rather than free fatty acids, which do. To compare, in sprue, the presence of fatty acids in the small intestine binds fat-soluble vitamins and calcium as soaps thereby facilitating the loss of these essential materials in the stool.

13.3 CREATORRHEA

The loss of nitrogen in the stool correlates with pancreatic trypsin output in the fashion that the loss of fat in the stool correlates with pancreatic lipase output. Creatorrhea occurs only when trypsin output is less than 10% of normal.[3] In chronic pancreatitis, pancreatic trypsin output is somewhat better preserved than is lipase output, and loss of nitrogen in the stool is not as serious a problem as loss of fat in the stool.[11]

13.4 DIABETES MELLITUS

The development of diabetes mellitus implies severe chronic pancreatitis. It is for this reason that diabetes, like steatorrhea, is more common in calcific than noncalcific pancreatitis.[12-14] In one report, overt diabetes was present in 30% of noncalcific and 70% of calcific pancreatitis[12]; in another, 61% of patients with chronic pancreatitis (mostly chronic calcific pancreatitis) were found to have overt diabetes.[14] The incidence of diabetes mellitus increases to 50% for noncalcific and 90% for calcific pancreatitis if the diagnosis rests with an abnormal glucose tolerance test rather than overt diabetes[10]; the figures are 75% for noncalcific and 98% for calcific pancreatitis if a low insulin reserve is used to define the diabetic state.[10]

The relative incidence of diabetes mellitus and steatorrhea in chronic pancreatitis depends to some extent on the definition of the diabetic state. It appears that glucose intolerance is more common than steatorrhea.[2,13-16] This suggests that the development of diabetes mellitus need not imply coexisting steatorrhea but that the development of steatorrhea does indicate that diabetes mellitus has also occured. One reason for this dichotomy may be that the diabetic state can be induced in the experimental animal if greater than 70% of the pancreas is resected,[17] whereas steatorrhea does not take place until enzyme output is less than 10% of normal.[3]

The diabetic state in chronic pancreatitis is extremely brittle.[12,13,18] This tendency to hypoglycemia has as its basis some important metabolic disturbances involving both insulin and glucagon. By way of comparison, adult-type and juvenile-type diabetes are both associated with inappropriate elevations in serum glucagon levels that contribute to the diabetic status.[19] In chronic pancreatitis, basal glucagon and insulin levels may be normal, but there is deficient glucagon and insulin reserve.[12,18] The diabetes of genetic origin can be distinguished from that of chronic pancreatitis by an increase of glucagon secretion in response to alanine in the former compared to an impairment in glucagon secretion in response to the stimulus in the latter.[18] In chronic pancreatitis, if exogenous insulin causes hypoglycemia, the deficiency in glucagon reserve prevents the restoration of serum glucose to normal. An induced state of hypoglycemia may therefore persist because of the absence of glucagon and represent a threat to the patient's life.

The physiologic importance of somatostatin is unclear. This hormone is present in islet cells, and has been shown to inhibit release of growth hormone, insulin, and glucagon.[20] A role for this hormone in glucose homeostasis in chronic pancreatitis has not as yet been defined.

Another feature of diabetes mellitus in chronic pancreatitis is the virtual absence of diabetic ketoacidosis. A deficiency in glucagon secretion, which may be catastrophic by prolonging severe hypoglycemia, appears to be protective by preventing ketoacidosis. The reason for this is that glucagon accelerates the development of ketonemia in insulin deficiency.[21,22] A deficiency in glucagon therefore prevents this effect presumably by reducing the liver's capacity to convert free fatty acids from adipose tissue into acetoacetic and β-hydroxybutyric acids.[22]

Other complications of diabetes mellitus in association with chronic pancreatitis occur very infrequently. Diabetic retinopathy and nephropathy are uncommon and tend not to be of clinical significance.[12,23] The rarity of vascular complications in pancreatic diabetes has not been fully explained. One suggestion is that fasting levels of serum cholesterol (but not triglycerides) tend to be lower than normal in chronic pancreatitis, and may retard the development of diabetic microangiopathy.[24]

The incidence of diabetic neuropathy has been estimated at 30% among patients with chronic pancreatitis caused by alcohol.[12] The neuropathy may be quite painful and includes both sensory and motor dysfunction. Neuropathy is found most characteristically among patients with symptomatic diabetes. Contributory factors may be alcohol abuse and malnutrition.[12]

REFERENCES

1. Marks IN, Bank S: The aetiology, clinical features and diagnosis of pancreatitis in the South Western Cape. A review of 243 cases. *S Afr Med J* 37:1039–1053, 1963.
2. Strum WB, Sprio HM: Chronic pancreatitis. *Ann Intern Med* 74:264–277, 1971.
3. DiMagno EP, Go VLW, Summerskill WHJ: Relations between pancreatic enzyme outputs and malabsorption in severe pancreatic insufficiency. *N Engl J Med* 288:813–815, 1973.
4. Regan PT, Malagelada JR, DiMagno EP, et al: Comparative effects of antacids, cimetidine and enteric coating on the therapeutic response to oral enzymes in severe pancreatic insufficiency. *N Engl J Med* 297:854–858, 1977.
5. Thompson JB, Ringrose RE, Welsh JD: Fecal triglycerides. II. Digestive versus absorptive steatorrhea. *J Lab Clin Med* 73:521–530, 1969.
6. Hofmann AF: Fat absorption and malabsorption: Physiology, diagnosis, and treatment. *Viewpoints on Digestive Diseases* 9:1977.
7. Kim YS, Spritz N: Hydroxy acid excretion in steatorrhea of pancreatic and nonpancreatic origin. *N Engl J Med* 279:1424–1426, 1968.
8. Coyne MJ, Bonorris GG, Chung A, et al: Propranolol inhibits bile acid and fatty acid stimulation of cyclic AMP in human colon. *Gastroenterology* 73:971–974, 1977.
9. Bright-Asare P, Binder HJ: Stimulation of colonic secretion of water and electrolytes by hydroxy fatty acids. *Gastroenterology* 64:81–88, 1973.
10. Taubin HL, Spiro HM: Nutritional aspects of chronic pancreatitis. *Am J Clin Nut* 26:367–373, 1973.

11. DiMagno EP, Malagelada JR, Go VLW: Relationship between alcoholism and pancreatic insufficiency. *Ann NY Acad Sci* 252:200–207, 1975.
12. Bank S, Marks IN, Vinik AI: Clinical and hormonal aspects of pancreatic diabetes. *Am J Gastroenterol* 64:13–22, 1975.
13. Bank S, Marks IN, Lurie B, et al: Precalcific pancreatitis. *S Afr Med J* 46:2093–2097, 1972.
14. Linde J, Nilsson L, Barany FR: Diabetes and hypoglycemia in chronic pancreatitis. *Scand J Gastroenterol*: 12:369–373, 1977.
15. Read G, Braganza JM, Howat HT: Pancreatitis—a retrospective study. *Gut* 17:945–952, 1976.
16. Joffe BI, Jackson WPU, Bank S, et al: Effect of oral hypoglycaemic agents on glucose tolerance in pancreatic diabetes. *Gut* 13:285–288, 1972.
17. Yasugi H, Mizumoto R, Sakurai H, et al: Changes in carbohydrate metabolism and endocrine function of remnant pancreas after major pancreatic resection. *Am J Surg* 132:577–580, 1976.
18. Donowitz M, Hendler R, Spiro HM, et al: Glucagon secretion in acute and chronic pancreatitis. *Ann Intern Med* 83:778–781, 1975.
19. Muller WA, Faloona GR, Aguilar-Parada E, et al: Abnormal alpha-cell function in diabetes. Response to carbohydrate and protein ingestion. *N Engl J Med* 283:109–115, 1970.
20. Konturek SJ: Somatostatin and the gastrointestinal secretions. *Scand J Gastroenterol* 11:1–4, 1976.
21. Barnes AJ, Bloom SR, Alberti GMM, et al: Ketoacidosis in pancreatectomized man. *N Engl J Med* 296:1250–1253, 1977.
22. McGarry JD, Foster DW: Hormonal control of ketogenesis. Biochemical considerations. *Arch Intern Med* 137:495–501, 1977.
23. Sevel D, Bristow JH, Bank S, et al: Diabetic retinopathy in chronic pancreatitis. *Arch Ophthalmal* 86:245–250, 1971.
24. Joffe BI, Krut L, Bank S, et al: Serum lipid levels in diabetes secondary to chronic pancreatitis. *Metabolism* 19:87–90, 1970.

Diagnosis of Chronic Pancreatitis

14.1 BASIC LABORATORY TESTS

During a relapse of chronic pancreatitis, serum amylase and lipase are minimally increased or are completely normal if there is severe destruction of acinar tissue. In far advanced chronic relapsing pancreatitis, these values tend to be uniformly normal. In these circumstances, pain may reflect perineural inflammation or marked ductal distention rather than a severe interstitial inflammatory process. Measurement of the amylase-creatinine clearance ratio is probably not of great help in long-standing pancreatitis especially if the serum amylase is normal. In severe chronic pancreatitis, serum isoamylase determination may show a deficiency of pancreatic amylase (p-amylase) indicative of pancreatic insufficiency (see Chapter 6).

Serum calcium may be decreased on the basis of hypoalbuminemia, hypomagnesemia, or possibly malabsorption.

Serum glucose level and glucose tolerance tests often show evidence of diabetes mellitus.

14.2 RADIOLOGIC STUDIES

14.2.1 Conventional Studies

A plain film of the abdomen should be obtained and inspected carefully for the presence of intraductal calcification. Calcification may be present in diffuse fashion throughout the gland either as relatively large concretions or small scattered stones (Figure 7). It is important to be certain that calcifications reside within the pancreas itself rather than in an adjacent structure. An oblique or lateral projection can be of great help in confirming that the calcification is situated in the retroperitoneum behind the stomach. The precise site of calcification within the pancreas is variable. At times, stones are first visible in the head of the pancreas to the right of the spine and then as time goes on more diffusely throughout the gland. Less often calcification is first visible in the tail of the pancreas. It is not uncommon to search for calcification for several years before noting its appearance. The radiologic findings may then remain stable for an indefinite period of time, or as time goes on, additional stones become visible and the preexisting concretions appear to become larger. Once stones develop, they do not disappear. A presumed reduction in calcification would be best explained by an alteration of radiologic technique so that stones are simply not as well seen. Actual disappearance of stones could mean the very rare complication of a carcinoma eroding the stones or, in the presence of a pancreaticojejunostomy, the evacuation of intraductal stones into the jejunum.

A gastrointestinal series may show a variety of abnormalities in chronic pancreatitis. Pancreatic calcification within the head of the pancreas is easily visualized if the clinician focuses on the inner aspect of the duodenal sweep. The mucosal folds in this area appear splayed and fixed indicating tethering by severe fibrosis in the head of the pancreas. The tethering of folds and encroachment by a fibrotic head of the pancreas may give rise to a variety of radiologic changes in the duodenal bulb and descending duodenum including one or more collections of barium simulating duodenal ulcers, extrinsic compression of the duodenal bulb, and marked duodenal narrowing associated at times with obstruction of the postapical duodenum. (Figure 32).[1] Encroachment on the duodenum may cause mucosal fold abnormalities and nodularity severe enough to lead to an erroneous diagnosis of carcinoma of the pancreas invading the duodenum.[2] At times, hypotonic duodenography is useful in clarifying the basic disease process, but even this technique may fail to distinguish carcinoma from chronic pancreatitis.

In chronic pancreatitis and especially chronic calcific pancreatitis, the distal common bile duct that passes through the substance of the head of the pancreas may become circumferentially stenotic giving rise to a stricture with proximal dilatation (Figure 22). This can be identified with the use of intravenous cholangiography, "skinny needle" transhepatic cholangigraphy, or ERCP. Tomographic views obtained during intravenous cholangiogram may reveal calcification of the head of the pancreas that is not visible by conventional x-ray methods. This discovery may

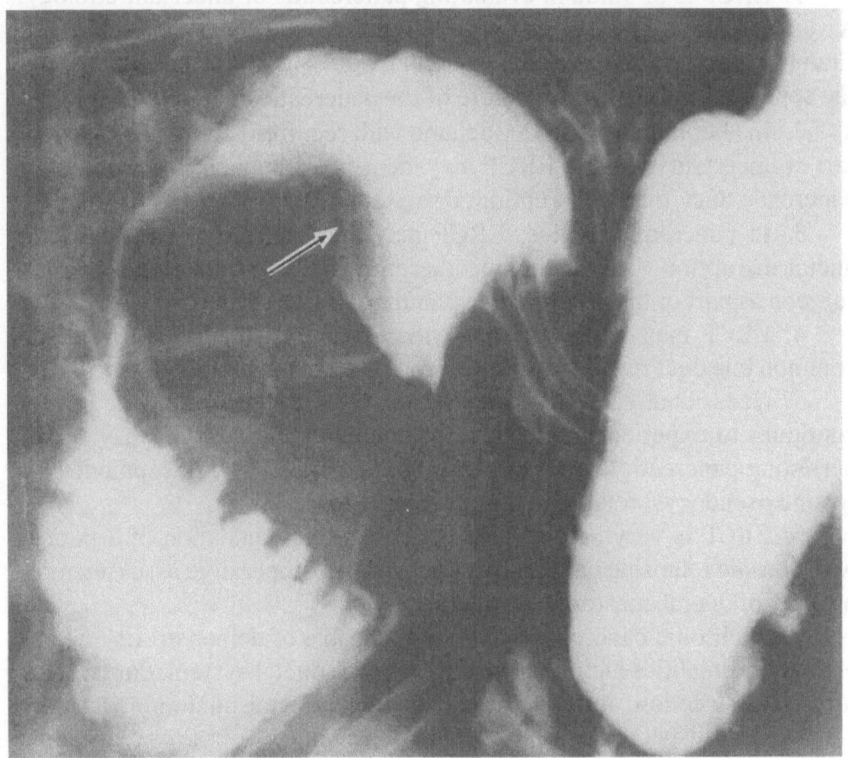

FIGURE 32 Duodenal Narrowing in Chronic Pancreatitis. Barium meal examination shows marked stenosis of postapical duodenum associated with a mass that deflects and stretches the greater curvature aspect of the duodenal bulb (arrow). At surgery, this patient with severe alcoholic pancreatitis had marked inflammation of the head of the pancreas with contiguous involvement of the postapical duodenum. A gastrojejunostomy was performed because of severe obstruction. Interestingly, there was no evidence of common bile duct obstruction.

alert the clinician for the first time to the pancreatic basis of puzzling abdominal pain.

14.2.2 Endoscopic Retrograde Cholangiopancreatography

The technique of endoscopic retrograde cholangiopancreatography (ERCP) has already been mentioned many times as an important diagnostic tool in the diagnosis and treatment of pancreatitis. It is worthwhile here to summarize indications for its use.

1. ERCP is of value in evaluating pancreatitis of uncertain etiology. A variety of unsuspected or unproven abnormalities may be found, including biliary tract gravel, choledochal cyst, structural abnormality of the sphincter of Oddi, and stricture of the pancreatic duct (see Chapter 2).

2. In abdominal trauma associated with recurrent abdominal discomfort of uncertain etiology, ERCP may identify a traumatic stricture of the pancreatic duct, ductal disruption, or a pseudocyst.

3. In pancreatic ascites, ERCP may demonstrate a pseudocyst or ductal disruption. This technique therefore has great usefulness to the surgeon as part of his preoperative planning (Figure 29).

4. ERCP may reveal the presence of severe stenosis of the distal common bile duct responsible for episodes of abdominal pain.

5. Occasionally, after surgery for pancreatic pseudocyst, the patient continues to experience episodes of abdominal pain. ERCP may reveal persisting pancreatic ductal stenosis and at times the development of a second pseudocyst related to this stenosis (Figure 33).

6. ERCP is very helpful in the preoperative evaluation of a patient with chronic relapsing pancreatitis and in the postoperative assessment of patency of ductal anastomosis to jejunum.

7. In chronic pancreatitis, ERCP is capable of demonstrating a variety of abnormalities including distortion of the ductal system, ductal stricture or obstruction, intraductal calcification, ductal dilatation, pseudocyst, and unsuspected carcinoma (Figures 19 and 20).[3-7] Pancreatic fluid can be aspirated for cytology, carcinoembryonic antigen (CEA), bicarbonate, and enzymes.[3] Abnormalities that are of help to the surgeon include significant ductal dilatation and a pancreatic pseudocyst. Surgical options are discussed in detail in Chapter 15. The presence of significant ductal dilatation enables the surgeon to consider a lateral pancreaticojejunostomy. On the other hand, marked stenosis of the pancreatic duct requires a major pancreatic resection. Finally, absence of significant ductal pathology or pseudocyst raises the important question as to whether any operative manipulation would yield a favorable clinical result.

14.2.3 Diagnostic Ultrasound and C-T Scan

Diagnostic ultrasound is capable of visualizing the size of the pancreas, calcifications within the pancreas, a pancreatic psuedocyst, and dilatation of the common bile duct. In an early stage of chronic pancreatitis associated with some degree of active inflammation, the pancreas may be swollen; in severe chronic pancreatitis, the gland may be severely fibrotic and small.

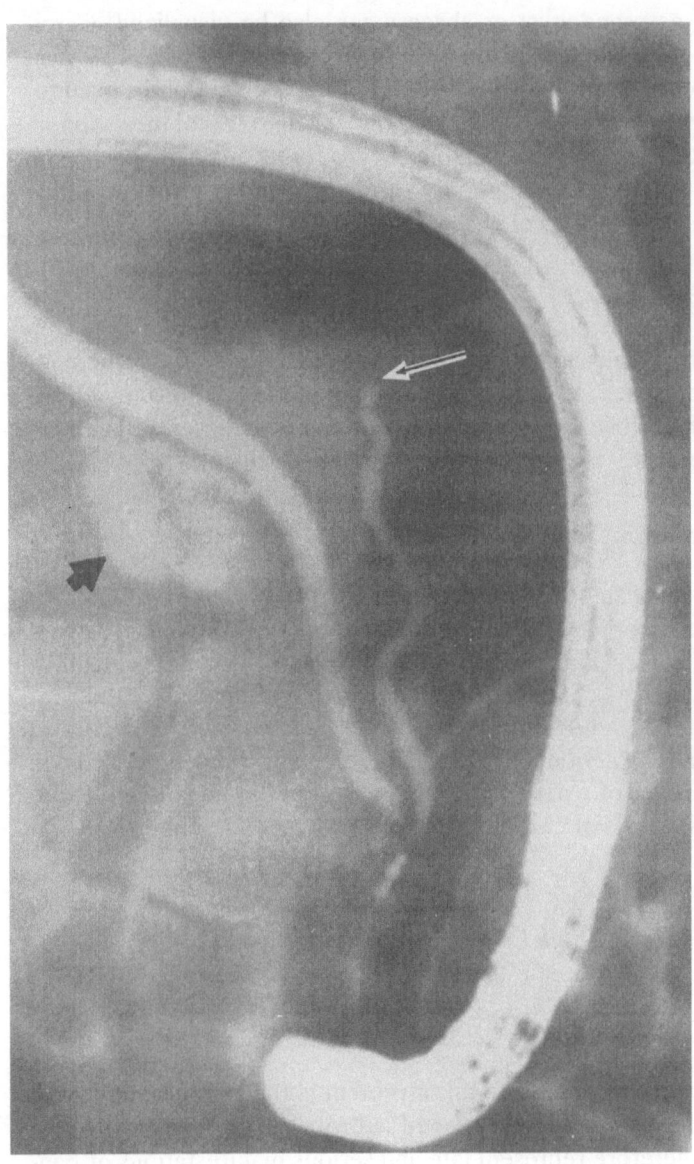

FIGURE 33 ERCP: Pancreatic Ductal Stenosis. This patient had previously undergone drainage of a pancreatic pseudocyst but continued to have abdominal pain. ERCP shows retrograde flow of contrast material into a normal-appearing pancreatic duct with abrupt termination of flow in the body of the pancreas (vertical arrow). The common bile duct and gallbladder (black arrow) are also visualized. At re-exploration, marked ductal stenosis was visualized in the body of the pancreas with evidence of acute and chronic inflammation of the distal body and tail of the pancreas. A pancreatic resection of the distal pancreas was performed. This case shows that if pancreatic ductal narrowing does not resolve following drainage of a pseudocyst, additional episodes of pancreatitis may occur. (Courtesy of Dr. R. Norton.)

The role of C-T scan in chronic pancreatitis is not fully established (Chapter 6). Pancreatic ductal calcification and at times pancreatic ductal dilatation can be visualized with this technique (Figures 17 and 18).[8] Complications such as pseudocyst or abscess can also be visualized. Carcinoma may be very difficult to distinguish from pancreatitis. The C-T scan may be extremely helpful if it shows severe ductal dilatation or pseudocyst at a time when diagnostic ultrasound has failed to reveal these abnormalities and ERCP is either unavailable or fails for technical reasons. The appearance on C-T scan of a markedly shrunken gland is visual evidence of the severity of some cases of chronic pancreatitis (Figure 18).

14.2.4 Angiography

Angiography is occasionally helpful in the diagnosis of chronic pancreatitis. The presence of aneurysms in peripancreatic arteries in pancreatitis, and their absence in carcinoma of the pancreas, has been reported to be a specific way to make this important distinction.[9]

14.2.5 Radioisotopic Scan

Radioisotopic scan of the pancreas is considered useful by some but of limited value by others. The usual technique is to combine [^{75}Se]selenomethionine, which is extracted by both liver and pancreas, with a second isotope such as colloidal gold-198, which is extracted by the liver but not pancreas. A radioisotope scan of the pancreas can be produced with the use of a subtraction technique. This technique may have a role in defining the presence of a pancreatic carcinoma but has had limited applicability in the diagnosis of chronic pancreatitis.

14.3 TESTS OF EXOCRINE DEFICIENCY

14.3.1 Stool Examination

The appearance of excessive fat or protein in the stool means that at least 90% of the pancreatic reserve of enzymes has been destroyed. These findings therefore represent late and serious manifestations of pancreatic insufficiency.

The diagnosis of steatorrhea is suggested by the passage of bulky, greasy, and offensive stools. The greasy quality can be best appreciated by smearing a portion of the stool on a piece of filter paper. A smear of fecal material can also be placed on a slide, dispersed in normal saline, and stained with Sudan-3. A microscopic finding of at least six fat globules per low-power field indicates significant steatorrhea. If 36% acetic acid is added and the slide is heated, soaps (which do not stain with Sudan-3) reconvert to fatty acids and appear as orange globules. On cooling, crystalization takes place which can be identified under low power by a characteristic spiculated appearance. Since the stool contains a mixture of both neutral fat, which stains with Sudan-3, and soaps, which do not, both procedures should be carried out. A mixture appears in the stool because bacterial lipases in the colon convert triglyceride to free fatty acids with formation of soaps. Therefore, pancreatic insufficiency cannot be distinguished from other causes of malabsorption by the proportions of triglyceride and fatty acid in the stool.[10]

Microscopic examination of a fecal smear may also visualize partially digested meat fibers indicating deficient protease secretion by the pancreas. While microscopic examination of stool for fat and meat fibers may readily yield convincing evidence of malabsorption in far-advanced pancreatic insufficiency, these tests may be equivocal in milder degrees of steatorrhea.

The most important and accurate examination of the stool in chronic pancreatitis is a quantitative chemical determination of fecal fat. The patient should be placed on a 100 gm fat intake for at least 2 to 3 days prior to the collection of stool for 72 hr. It is important to ascertain in advance from the laboratory the proper method of collection and storage of stool. It is not uncommon to learn, after a tedious 72-hr collection, that the laboratory refuses to process the stool because of the use of improper receptacles that make retrieval without spillage impossible for the wary technician. It is also important to enlist the services of a dietitian to be absolutely sure of the amount of fat consumed each day. If the patient consumes approximately 100 gm of fat per day for at least 2 to 3 days prior to the test and for a full 3 days during which all stool is collected, approximately 94 gm should be absorbed each day and no more than 6 gm recovered in the stool. This gives a coefficient of fat absorption of 94%. Attempts have been made to diagnose pancreatic exocrine sufficiency by measurement of fecal chymotrypsin activity.[11] This may be useful in demonstrating malabsorption in severe pancreatic insufficiency, but does not appear to offer any advantage to measurements of fecal fat.

14.3.2 Urinary Tests

An imaginative method has been developed to document the presence of steatorrhea by measurement of urinary p-aminobenzoic acid

(PABA) after the oral administration of a synthetic peptide that contains PABA. The cleavage of PABA from the peptide depends on intraluminal pancreatic chymotrypsin. Thus far, in two studies, urinary levels of PABA were markedly decreased in chronic pancreatitis associated with steatorrhea.[12,13] In one study, the severest forms of steatorrhea were associated with the greatest reductions in urinary PABA, and, appropriately, lesser degrees of steatorrhea were associated with more normal recovery of PABA in urine.[12] This test appears to be very promising in documenting exocrine pancreatic insufficiency and certainly easier than assay of a 72-hr stool for fat. It has not yet been ascertained whether this test reliably documents mild pancreatic insufficiency.

14.3.3 Aspiration of Duodenal Contents

(a) Secretin Test. The purpose of the secretin test is to detect abnormalities of pancreatic secretion that are diagnostic of pancreatic disease. Two diseases for which the secretin test has had the greatest applicability are chronic pancreatitis and carcinoma of the pancreas.

The methodology involves the peroral passage of a double lumen tube and localization by fluoroscopic control such that the apertures of one tube rest in the stomach and the apertures of the other in the duodenum. A Dreiling tube (Davol Rubber Company) is ideal for this purpose and is not difficult to maneuver into position with fluoroscopic control. The proximal two ends of the double lumen tube are attached to separate receptacles for collection of gastric and duodenal fluid. Gentle negative suction can be achieved with a Gomco apparatus. According to methodology at Mount Sinai Hospital in New York,[14,15] secretin is administered intravenously in a dosage of 1 unit per kilogram body weight, duodenal fluid is aspirated continuously for a total of 80 min (four collections of 10 min each and two collections of 20 min each), and measurements are made of volume output, bicarbonate concentration, and amylase concentration. The characteristic secretory profile of chronic pancreatitis is a normal volume output, a reduction in bicarbonate concentration, and a normal or reduced amylase concentration. The characteristic profile of a carcinoma of the pancreas is a decrease in volume, a normal bicarbonate concentration, and a normal amylase concentration.[14,15] On rare occasions, if chronic pancreatitis is particularly severe or if a carcinoma of the head of the pancreas blocks essentially all pancreatic secretion, volume, bicarbonate concentration, and amylase concentration are all reduced.

Proper localization of the double lumen tube with fluoroscopic control is essential. If the tube is advanced too far into the duodenum, apertures intended for the recovery of only gastric juice are now situated in the proximal duodenum and are likely to aspirate some pancreatic fluid into the "gastric receptacle" thereby reducing the volume of fluid aspirated through the duodenal apertures into the "pancreatic receptacle." A reduction in volume in the pancreatic receptacle would suggest a carcinoma of the pancreas. On the other hand, if the double lumen tube is not advanced far enough into the duodenum, duodenal apertures will straddle the pylorus. When this occurs, some pancreatic juice may escape distally beneath the lowermost duodenal apertures causing a deficit in volume in the pancreatic receptacle. Furthermore, some of the duodenal apertures lying in the distal antrum may aspirate gastric acid thereby reducing bicarbonate concentration.

Diagnostic accuracy of the secretin test in chronic pancreatitis has been excellent.[14-16] Attempts have been made to improve diagnostic accuracy further by utilizing larger amounts of secretin,[16,17] but it is not clear whether this modification is necessary. Another modification of the standard methodology has been the use of intravenous cholecystokinin-pancreozymin (CCK-PZ) either before, with, or following the injection of secretin. There is no strong evidence thus far that the addition of CCK-PZ adds to the diagnostic usefulness of secretin test for clinical purposes.[14]

The performance of a secretin test can be somewhat tedious for both patient and clinician. If the test were no more sensitive than a 72-hr stool for fat, its usefulness would be limited. The greater sensitivity of a secretin test can best be appreciated by the following data. All patients with steatorrhea, a hallmark of severe chronic pancreatitis, can also be expected to have characteristic secretory abnormalities on secretin test.[12,18-22] On the other hand, in an earlier stage of chronic pancreatitis when steatorrhea is absent, the secretin test may show a decrease in bicarbonate concentration indicative of chronic pancreatitis.[12,19,22]

The secretin test has given us many valuable insights into the natural history of chronic pancreatitis and the physiology of the pancreas. Studies have shown that calcific pancreatitis, indicative of a very severe form of chronic pancreatitis, is associated with greater deficits of pancreatic function than noncalcific pancreatitis.[23,24] These observations have been made on patients with either calcific or noncalcific pancreatitis, and the presumption is that pancreatic function deteriorates as noncalcific pancreatitis progresses in time to calcific pancreatitis. Surprisingly, there are very little data on the natural history of pancreatic function among individual patients with alcoholic pancreatitis studied for many years.

Various abnormalities of pancreatic secretion have been documented in chronic pancreatitis. The characteristic secretory abnormality of well-established chronic pancreatitis is a decrease in bicarbonate concentration. Later in the course of chronic pancreatitis, there may also be decreases in enzyme concentration or decreases in both enzyme concentration and volume output. A recently discovered pattern early in chronic pancreatitis is an increase in volume associated with either a normal or only slightly reduced bicarbonate concentration. The cause of the increased volume output may be ductal hypertrophy and hyperplasia.[15]

On rare occasions, in illnesses characterized by malnutrition in the United States, only the enzyme concentration is reduced. In adult patients with protein-calorie malnutrition in India, pancreatic function testing with intravenous CCK-PZ followed by intravenous secretin has revealed a reduction in bicarbonate concentration and enzyme secretion with preservation of a normal volume response.[25] Exocrine pancreatic function recovered promptly following dietary therapy so that bicarbonate concentration and several of the enzyme deficiencies return to normal within 2 to 12 weeks.[26,27] Improvement in pancreatic secretion has also been noted among patients with chronic alcoholism once protein intake returned to normal.[28] Since the secretory abnormality in both chronic pancreatitis and protein-calorie malnutrition is qualitative (a reduction in bicarbonate concentration with normal volume output), it is possible that some patients thought to have chronic pancreatitis because of a decreased bicarbonate concentration actually have protein-calorie malnutrition. For this reason a dietary history is essential for the proper interpretation of a secretin test.

In calcific pancreatitis in India, an unexpected profile was a normal bicarbonate concentration and reduction in volume flow.[29] This may imply that the basic pathophysiology of calcific pancreatitis in India is different from that of chronic calcific pancreatitis secondary to alcohol in other parts of the world.

One imperfection of the secretin test is the fact that duodenal fluid obtained in response to secretin is a mixture of pancreatic secretion, bile, and small intestinal fluid. Now that ERCP has become available, it is possible to obtain pure pancreatic juice. In one study performed by this technique, bicarbonate concentration of pancreatic secretion was decreased as would be expected in chronic pancreatitis.[5]

(b) Lundh Test Meal. The Lundh test meal requires positioning of a radiopaque tube fluoroscopically in the distal duodenum. The tube has numerous collecting holes in its distal portion and is weighted at the end by a mercury bag. The standard test meal is then swallowed, and duodenal contents are gently aspirated for 2 hr in four consecutive 30-min samples. Enzyme concentration, usually trypsin, is determined on each sample.

An advantage of this test is that there is no need for intravenous administration of an expensive hormone such as secretin. A major disadvantage is that measurement of the concentration of enzyme in the duodenum is influenced not only by capacity of the pancreas to secrete that enzyme but also rate of gastric emptying, rate of absorption of the test meal by the small intestine, and dilution of pancreatic secretion by both biliary and small intestinal secretion. For these reasons, unless dilution indicators are utilized, one in the test meal to measure dilution and a second to assess the completeness of recovery of duodenal fluid, there are likely to be inaccuracies. Despite these limitations, the Lundh test meal is considered to be of value as a test of pancreatic function.[30-36] Extensive parallel studies of sensitivity of the Lundh test meal and the secretin test are lacking. The suggestion has been made that the two tests are comparable,[37] although the secretin test may be more sensitive in mild chronic pancreatitis.[34]

(c) Duodenal Perfusion. With the use of a dilution indicator, a very accurate method has been developed to measure pancreatic enzyme output in response to either the intravenous administration of CCK-PZ or the intraduodenal perfusion of a stimulant of pancreatic secretion (either essential amino acids or emulsified fat).[38] This technique has demonstrated that decreases in trypsin and lipase secretion in chronic pancreatitis do not cause significant creatorrhea or steatorrhea until the outputs of these enzymes are reduced to less than 10% of normal.[38] This is another example of a test of pancreatic function revealing impairment in pancreatic secretion prior to the development of steatorrhea. The methodology of duodenal perfusion has led to many important physiologic discoveries but is currently too complex for routine clinical use.

14.3.4 Miscellaneous Laboratory Tests

Various other laboratory tests have been utilized to assess pancreatic function in suspected chronic pancreatitis.[38,39] These include fecal excretion of ^{131}I-labeled triolein, and a variety of tolerance tests including gelatin, starch, ^{131}I-labeled triolein, and oleic acid. These tests have major drawbacks, including lack of accuracy, specificity, and sensitivity.[38]

In the differential diagnosis of steatorrhea of uncertain etiology, tests of small bowel function are frequently required, including D-xylose absorption study, measurement of serum carotene, small-bowel barium x-ray, and small-bowel biopsy.

14.4 TESTS OF ENDOCRINE DEFICIENCY

In chronic pancreatitis a glucose tolerance test may give evidence of diabetes mellitus. Serum insulin levels may reflect a deficiency of insulin secretion as a result of destruction of islet cells. Serum glucagon levels may also be reduced for the same reason. It is this reduction in glucagon secretion that renders the diabetes of chronic pancreatitis extremely brittle.[40]

14.5 SUMMARY OF TESTS

The following tests are recommended in the evaluation of a patient with suspected chronic pancreatitis. In addition to the usual chemical testing, blood tests should include serum amylase, lipase, 1-hr postprandial blood sugar, and possibly a glucose tolerance test. Radiologic studies should include a plain film of the abdomen, gastrointestinal series, oral cholecystogram, and if obstruction of the common bile duct is suspected, an intravenous cholangiogram. A 72-hr stool for fat content should be collected if steatorrhea is suspected. If available, a secretin test should be performed to detect abnormalities of pancreatic secretion in a relatively early stage of chronic pancreatitis.

REFERENCES

1. Farman J, Werbeloff L, Marks IN, et al: Proximal duodenal deformities due to chronic pancreatitis. *Br J Radiol* 39:662–668, 1966.
2. Blackstone MO, Mizuno H: Reactive duodenal changes in chronic pancreatitis simulating the contiguous spread of pancreatic carcinoma. *Am J Dig Dis* 22:658–661, 1977.
3. Steward EP, Vennes JA, Geenan HE (editors): *Atlas of Endoscopic Retrograde Cholangiopancreatography*. Mosely and Company, 1977.
4. Rohrmann CA, Jr., Silvis SE, Vennes JA: The significance of pancreatic ductal obstruction in differential diagnosis of the abnormal endoscopic retrograde pancreatogram. *Radiology* 121:311–314, 1976.
5. Kawanishi H, Sell JE, Pollard HM: Combined endoscopic pancreatic fluid collection and retrograde pancreatography in the diagnosis of pancreatic cancer and chronic pancreatitis. *Gastrointest Endos* 22:82–85, 1975.
6. Varley PF, Rohrmann CA, Jr., Silvis SE, et al: The normal endoscopic pancreatogram. *Radiology* 118:295–300, 1976.
7. Paul RE, Jr., Norton RA: Endoscopic retrograde cholangiopancreatography. In *Radiologic Contrast Agents*, Roscoe E. Miller and Jovitas Skucas (eds). University Park Press, Baltimore, 1977, pp 261–273.
8. Haaga JR, Alfidi RJ, Zelch MG, et al: Computed tomography of the pancreas. *Radiology* 120:589–595, 1976.
9. White AF, Baum S, Buranasir S: Aneurysms secondary to pancreatitis. *Am J Roentgenol* 127:393–396, 1976.
10. Moore JG, Englert E, Jr., Bigler AH, et al: Simple fecal tests of absorption. A prospective study and critique. *Am J Dig Dis* 16:97–105, 1971.

11. Moeller DD, Dunn GD, Klotz AP: Diagnosis of pancreatic exocrine insufficiency by fecal chymotrypsin activity. *Am J Dig Dis* 18:792–796, 1973.
12. Greenberger AC: A tubeless test of exocrine pancreatic function. *Lancet* 1:663–666, 1976.
13. Gyr K, Stalder GA, Schiffmann I, et al: Oral administration of a chymotrypsin-labile peptide—a new test of exocrine pancreatic function in man (PFT). *Gut* 17:27–32, 1976.
14. Dreiling DA, Janowitz HD, and Perrier C: The diagnosis of pancreatic disease. In *Pancreatic Inflammatory Disease.* (Hoeber) Harper and Row, New York, 1964, pp 129–147.
15. Dreiling DA: Pancreatic secretory testing. *Gut* 16:653–657, 1975.
16. Bordalo O, Noronha M, Lamy J, et al: Standard and augmented secretin testing in chronic pancreatic alcoholic disease. *Am J Gastroenterol* 64:125–132, 1975.
17. Petersen H, Myren J: Secretin dose response in health and chronic pancreatic inflammatory disease. *Scand J Gastroenterol* 10:851–861, 1975.
18. Marks IN, Bank S, Airth EM: Pancreatic replacement therapy in the treatment of pancreatic steatorrhea. *Gut* 4:217–222, 1963.
19. Cerda JJ, Brooks FP: Relationships between steatorrhea and an insufficiency of pancratic secretion in the duodenum in patients with chronic pancreatitis. *Am J Med Sci* 253:38–44, 1967.
20. Marin GA, Clark ML, Senior JR: Studies of malabsorption occurring in patients with Laennec's cirrhosis. *Gastroenterol* 56:727–736, 1969.
21. Sun DCH, Albacete RA, Chen JK: Malabsorption studies in cirrhosis of the liver. *Arch Intern Med* 119:567–572, 1967.
22. Lippe GVD, Andersen K-J, Schionsby H: Intestinal absorption of vitamin B-12 in patients with chronic pancreatic insufficiency and the effect of human duodenal juice on the intestinal uptake of vitamin B-12. *Scand J Gastroenterol* 11:689–695, 1976.
23. Janowitz HD, Dreiling DA: Is there pancreatic ductal obstruction in chronic pancreatitis? An analysis of the functional trans-sphincteric pancreatic and biliary flow in patients with and without pancreatic disease. *Gastroenterology* 36:12–16, 1959.
24. Vagne M, Descos L: Pancreatic secretion of bicarbonate in patients with chronic pancreatitis. *Digestion* 3:350–356, 1970.
25. Tandon BN, George PK, Sama SK, et al: Exocrine pancreatic function in protein calorie malnutrition disease of adults. *Am J Clin Nutr* 22:1476–1482, 1969.
26. Tandon BN, Banks PA, George PK, et al: Recovery of exocrine pancreatic function in adult protein-calorie malnutrition. *Gastroenterology* 58:358–362, 1970.
27. Kumar R, Banks PA, George PK, et al: Early recovery of exocrine pancreatic function in adult protein calorie malnutrition. *Gastroenterology* 68:1593–1595, 1975.
28. Mezey E, Jow E, Slavin RE, et al: Pancreatic function and intestinal absorption in chronic alcoholism. *Gastroenterology* 59:657–664, 1970.
29. George PK, Banks PA, Pai KN, et al: Exocrine pancreatic function in calcific pancreatitis in India. *Gastroenterology* 60:858–863, 1971.
30. Gyr K, Agrawal NM, Felsenfeld O, et al: Comparative study of secretin and Lundh tests. *Am J Dig Dis* 20:506–512, 1975.
31. Zeitlin IJ, Sircus W: Factors influencing duodenal trypsin levels following a standard test meal as a test of pancreatic function. *Gut* 15:173–179, 1974.
32. Mottaleb A, Kapp F, Noguera ECA, et al: The Lundh test in the diagnosis of pancreatic disease: A review of five years' experience. *Gut* 14:835–841, 1973.
33. Youngs GR, Agnew JE, Levin GE, et al: A comparative study of four tests of pancreatic function in the diagnosis of pancreatic disease. *Q J Med* XLII :597–618, 1973.
34. James O: Progress report. The Lundh test. *Gut* 14:582–591 1973.
35. Waller SL: The Lundh test in the diagnosis of pancreatic disease. *Gut* 16:657–658, 1975.

36. Ihs EI, Arnesjo B, Kugelberg C, et al: Intestinal activities of trypsin, lipase, and phospholipase after a test meal. *Scand J Gastroent* 12:663–668, 1977.
37. Lurie B, Brom B, Bank S, et al: Comparative response of exocrine pancreatic secretion following a test meal and secretin-pancreozymin stimulation. *Scand J Gastroent* 8:27–32, 1973.
38. Di Magno EP, Go VLW: The clinical application of exocrine pancreatic function tests. *Dis Mon* September: 3–36, 1976.
39. Brooks FP: Testing pancreatic function. *N Engl J Med* 286:300–303, 1972.
40. Donowitz N, Hendler R, Spiro HM, et al: Glucagon secretion in acute and chronic pancreatitis. *Ann Int Med* 83:778–781, 1975.

Treatment of Chronic Pancreatitis

15.1 MEDICAL TREATMENT

15.1.1 Abdominal Pain

The treatment of chronic relapsing pancreatitis as typified by alcoholic pancreatitis follows the same therapeutic efforts outlined in Chapter 8 for treatment of acute pancreatitis. If a relapse is associated with minimal discomfort, the nasogastric tube can be omitted or removed after only 1 or 2 days. Proper attention must still be directed to fluid and electrolyte balance, and the use of a metabolic flow sheet is strongly urged in all instances of pancreatitis whether clinically mild or severe.

With each apparent relapse of pancreatitis, the clinician should review three areas of differential diagnosis: (1) Other causes of abdominal pain, such as penetrating duodenal ulcer, cholecystitis, and even malingering in an effort to receive additional amounts of narcotic agents. (2) Other causes of pancreatitis. On rare occasions, measurement of serum calcium or triglyceride level reveals an abnormality of diagnostic significance. A marked elevation in serum triglyceride caused by alcohol may occasionally cause a relapse of pancreatitis (Chapter 2). The gallbladder should also be viewed with suspicion. It is extremely important that oral cholecystography or diagnostic ultrasound, or both, be carried out to confirm that the patient does not have cholelithiasis. If gallstones are visualized, careful clinical evaluation is necessary to determine whether the pancreatitis is caused by passage of gallstones or represents a typical relapse from alcohol. Documentation of gallstones in the common bile duct on intravenous or endoscopic cholangiography is reasonably strong evidence that gallbladder disease is symptomatic and deserving of surgical therapy. The best way at present to be certain that a recurrence of pancreatitis is caused by the passage of gallstones is the recovery of gallstones in the stool. (3) A complication of pancreatitis, such as pancreatic pseudocyst or stricture of the distal common bile duct.

One of the most difficult problems in chronic pancreatitis is abdominal pain that persists indefinitely with minor fluctuations. There are several possible causes: (1) Smoldering pancreatic inflammation may cause pain which lasts for several days and even several weeks. (2) Distention and pressure from one or more pancreatic pseudocysts may lead to chronic pain. (3) Chronic perineural inflammation and fibrosis may lead to pain which persists indefinitely despite the use of narcotic agents. (4) There is the pain of ductal obstruction owing to intraductal stones or strictures, which develops promptly after a meal and lasts several hours, associated at times with nausea and vomiting.

There are several therapeutic efforts that are worth pursuing. These have been described in detail in Chapter 8. The patient should be instructed to avoid large meals rich in protein and fat. The use of a liquid antacid preparation 1 and 3 hr after meals as well as at bedtime will reduce the delivery of acid into the duodenum. If this fails to effect clinical improvement, and if acid secretory studies reveal marked hypersecretion of acid, Cimetidine may be beneficial, especially if used in conjunction with a liquid antacid preparation or Probantheline to reduce the delivery of gastric acid into the duodenum even further. A liquid elemental diet may be tried to maintain nutrition and prevent an exacerbation of pain. This diet seemingly has the advantage of containing modest amounts of protein, negligible or modest amounts of fat, and an abundance of carbohydrate. It must be stressed, however, that there has been no carefully controlled clinical study which compares the efficacy of an elemental diet with dietary foods in preventing an exacerbation of pain. Medium-chain triglycerides may be preferable to dietary fat as a source of nourishment because they are less of a stimulant of pancreatic secretion. The usefulness of pancreatic extracts in preventing relapses of pain requires more careful study. Theoretically, there may be a negative feedback mechanism in the small intestine such that the administration of pancreatic extracts by mouth inhibits the synthesis of pancreatic enzymes.

An intensive effort must be made to persuade the patient to discontinue alcohol completely. All members of the health team including psychiatrist, social worker, self-help group, and the constant helpful and supportive presence of the primary physician are indispensable in this effort. Occasionally, once total abstinence from alcohol is achieved, there is marked clinical improvement and even cessation of relapses of pancreatitis. Altogether too frequently, however, additional relapses are inevitable. It is likely that the severe anatomic derangement caused by alcohol, including pancreatic ductal obstruction and lymphatic obstruction, causes both clinical relapses and further histologic deterioration.

15.1.2 Steatorrhea

Since a wide variety of commercial pancreatic supplements is available,[1,2] the treatment of steatorrhea in chronic pancreatitis should be relatively straightforward, yet there are many problems and a variety of therapeutic approaches.[3–6]

One problem is the marked variability in the potency of commercially available preparations and even in the potency of batches of pancreatic extracts marketed by the same company. Further, because there are differences in techniques utilized to test pancreatic extracts, the same product may be accorded different potencies by different investigators.[1,2]

Another problem is that the use of even potent pancreatic extracts improves but does not eliminate steatorrhea completely.[7–12] By way of review, it should be restated that steatorrhea does not occur until pancreatic secretion of lipase is reduced to less than 10% of normal.[13] This correlates well with surgical information that steatorrhea occurs with a greater than 80% resection of pancreas,[8,14] but either does not occur[8] or is clinically insignificant[14] with less than 80% resection. The inability of pancreatic extracts to correct steatorrhea entirely has led to a variety of techniques to enhance their effectiveness. One has been to administer pancreatic extracts on an hourly basis rather than simply with meals. Although one study has reported a greater improvement in steatorrhea by this schedule,[10] there is generally no particular advantage of one schedule over another,[7,8] and steatorrhea is not completely abolished whether pancreatic replacement is given by either schedule.[7–12]

The reason for the relative ineffectiveness of pancreatic extracts is the fact that pancreatic enzymes are inactivated by hydrochloric acid and pepsin. It has recently been determined that lipase is inactivated by acid but not pepsin whereas trypsin and chymotrypsin are inactivated by pepsin but not hydrochloric acid.[15] At a pH of 3.5 or below, lipase is completely inactivated by acid.[15] The administration of pancreatic extracts with antacids[8,9] or sodium bicarbonate[9,16] in an effort to neutralize gastric juice corrects steatorrhea only partially and no more so than when the pancreatic extract is administered by itself.[9] The ineffectiveness of bicarbonate, and presumably antacids as well, is explained by the persistence of gastric and duodenal pHs in an acid range despite their use.[7,9] As a result, almost all pancreatic enzymes administered by mouth are rapidly inactivated by gastric acid, and only very small amounts reach the duodenum in active form.

One might predict that if sufficient amounts of potent antacids are given frequently enough, gastric and duodenal pH will remain relatively neutral, and pancreatic extracts will be more effective in reducing steatorrhea. One difficulty is that antacids cause additional secretion of gastric acid which, even if buffered substantially by periodic amounts of liquid antacid, dilutes pancreatic enzymes to ineffective concentrations and thereby impairs hydrolysis of fat.[17]

The use of enteric coating of pancreatic extracts to protect enzymes until the capsule reaches the duodenum also fails to enhance the effectiveness of a pancreatic extract in correcting steatorrhea.[9] This effort probably fails because the coating dissolves prematurely in the stomach or tardily in the colon, or because the capsules are retained in the stomach until most of the food has already left the stomach and small intestine.[3]

The only way that has been found thus far to enhance the effectiveness of a pancreatic extract and eliminate steatorrhea altogether has been the use of Cimetidine, which inhibits gastric acid secretion.[9] The use of this medication is recommended when a potent pancreatic extract fails to achieve a gain in weight and improvement in nutritional status.

The following recommendation should be helpful for the bewildered clinician looking for guidance in the treatment of steatorrhea. He should choose a pancreatic extract that is very potent. Published data that compare enzyme activities in pancreatic supplementations indicate that Ilozyme (Warren-Teed), Cotazym (Organon), and Viokase (Viobin) among preparations readily available in the United States contain very high lipase activities.[1,2] It is reasonable to initiate therapy by providing 3 tablets of a potent pancreatic extract with each meal and noting whether the patient gains weight. My instructions are usually to swallow 1 tablet before, 1 during, and 1 after each meal. It may be equally therapeutic to swallow all 3 tablets at the same time. If the clinical response is not satisfactory, the number of tablets can be increased to 6 to 8 with each of three meals (a total of 18 to 24 tablets daily). Alternatively, a total of 18 to 24 tablets can be administered at frequent intervals during the day, such as 1 to 2 tablets every hour while awake. Although in one study there was no difference in therapeutic response when hourly administration was compared with pancreatic replacement at mealtimes,[7] nonetheless, steatorrhea may possibly be better controlled in selected instances with frequent administration of pancreatic extracts.

One criterion to gauge clinical response is to calculate a 72-hr stool for fat before and after a therapeutic endeavor. A much easier and entirely reasonable procedure is simply to determine whether the patient is gaining weight and having fewer offensive stools. From a practical stand-point, a favorable clinical response is as good as documentation of reduction of a 72-hr stool for fat.

If the clinical response is satisfactory, no additional therapy is required even if steatorrhea has not been fully eliminated. If clinical response is unsatisfactory as evidenced by a failure to gain weight and improve nutritionally, liquid antacid can be administered 1 and 3 hr after each meal, but probably will not be helpful. Cimetidine can then be administered for 6 to 8 weeks in order to achieve a gain in weight. It has been my practice to obtain an acid secretory study prior to the use of Cimetidine, but this is probably optional. If the clinical response remains unfavorable after the administration of Cimetidine, an acid secretory study would then be essential to document whether acid secretion is considerable. Under these circumstances, the combination of Cimetidine and Propantheline should be administered in view of evidence that the combination of these medications achieves a greater reduction of acid secretion than either alone.[18]

Additional dietary support can be provided with medium-chain-tri-glyceride (MCT) oil. This preparation has several advantages. It is hydro-lyzed more rapidly than dietary fat by available lipase, is absorbed intact through the mucosa of the small intestine without the need for hydrolysis, and does not stimulate pancreatic enzyme secretion as readily as dietary fats. There are many ways that MCT oil can be incorporated into the diet in a palatable fashion. Most dietitians are familiar with recipes to achieve this goal. Another dietary measure is an elemental diet, which furnishes additional calories in a reasonably palatable fashion.

Excessive steatorrhea can be reduced by restricting the amount of dietary fat that is consumed. Dietary fat should be offered in small meals consumed four to six times per day. Pancreatic enzyme replacement helps not only in the digestion of fat, but perhaps in a second way. In pancreatic insufficiency, fatty meals are emptied by the stomach at an excessive rate. Pancreatic extracts tend to retard gastric emptying of fatty meals and by doing so perhaps permit more complete digestion in the small intestine.[19]

Some pancreatic extracts are marketed in the form of a powder as well as tablets. Since powder tends to be less palatable than the tablets, its use should be reserved for a situation in which the tablet is likely to be ineffective in correcting steatorrhea. An example of this might be a patient with a gastrojejunostomy. The tablet could pass rapidly into the distal small intestine before disintegration. Since the presence of acid would rapidly inactivate enzymes in the form of powder, an acid secretory study is desirable before instituting this therapy.

One question difficult to answer is the number of tablets that should be administered in an effort to correct steatorrhea. A possible drawback to excessive amounts of pancreatic extract is the possibility of hyperuricosuria caused by the high purine content of presently available pancreatic extracts.[20]

15.1.3 Creatorrhea

Loss of nitrogen in the stool is not as significant a problem as loss of fat. First, in chronic pancreatitis, trypsin output is maintained at a more normal level than lipase output.[21] Second, a potent pancreatic extract is capable of eliminating excessive fecal nitrogen excretion even when steatorrhea is only partially corrected.[9] Its greater efficacy in correcting creatorrhea is not fully understood, but may relate to the fact that proteases are not inactivated by acid but lipase is.[15]

15.1.4 Diabetes Mellitus

Since the diabetic state in chronic pancreatitis is quite brittle and since elevations in serum glucose are usually well tolerated and not ordinarily complicated by diabetic ketoacidosis, the precise regulation of blood sugar may be a hazardous undertaking (Chapter 13). An initial attempt may be made to regulate blood sugar with oral hypoglycemic agents which in selected instances may improve glucose tolerance.[22] If insulin is required, it should be administered with extreme caution. Very small amounts of subcutaneous insulin, sometimes only 10 to 15 units of regular insulin, may reduce an extremely high blood sugar of 600 to 700 mg % to less than 100 mg % owing to the deficiency of glucagon in chronic pancreatitis. Precautions to be observed to avoid the dangers of hypoglycemia include thorough instruction of the patient in the symptoms of hypoglycemia and the use of an "alert" bracelet or chain indicating that the patient is a diabetic on insulin. Reliability of the patient is indispensable if insulin is to be administered. Periodic measurements should be made of urinary sugar and blood sugar. The patient should always have on his person a source of carbohydrate such as powdered sugar or a sugar-coated candy. A dietician can be extremely helpful in standardizing diet in a way that renders diabetic management somewhat easier.

15.2 SURGICAL TREATMENT

Consideration of surgical treatment of chronic pancreatitis depends on at least two distinct indications. The first is a complication such as pseudocyst or abscess, as discussed in Chapter 8, and the second is intractable pain leading to narcotic addiction, loss of weight, and generalized debility. Almost all cases of chronic pancreatitis requiring surgery are caused by alcohol. Since the majority of patients continue to drink after surgery and many are lost to follow-up, it is extremely difficult to judge the results of surgical therapy. This difficulty is compounded by the fact that there have been no randomized prospective clinical trials comparing surgical with medical therapy and contrasting the various surgical procedures to control pain.

Operations on the biliary system are not helpful unless symptoms are clearly from passage of gallstones.[23] Sphincterotomy of the ampulla of Vater, once considered a proper approach for chronic pancreatitis,[24] has generally been abandoned as worthless by itself. Splanchnicectomy has been reported to relieve pain on a temporary basis but does not provide permanent relief.[25,26] Splanchnicectomy, vagotomy, and either antrectomy with Bilroth II anastomosis or gastroenterostomy was reported beneficial in 5 patients, but the period of follow-up was less than 2 years,[27] and this procedure seems unlikely to afford permanent help. Ligation of the pancreatic duct in a small group of patients has led to apparent relief of pain.[28] Ductal obstruction has also been produced with an acrylate glue in 3 patients with apparent relief of pain.[29] The efficacy and safety of ductal obstruction requires much more extensive evaluation before the technique can be endorsed.

The surgical procedures that have received the most attention have involved either resection of a portion of the pancreas[8,14,30-34] or decompression of the main pancreatic duct utilizing an anastomosis with a loop of jejunum.[25,26,35-40]

The type of resection that was first recommended was a distal 95% pancreatectomy.[30] More recently, the same authors hav reported that a 40% to 80% distal pancreatectomy is preferable to an 80% to 95% distal resection in that diabetes and steatorrhea are less severe, operative mortality is decreased, and clinical results are in general more favorable.[14] Since islet cells are more concentrated in the tail of the pancreas than in the head and body, preservation of as much pancreatic tissue as possible would ameliorate postoperative diabetes.[41] Other types of pancreatic resection represent relatively unusual special situations. If severe pancreatitis is restricted to the head of the pancreas and is associated with severe inflammation of the duodenum or a pseudocyst, a proximal resection (pancreaticoduodenectomy) may be required.[8,14,31-34] On very rare occasions, a total pancreatectomy may be the procedure of choice.[32-34]

Drainage of the main pancreatic duct has been advocated if there is severe dilatation of the main pancreatic duct or multiple strictures associated with severe dilatation in a chain-of-lakes appearance. All drainage procedures involve an anastomosis with a loop of jejunum which has been defunctionalized with a Roux-en-Y anastomosis. One technique involves amputation of the tail of the pancreas and an anastomosis of the dilated pancreatic duct in an "end-to-end" fashion to the mucosa of the jejunum.[40] Another technique involves the anastomosis of almost the entire main pancreatic duct to the jejunum and is called a "lateral" pancreaticojejunostomy. The incision of the main pancreatic duct extends from approximately 1 cm from the duodenum to approximately 1 to 3 cm from the tail of the pancreas. Once the main pancreatic duct has been fully exposed, areas of strictures incised, and intraductal calculi have been plucked from the main pancratic duct and the orifices of the secondary pancreatic duct, a Roux-en-Y loop of jejunum is then brought into approximation in a lateral orientation and anastomosed side-to-side.[35,36,38,39] Most surgeons prefer the lateral pancreaticojejunostomy because if the pancreatic duct near the tail is simply joined in an "end-to-end" fashion with a loop of jejunum, stricturing of this single aperture representing the anastomosis results in poor drainage. Indeed, the use of ERCP following pancreaticojejunal shunts have indicated patent anastomoses in instances of lateral pancreaticojejunostomy but possible occlusion following end-to-end (caudal) pancreaticojejunostomy.[42,43]

Surgical results are difficult to appraise in the absence of randomized clinical trials. Since alcoholic pancreatitis involves obstruction of small pancreatic ducts as well, it could be reasoned that any surgical procedure short of major pancreatic resection would fail to control pain on a permanent basis. On the other hand, a strong case can be made for lateral pancreaticojejunostomy as an initial procedure for a patient with a dilated main pancreatic duct especially if there are intraductal calculi. First, when a pancreatic duct is opened, pancreatic juice can frequently be seen to spurt into the surgical field indicating that there is high intraductal pressure which has contributed to at least some of the chronic pain. Further, it is not uncommon for the patient to indicate within 1 or 2 days of surgery that there has been marked relief of discomfort. Third, additional stones that are lodged in the secondary pancreatic ducts are then liberated and drop through the anastomosis into the jejunum thereby decompressing some of the smaller ducts as well. This phenomenon occurs only rarely, but can be documented on periodic plain films of the abdomen which show progressive disappearance of calcification. Finally, a lateral pancreaticojejunostomy is less apt to be associated with severe diabetes and steatorrhea than a major pancreatic resection. If clinical improvement is not forthcoming, a pancreatic resection can always be offered. Nutritional and metabolic status of patients has not been appraised in detail following lateral pancreaticojejunsotomy. Once there is more effective drainage of pancreatic secretion into the jejunum, there could be amelioration of steatorrhea.

In general, the operative approach depends largely on the skill and experience of the surgeon. Favorable results are generally reported in the majority of cases for both lateral pancreaticojejunostomy and pancreatic resection. A limiting factor in prognosis is the continued use of alcohol which makes the long-term prognosis considerably less favorable. [14,25,26,31]

The decision to attempt corrective surgery is most important. The timing is subject to a number of variables including narcotic addiction, general nutrition, impact of intractable pain on socioeconomic factors, and the willingness of the patient to help in his own rehabilitation by the discontinuation of alcohol.

REFERENCES

1. Graham DY: Enzyme replacement therapy of exocrine pancreatic insufficiency in man. Relation between vitro enzyme activities and in vivo potency in commercial pancreatic extracts. *N Engl J Med* 296:1314–1317, 1977.
2. Pairent FW, Howard JM: Pancreatic exocrine insufficiency. IV. The enzyme content of commercial pancreatic supplements. *Arch Surg* 110:739–741, 1975.
3. Meyer JH: The ins and outs of oral pancreatic enzymes. *N Engl J Med* 296:1347–1348, 1977.
4. Pancreatic extracts. *Lancet* 2:73–74, 1977.
5. Littman A, Hanscom DH: Pancreatic extracts. *N Engl J Med* 281:201–204, 1969.
6. Saunders JHB, Wormsley KG: Pancreatic extracts in the treatment of pancreatic exocrine insufficiency. *Gut* 16:157–162, 1975.
7. DiMagno EP, Malagelada JR, Go VLW, et al: Fate of orally ingested enzymes in pancreatic insufficiency. Comparison of two dosage schedules. *N Engl J Med* 296:1318–1322, 1977.
8. Kalser MH, Leite CA, Warren WD: Fat assimilation after massive distal pancreatectomy. *N Engl J Med* 279:570–576, 1968.
9. Regan PT, Malagelada JR, DiMagno EP, et al: Comparative effects of antacids, cimetidine and enteric coating on the therapeutic response to oral enzymes in severe pancreatic insufficiency. *N Engl J Med* 297:854–858, 1977.
10. Jordan PH, Grossman MI: Effect of dosage schedule on the efficacy of substitution therapy in pancreatic insufficiency. *Gastroenterology* 36:447–451, 1959.
11. Marks IN, Bank S, Airth EM: Pancreatic replacement therapy in the treatment of pancreatic steatorrhea. *Gut* 4:217–222, 1963.
12. Roller RJ, Kern F, Jr: Minimal bile acid malabsorption and normal bile acid breath tests in cystic fibrosis and acquired pancreatic insufficiency. *Gastroenterology* 72:661–665, 1977.
13. DiMagno EP, Go VLW, Summerskill WHJ: Relations between pancreatic enzyme outputs and malabsorption in severe pancreatic insufficiency. *N Engl J Med* 288:813–815, 1973.

14. Frey CF, Child CG, III, Fry W: Pancreatectomy for chronic pancreatitis. *Ann Surg* 184:403–414, 1976.
15. Lebenthal E, Krasner J, Hatch TF, et al: The effect of hydrochloric acid and pepsin on the exocrine pancreatic enzymes. Presented at the annual meeting of the American Pancreatic Association, Chicago, November, 1977.
16. Veeger W. Abels J, Hellemans N, et al: Effect of sodium bicarbonate and pancreatin on the absorption of vitamin B-12 and fat in pancreatic insufficiency. *N Engl J Med* 267:1341–1344, 1962.
17. Regan PT, Malagelada J-R, DiMagno EP, et al: Cimetidine as an adjunct to oral enzymes in the treatment of malabsorption due to pancreatic insufficiency. *Gastroenterology* 74:468–469, 1978.
18. Feldman M, Richardson CT, Peterson WL, et al: Effective low-dose Propantheline on food-stimulated gastric acid secretion. *N Engl J Med* 297:1427–1430, 1977.
19. Long WB, Weiss JB: Rapid gastric emptying of fatty meals in pancreatic insufficiency. *Gastroenterology* 67:920–925, 1974.
20. Stapleton FB, Kennedy J, Nousia-Arvanitakis S, et al: Hyperuricosuria due to high-dose pancreatic extract therapy in cystic fibrosis. *N Engl J Med* 295:246–248, 1976.
21. DiMagno EP, Malagelada JR, Go VLW: Relationship between alcoholism and pancreatic insufficiency. *Ann NY Acad Sci* 252:200–207, 1975.
22. Joffe BI, Jackson WPU, Bank S, et al: Effect of oral hypoglycaemic agents on glucose tolerance in pancreatic diabetes. *Gut* 13:285–288, 1972.
23. Way LW, Gadacz T, Goldman L: Surgical treatment of chronic pancreatitis. *Am J Surg* 127:202–209, 1974.
24. Doubilet H and Mulholland JH: Surgical treatment of chronic pancreatitis. *JAMA* 175:177–182, 1961.
25. Leger L, Lenriot JP, Lemaigre G: Five to twenty year followup after surgery for chronic pancreatitis in 148 patients. *Ann Surg* 180:185–191, 1974.
26. White TT, Keither RG: Long term follow-up study of fifty patients with pancreaticojejunostomy. *Surg Gynecol Obstet* 136:353–358, 1973.
27. Cahow CE, Hayes MA: Operative treatment of chronic recurrent pancreatitis. *Am J Surg* 125:390–398, 1973.
28. Madding GF, Kennedy PA: Chronic alcoholic pancreatitis. Treatment by ductal obstruction. *Am J Surg* 125:538–541, 1973.
29. Little JM, Lauer C, Hogg J: Pancreatic duct obstruction with an acrylate glue: A new method for producing pancreatic exocrine atrophy. *Surg* 81:243–249, 1977.
30. Fry WJ, Child CG, III: Ninety-five percent distal pancreatectomy for chronic pancreatitis. *Ann Surg* 162:543–549, 1965.
31. Guillemin G, Cuilleret J, Michel A, et al: Chronic relapsing pancreatitis. Surgical management including sixty-three cases of pancreaticoduodenectomy. *Am J Surg* 122:802–807, 1971.
32. Morgan JE, Robbins AH, Matsumoto G, et al: Total pancreatectomy for recurrent medullary fat necrosis. *Arch Surg* 111:1394–1398, 1976.
33. Warren KW, Mountain JC: Comprehensive management of chronic relapsing pancreatitis. *Surg Clin North Am* 51:693–710, 1971.
34. Warren KW: Surgical management of chronic relapsing pancreatitis. *Am J Surg* 117:24–32, 1969.
35. Cox WD, Gillesby WJ: Longitudinal pancreaticojejunostomy in alcoholic pancreatitis. *Arch Surg* 94:469–475, 1967.
36. Silen W, Baldwin J, Goldman L: Treatment of chronic pancreatitis by longitudinal pancreaticojejunostomy. *Am J Surg* 106:243–258, 1963.

37. Anderson MC: Surgical approach to pancreatic inflammatory disease. *Arch Surg* 107:340–347, 1973.
38. Jordan GL, Jr., Strug BS, Crowder WE: Current status of pancreatojejunostomy in the management of chronic pancreatitis. *Am J Surg* 133:46–51, 1977.
39. Puestow CB, Gillesby WJ: Retrograde surgical drainage of pancreas for chronic relapsing pancreatitis. *AMA Arch Surg* 76:898–907, 1958.
40. DuVal MK, Jr., Enquist IF: The surgical treatment of chronic pancreatitis by pancreaticojejunostomy: an 8-year reappraisal. *Surg* 50:965–969, 1961.
41. Wittingen J, Frey CF: Islet concentration in the head, body, tail and uncinate process of the pancreas. *Ann Surg* 179:412–414, 1974.
42. Kugelberg C, Wehlin L, Arnesjo B, et al: Endoscopic pancreatography in evaluating results of pancreaticojejunostomy. *Gut* 17:267–272, 1976.
43. Miller EW, Goldberg HI, Goldberg SB, et al: Radiographic evaluation of pancreaticojejunal shunts. *Gut* 17:439–443, 1976.

16

Complications of Chronic Pancreatitis

16.1 METABOLIC CONSEQUENCES

In chronic pancreatitis associated with steatorrhea, clinically significant deficiencies of fat-soluble vitamins (vitamins A, D, and K) do not
generally occur (Chapter 13). One important reason is that the composition of dietary fat in the small intestine in pancreatic insufficiency is
mostly triglycerides, which do not complex with fat-soluble vitamins,
calcium, or magnesium, whereas in diseases of the small intestine, dietary
fat is hydrolyzed by pancreatic lipase to free fatty acids, which do complex with these vitamins and cause deficiencies of prothrombin, calcium
and magnesium, and vitamin A. Deficiency in vitamin E has been noted in
chronic pancreatitis, and has been associated with a variety of histologic
changes including ceroid pigmentation of smooth muscle without clinical
signs or symptoms of vitamin deficiency.[1] Subclinical abnormalities in
retinal function appear to correlate with zinc deficiency rather than vitamin A deficiency or steatorrhea.[2] Some patients with pancreatic insufficiency have decreased absorption of vitamin B-12, at least by the Schilling test.[3] B-12 malabsorption does not appear to be related to the presence
or absence of steatorrhea or any other variable that has been tested thus
far. A single dose of a potent pancreatic extract is nonetheless able to
correct vitamin B-12 malabsorption, but only in vitamin B-12 malabsorption associated with pancreatic insufficiency, and not in pernicious anemia. There is no known method other than the administration of pancreatic extracts to correct this problem.[3,4] The mechanism of vitamin B-12
malabsorption in pancreatic insufficiency has been clarified with the discovery that the incubation of gastric intrinsic factor with pancreatic pro-

teases enhanced the absorption of vitamin B-12 whereas intrinsic factor without pancreatic proteases did not.[5] It appears that the correction of vitamin B-12 malabsorption is not on the basis of either tryptic or chymo-tryptic activity but depends on a low molecular weight protein contained within the protease preparations.[6] This protein, secreted in pancreatic juice without recognizable protease activity, promotes vitamin B-12 absorption by influencing the intrinsic factor–vitamin B-12 complex. Despite the abnormal Schilling test, patients rarely develop clinically significant vitamin B-12 deficiency.[7,8]

Several patients with chronic pancreatitis and steatorrhea have been found to have increased urinary secretion of oxalate.[9,10] Hyperoxaluria would subject such patients to the risk of developing calcium oxalate urolithiasis, but thus far there have been no reported cases of oxalate stones in chronic pancreatitis. For hyperoxaluria to take place in chronic pancreatitis, it would appear that steatorrhea of some degree must be present in order that lipolytic enzymes of colonic bacteria have the opportunity to hydrolyze triglycerides to free fatty acids. Intraluminal calcium would then bind fatty acids in the colon thereby increasing the solubility of oxalate and enhancing its absorption through colonic mucosa.[10] By way of contrast, gastrointestinal disorders associated with defective reabsorption of bile salts, such as ileal resection for regional enteritis, lead to hyperoxaluria in the absence of statorrhea since bile salts enhance oxalate absorption directly by increasing the permeability of the colon to oxalate.[11] From a clinical standpoint, it is reasonable to measure 24 hr urinary oxalate levels, which are normally less than 45 mg/24 hr, in patients with steatorrhea. Excessive excretion of oxalate in urine can be reduced by either decreasing fat or oxalate in the diet or increasing dietary calcium.[9,10]

16.2 GASTROINTESTINAL COMPLICATIONS

The relationship between peptic ulcer disease and chronic pancreatitis has been summarized.[12] The bulk of evidence suggests that duodenal ulcer disease is distinctly uncommon among patients with alcoholic pancreatitis. This correlates well with the many studies that indicate a marked reduction of acid secretion in chronic pancreatitis. Despite all of this evidence, the precise incidence of peptic ulcer disease in patients with chronic pancreatitis remains uncertain. Various estimates include figures of 22%,[8] 13%,[13] and 2%.[14] Since fibrosis of the head of the pancreas may distort and fix duodenal bulb creating one or more crevices that resemble an ulcer niche, it is possible that some of the estimates of the incidence of duodenal ulcer disease are falsely elevated. A prospective study in which the presence of active duodenal ulcer disease is confirmed both by endoscopic visualization and by histologic verification would resolve these divergent figures.

In addition to an appearance that suggests duodenal ulcer disease, other abnormalities may occur as a result of fibrosis of the head of the pancreas including an appearance suggestive of nodular carcinoma,[15] and severe duodenal obstruction usually in the postapical duodenum (Figure 32). Distinction from gastric outlet obstruction such as from conventional peptic ulcer is best appreciated clinically first by the presence of an air-fluid level in both the duodenal bulb and body of the stomach on an upright plain x-ray of the abdomen and secondly by the recovery of bile on nasogastric aspiration, indicating reflux of duodenal contents into the stomach. The development of stenosis of the postapical duodenum in chronic pancreatitis should stimulate a differential diagnosis that includes cicatrization from a fibrotic head of the pancreas, an atypically located duodenal ulcer, carcinoma of the head of the pancreas, and pseudocyst of the head of the pancreas compressing the duodenum.

The incidence of cirrhosis in chronic alcoholic pancreatitis has been described in Chapter 9. It is not clear whether the risk of developing cirrhosis on the basis of heavy alcohol consumption is influenced by the presence or absence of chronic relapsing pancreatitis.

Common bile duct obstruction caused by fibrosis of the head of the pancreas has also been described in Chapter 9 (Figure 22). It should be emphasized that this entity may be confused with an exacerbation of pancreatitis, biliary sepsis, alcoholic hepatitis, and even secondary biliary cirrhosis. The techniques that are utilized to visualize the common bile duct include diagnostic ultrasound, IV cholangiography, ERCP, and "skinny needle" transhepatic cholangiography. Since a temporary narrowing of the common bile duct can be caused by the distorting force of the endoscope on this structure,[16] it is essential that multiple views of the common bile duct be obtained with the patient in a variety of positions and with the endoscope withdrawn from the duodenum in order to be sure that the endoscope itself has not caused compression.

Extrahepatic portal hypertension has also been described in Chapter 9. It has been emphasized that chronic pancreatitis and particularly chronic calcific pancreatitis may cause secondary thrombosis of portal vein, splenic vein, or both.[17,18] Important clinical features of this complication are gastrointestinal bleeding from either esophageal or gastric varices, splenomegaly, and absence of cirrhosis on liver biopsy. If the obstruction occurs solely in the splenic vein, splenectomy is usually sufficient. If the portal vein is obstructed, a shunting procedure such as mesocaval shunt or splenorenal shunt is necessary.

16.3 PANCREATIC CALCIFICATION

Pancreatic calcification occurs in approximately 40% to 60% cases of alcoholic pancreatitis,[8,19,20] and takes the form of intraductal stones. Intraductal stones are also commonly seen in hereditary pancreatitis and in chronic pancreatitis associated with hyperparathyroidism.

It should be stressed that abdominal calcification in the general vicinity of the pancreas need not indicate chronic calcific pancreatitis. One must be certain that the calcification is located within the pancreas and not in a nearby structure. Additional x-ray views including oblique and lateral views are often necessary to make this distinction. Once calcification has been confirmed as intrapancreatic, one must include in a proper differential diagnosis a variety of benign diseases of the pancreas including cysts and pseudocysts as well as malignant diseases including hemangioma, lymphangioma, cystadenoma, cystadenocarcinoma, and islet cell tumors.[21]

16.4 CARCINOMA OF THE PANCREAS

The suggestion has been made that chronic pancreatitis, and particularly chronic calcific pancreatitis, is a premalignant condition, since carcinoma of the pancreas has been documented on occasion among patients with alcoholic pancreatitis and chronic calcific pancreatitis of uncertain etiology.[14,22-26] The incidence of pancreatic carcinoma under these circumstances has not been established. A reasonable figure may be 2%.

In some instances, a carcinoma of the pancreas causes clinical symptoms of pancreatitis and by doing so misleads the clinician into thinking that the pancreatitis was present for an extended period of time.[27,28] The presence of intraductal calcification[27] need not be taken as evidence of chronic calcific pancreatitis especially in the absence of alcohol ingestion,[27] since ductal obstruction, whether caused by carcinoma or stricture, may give rise to calcifications.[29] It may be impossible to decide between the alternatives of chronic pancreatitis predisposing to carcinoma or carcinoma leading to pancreatic inflammation.[30]

Carcinoma of the pancreas should be suspected in a patient with chronic pancreatitis if there is increasing abdominal discomfort, progressive weight loss, jaundice, radiologic evidence including nodularity of the duodenal sweep. On one occasion, pancreatic calcification was seen to recede presumably as a result of erosion of calcific deposits by the expanding carcinoma.[23] This is a unique occurrence, and usually when it is supected, variations in radiologic technique have been responsible for changes in appearance of calcific deposits. Confirmation of the presence of carcinoma may be quite difficult in chronic calcific pancreatitis. There are many tests that have proven helpful in detecting the presence of carcinoma of the pancreas. The ones that are most readily available include diagnostic ultrasound,[31] ERCP,[31,32] and hypotonic duodenography. C-T scan[33,34] and arteriography[31,35] are also helpful, but require advanced technological skill. Percutaneous pancreatic biopsy[36,37] and transduodenal aspiration biopsy using an endoscope[38] are newer techniques that offer promise of nonoperative confirmation of carcinoma. Pancreatic function tests with intravenous cholecystokinin-pancreozymin associated with pancreatic cytology[31] and pancreatic function test with intravenous secretin[39] also yield diagnostic information but require specialized laboratories devoted to these techniques. Carcinoma associated with hereditary pancreatitis represents a particularly difficult problem (see Chapter 2). There is speculation that not only patients with hereditary pancreatitis but also their relatives have a higher than normal incidence of carcinoma of the pancreas.

In the evaluation of a patient with suspected carcinoma, it is worth considering whether difficult studies should be pursued to prove a diagnosis that uniformly has a most unfavorable prognosis. A common clinical dilemma is a patient with recurrent pancreatitis and evidence suggestive of carcinoma. Under these circumstances, my suggestion would be to pursue a vigorous diagnostic course in order to distinguish between carcinoma and a benign complication of pancreatitis that can be helped surgically, such as an obstruction of the main pancreatic duct or a pseudocyst. If the distinction cannot be made with certainty without surgery, my recommendation would be a laparotomy for this purpose.

16.5 MISCELLANEOUS

Hemorrhagic pancreatitis is less common with each succeeding episode of pancreatitis because of increasing destruction of acinar tissue. Complications such as pseudocysts and abscess, which reflect significant pancreatic necrosis, might also be expected to be less common with each episode, but data in support of this concept are lacking. A pseudocyst may occur in far advanced chronic pancreatitis on the basis of severe ductal obstruction rather than pancreatic necrosis.

Pancreatic ascites, caused by either a ductal disruption or a leaking pancreatic pseudocyst, may occur at various intervals following the onset of symptomatic pancreatitis and can develop with no features suggestive of a preceding acute episode of pancreatitis.

REFERENCES

1. Braunstein H: Tocopherol deficiency in adults with chronic pancreatitis. *Gastroenterology* 40:224–231, 1961.
2. Toskes P, Curington C, Levy N, et al: Abnormalities in retinal function in patients with chronic pancreatitis. Presented at the annual meeting of the American Pancreatic Association, Chicago, November, 1977.
3. Toskes PP, Hansel J, Cerda J, et al: Vitamin B-12 malabsorption in chronic pancreatic insufficiency. Studies suggesting the presence of a pancreatic "intrinsic factor." *N Engl J Med* 284:627–632, 1971.
4. Specificity of the correction of vitamin B-12 malabsorption by pancreatic extract and its clinical significance. *Gastroenterology* 65:199–204, 1973.
5. Toskes PP, Smith GW, Francis GM, et al: Evidence that pancreatic proteases enhance vitamin B-12 absorption by acting on crude preparations of hog gastric intrinsic factor and human gastric juice. *Gastroenterology* 72:31–36, 1977.
6. Toskes P, Smith G: Isolation of a low molecular weight vitamin B-12-promoting protein from preparations of trypsin and chymotrypsin. *Gastroenterology* 74:1106, 1978.
7. Jeffries GH: The pancreas and vitamin B-12 absorption. *N Engl J Med* 284:666–667, 1971.
8. Strum WB, Spiro HM: Chronic pancreatitis. *Ann Intern Med* 74:264–277, 1971.
9. Stauffer JQ, Steward RJ, Bertrand G: Acquired hyperoxaluria: Relationship to dietary calcium content and severity of steatorrhea. *Gastroenterology* 66:783, 1974.
10. Dobbins JW, Binder HJ: Importance of the colon in enteric hyperoxaluria. *N Engl J Med* 296:298–301, 1977.
11. Fairclough PD, Feest TG, Chadwick VS, et al: Effect of sodium chenodeoxycholate on oxalate absorption from the excluded human colon—a mechanism for "enteric" hyperoxaluria. *Gut* 18:240–244, 1977.
12. Banks PA, Janowitz HD: Some metabolic aspects of exocrine pancreatic disease. *Gastroenterology* 56:601–617, 1969.
13. Dreiling DA, Naqui MA: Peptic ulcer diathesis in patients with chronic pancreatitis. *Am J Gastroenterol* 51:503–510, 1969.
14. Sarles H, Sahei J: Pathology of chronic calcifying pancreatitis. *Am J Gastroenterol* 66:117–139, 1976.
15. Blackstone MO, Mizuno H: Reactive duodenal changes in chronic pancreatitis simulating the contiguous spread of pancreatic carcinoma. *Am J Dig Dis* 22:658–661, 1977.
16. Falkenstein DB, Hsu KD, Abrams RM, et al: Influence of endoscopic manipulation and patient position on cholangiographic interpretation in endoscopic retrograde cholangiopancreatography. *Radiology* 122:836–838, 1977.

17. Longstreth GF, Newcomer AD, Green PA: Extrahepatic portal hypertension caused by chronic pancreatitis. *Ann Intern Med* 75:903–908, 1971.
18. Rignault D, Mine J, Moine D: Splenoportographic changes in chronic pancreatitis. *Surg* 63:571–575, 1968.
19. Read G, Braganza JM, Howat T: Pancreatitis—a retrospective study. *Gut* 17:945–952, 1976.
20. Johnson JR, Zintel HA: Pancreatic calcification and cancer of the pancreas. *Surg Gynecol Obstet* 117:585–588, 1963.
21. Ring EJ, Eaton B, Jr., Ferrucci JT, et al: Differential diagnosis of pancreatic calcification. *Am J Roentgenol Radium Ther Nucl Med* 117:446–452, 1973.
22. Lungh G, Nordenstam H: Pancreas calcification and pancreas cancer. *Acta Chir Scand* 136:493–496, 1970.
23. Tucker DH, Moor IB: Vanishing pancreatic calcification in chronic pancreatitis. A sign of pancreatic carcinoma. *N Engl J Med* 268:31–33, 1963.
24. Creutzfeldt W, Fehr H, Schmidt: Verlaufsbeobachtungen und diagnostische Verfahren bei der chronischrezidivierenden und chronischen Pankreatitis. *Schweiz Med Wochenschr* 100:1180–1189, 1970.
25. Geevarghese PJ: Pancreatic diabetes. G. R. Bhatkal for *Popular Prakashan*. Bombay, 1968.
26. Short WF: Duodenal narrowing associated with chronic pancreatitis. *Am J Dig Dis* 22:241–242, 1977.
27. Paulino-Netto A, Dreiling DA, Baronofsky ID: The relationship between pancreatic calcification and cancer of the pancreas. *Ann Surg* 151:530–537, 1960.
28. Gambill E: Pancreatitis associated with pancreatic carcinoma. *Mayo Clin Proc* 46:174–177, 1971.
29. Stobbe KC, ReMine WH, Baggenstoss AH: Pancreatic lithiasis. *Surg Gynecol Obstet* 131:1090–1099, 1970.
30. White TT, Keith RG: Long term follow-up study of fifty patients with pancreaticojejunostomy. *Surg Gynecol Obstet* 136:353–358, 1973.
31. DiMagno EP, Malagelada JR, Taylor WF, et al: A prospective comparison of current diagnostic tests for pancreatic cancer. *N Engl J Med* 297:737–742, 1977.
32. Freeny PC, Bilbao MK, Katon RM: "Blind" evaluation of endoscopic retrograde cholangiopancreatography (ERCP) in the diagnosis of pancreatic carcinoma: The "double duct" and other signs. *Radiology* 119:271–274, 1976.
33. Haaga JR, Alfidi RJ, Havrilla TR, et al: Definitive role of C-T scanning of the pancreas. *Radiology* 124:723–730, 1977.
34. Stanley RJ, Sagel SS, Levitt RG: Computed tomographic evaluation of the pancreas. *Radiology* 124:715–722, 1977.
35. White AF, Baum S, Buranasin S: Aneurysms secondary to pancreatitis. *Am J Roentgenol* 127:393–396, 1976.
36. Smith EH, Bartrum RJ, Jr., Cang YC, et al: Percutaneous pancreatic biopsy. *Gastroenterology* 69:1359–1365, 1975.
37. Hancke S, Holm HH, Koch F: Ultraconically guided percutaneous fine needle biopsy of the pancreas. *Surg Gynecol Obstet* 140:361–364, 1975.
38. Tsuchiya R, Henmi T, Kondo N, et al: Endoscopic aspiration biopsy of the pancreas. *Gastroenterology* 73:1050–1052, 1977.
39. Dreiling DA: Pancreatic secretory testing in 1974. *Gut* 16:653–657, 1975.

17

Prognosis of Chronic Pancreatitis

Prognosis in chronic pancreatitis must be viewed as guarded. In one series of 50 patients who were followed closely for periods up to 19 years, mortality was 56%.[1] More than half of the deaths were caused directly by alcohol. These included cirrhosis of the liver and a variety of pancreatic complications (including abscess, pseudocyst, and hemorrhagic necrosis). Other causes of death in chronic pancreatitis include general debilitation, varieties of infections including pneumonia and tuberculosis, narcotic addiction, and prolonged hypoglycemia caused by inappropriately large amounts of insulin.

Thus far, the exocrine and endocrine complications of chronic pancreatitis have not played a major prognostic role. On occasion, massive steatorrhea contributes to cachexia and susceptibility to infection, and would have prognostic significance. The vascular complications of diabetes, including retinopathy, nephropathy, and coronary artery disease, have not been demonstrated to have major prognostic significance.

Prognosis is more serious if a patient continues to drink alcohol. The deleterious effect of alcoholism is particularly striking following pancreatic surgery for intractable pain. Among patients who have discontinued the use of alcohol postoperatively, 10-year survival figures are in general higher than 80% and are associated with symptomatic improvement. Among patients who have continued to consume alcohol, 10-year survival figures are of the order of 25% to 60% and are associated with unsatisfactory clinical improvement.[2-5] Thus far, there are no controlled clinical trials which compare the prognosis of patients treated medically with those treated surgically.

REFERENCES

1. Strum WB, Spiro HM: Chronic pancreatitis. *Ann Intern Med* 74:264–277, 1971.
2. Frey CF, Child CG, Fry W: Pancreatectomy for chronic pancreatitis. *Ann Surg* 184:403–414, 1976.
3. White TT, Keith RG: Long-term follow-up study of 50 patients with pancreaticojejunostomy. *Surg Gynecol Obstet* 136:353–358, 1973.
4. Leger L, Lenriot JP, Lemaigre G: Five to twenty-year follow-up after surgery for chronic pancreatitis in 148 patients. *Ann Surg* 180:185–191, 1974.
5. Guillemin G, Cuilleret J, Michel A, et al: Chronic relapsing pancreatitis. *Am J Surg* 122:802–807, 1971.

Index